T0302070

Antipsychotic Trials in Schizophrenia

The CATIE Project

Antipsychotic Trials in Schizophrenia

The CATIE Project

Edited by

T. Scott Stroup MD, MPH
Department of Psychiatry, Columbia University, College of Physicians and Surgeons, New York, USA

Jeffrey A. Lieberman MD
Department of Psychiatry, Columbia University, College of Physicians and Surgeons,
New York State Psychiatric Institute, Lieber Center for Schizophrenia Research
New York Presbyterian Hospital & Columbia University Medical Center, New York, USA

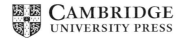

CAMBRIDGE
UNIVERSITY PRESS

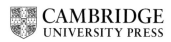

Shaftesbury Road, Cambridge CB2 8EA, United Kingdom

One Liberty Plaza, 20th Floor, New York, NY 10006, USA

477 Williamstown Road, Port Melbourne, VIC 3207, Australia

314–321, 3rd Floor, Plot 3, Splendor Forum, Jasola District Centre, New Delhi – 110025, India

103 Penang Road, #05–06/07, Visioncrest Commercial, Singapore 238467

Cambridge University Press is part of Cambridge University Press & Assessment,
a department of the University of Cambridge.

We share the University's mission to contribute to society through the pursuit of
education, learning and research at the highest international levels of excellence.

www.cambridge.org
Information on this title: www.cambridge.org/9780521895330

© Cambridge University Press & Assessment 2010

This publication is in copyright. Subject to statutory exception and to the provisions
of relevant collective licensing agreements, no reproduction of any part may take
place without the written permission of Cambridge University Press & Assessment.

First published 2010

A catalogue record for this publication is available from the British Library

Library of Congress Cataloging-in-Publication data
Antipsychotic trials in schizophrenia : the CATIE project / edited by
T. Scott Stroup, Jeffrey A. Lieberman.
    p. ; cm.
    Includes bibliographical references and index.
    ISBN 978-0-521-89533-0 (Hardback)
    1. CATIE Project.   2. Antipsychotic drugs–Testing.
3. Schizophrenia–Chemotherapy.   I. Stroup, T. Scott, 1960–
II. Lieberman, Jeffrey A., 1948–   III. Title.
    [DNLM: 1. CATIE Project.   2. Schizophrenia–drug therapy.
3. Antipsychotic Agents–standards.   4. Antipsychotic Agents–
therapeutic use.   5. Clinical Trials as Topic.   6. Drug Evaluation–
methods. WM 203 A633 2010]
    RM333.5.A58 2010
    616.89´8061–dc22

                                                    2009048606

ISBN   978-0-521-89533-0   Hardback

Cambridge University Press & Assessment has no responsibility for the persistence
or accuracy of URLs for external or third-party internet websites referred to in this
publication and does not guarantee that any content on such websites is, or will
remain, accurate or appropriate.

....

Every effort has been made in preparing this book to provide accurate and up-to-date
information which is in accord with accepted standards and practice at the time of
publication. Although case histories are drawn from actual cases, every effort has been
made to disguise the identities of the individuals involved. Nevertheless, the authors,
editors and publishers can make no warranties that the information contained herein
is totally free from error, not least because clinical standards are constantly changing
through research and regulation. The authors, editors and publishers therefore
disclaim all liability for direct or consequential damages resulting from the use of
material contained in this book. Readers are strongly advised to pay careful attention
to information provided by the manufacturer of any drugs or equipment that they plan
to use.

To the participants in the CATIE study
for their critical contribution to the effort
to better understand schizophrenia and its
treatment.

To Thelma and Meg with love: TSS

To my family in gratitude for their love, support,
and patience: JAL

Contents

Contributors

Paul Appelbaum, MD
Department of Psychiatry
Columbia University
College of Physicians and Surgeons
New York, USA

Robert R. Bies, PharmD, PhD
Department of Pharmaceutical Sciences
and Department of Psychiatry
University of Pittsburgh
Pittsburgh, Pennsylvania, USA

Kristin L. Bigos, PhD
Clinical Brain Disorders Branch
National Institute of Mental Health, NIH
Bethesda, Maryland, USA

Stanley N. Caroff, MD
University of Pennsylvania School
of Medicine and the Veterans
Affairs Medical Center
Philadelphia, Pennsylvania, USA

James J. Crowley, PhD
Department of Genetics
University of North Carolina at Chapel Hill
Chapel Hill, North Carolina, USA

Sonia M. Davis, DrPH
Quintiles Incorporated
Research Triangle Park,
North Carolina, USA
Department of Psychiatry
and Department of Biostatistics
University of North Carolina at Chapel Hill
Chapel Hill, North Carolina, USA

Vicki G. Davis, DrPH
Department of Biostatistics
University of North Carolina at Chapel Hill
Chapel Hill, North Carolina, USA

Donald C. Goff, MD
Department of Psychiatry
Harvard University
Schizophrenia Program
Massachusetts General Hospital
Freedom Trail Clinic,
Lindemann Mental Health Center
Boston, Massachusetts, USA

Richard Kaczynski, PhD
Department of Psychiatry
Yale University School of Medicine
New Haven, Connecticut, USA

Richard S. E. Keefe, PhD
Department of Psychiatry and
Behavioral Sciences
Duke University Medical Center
Durham, North Carolina, USA

Gary G. Koch, PhD
Department of Biostatistics
University of North Carolina at Chapel Hill
Chapel Hill, North Carolina, USA

Douglas L. Leslie, PhD
Department of Public Health Sciences
and Department of Psychiatry
Pennsylvania State University
Hershey, Pennsylvania, USA

Jeffrey A. Lieberman, MD
Department of Psychiatry
Columbia University
College of Physicians and Surgeons
New York State Psychiatric Institute
Lieber Center for Schizophrenia Research
New York Presbyterian Hospital &
Columbia University Medical Center
New York, USA

Joseph P. McEvoy, MD
Department of Psychiatry and
Behavioral Sciences
Duke University
Medical Center Durham,
North Carolina, USA
Clinical Research
John Umstead Hospital
Butner, North Carolina, USA

Stephen R. Marder, MD
Department of Psychiatry and
Biobehavioral Sciences
University of California at Los Angeles
Los Angeles, California, USA

Jonathan M. Meyer, MD
Department of Psychiatry
University of California, San Diego
Staff Psychiatrist,
VA San Diego Healthcare System
San Diego, California, USA

Del D. Miller, MD, PharmD
Department of Psychiatry
University of Iowa
Carver College of Medicine
Iowa City, Iowa, USA

John L. Olsen
Department of Psychiatry
University of Utah Medical Center
Salt Lake City, Utah, USA

Deborah A. Perlick, PhD
Department of Psychiatry
Mount Sinai School of Medicine
New York, USA

Bruce G. Pollock, MD PhD
Rotman Research Institute Centre for
Addiction and Mental Health
University of Toronto
Toronto, Canada
Department of Psychiatry
University of Pittsburgh
Pittsburgh, Pennsylvania, USA

Fred Reimherr, MD
Department of Psychiatry
University of Utah Medical Center
Salt Lake City, Utah, USA

Sandra G. Resnick, PhD
Department of Psychiatry
Yale School of Medicine
New Haven, Connecticut, USA

Robert A. Rosenheck, MD
Department of Psychiatry
Public Health, and the Child Study Center
Yale School of Medicine
New Haven, Connecticut, USA

T. Scott Stroup, MD, MPH
Department of Psychiatry
Columbia University
College of Physicians and Surgeons
New York, USA

Patrick F. Sullivan, MD, FRANZCP
Department of Genetics and
Department of Psychiatry
University of North Carolina at Chapel Hill
Chapel Hill, North Carolina, USA

Jeffrey Swanson, PhD
Department of Psychiatry and
Behavioral Sciences
Duke University School of Medicine
Durham, North Carolina, USA

Marvin S. Swartz, MD
Department of Psychiatry and
Behavioral Sciences
Duke University School of Medicine
Durham, North Carolina, USA

Richard Van Dorn, PhD
Department of Mental Health
Law and Policy
Louis de la Parte Florida
Mental Health Institute
University of South Florida
Tampa, Florida, USA

Acknowledgments

We are indebted to the leadership and staff of NIMH for their support of the CATIE project. In particular, we thank John Hsiao and Joanne Severe for their enduring commitment to the success of the project. Also of critical importance were Barry Lebowitz, Grayson Norquist, Louise Ritz, Jean Baum, Steve Hyman, and Tom Insel.

At Quintiles, we are grateful for the help and support of Paula Stafford-Brown, Paula Butler, Sonia Davis, Barbra Laplante, and Nancy Mitchell.

At UNC-Chapel Hill, we are extremely grateful to Ingrid Rojas and Janice Linn.

The Schizophrenia Trials Network Executive Committee, including Ed Davis, Sonia Davis, Richard Keefe, Joe McEvoy, Diana Perkins, Bob Rosenheck, and Marvin Swartz made immeasurable contributions to the study and to this volume.

We also thank the investigators at the following research sites where the study was conducted:

L. Adler, Clinical Insights, Glen Burnie, Md.; M. Bari, Synergy Clinical Research, Chula Vista, Calif.; I. Belz, Tri-County/Mental Health and Mental Retardation Services, Conroe, Tex.; R. Bland, Southern Illinois University School of Medicine, Springfield; T. Blocher, Mental Health and Mental Retardation Authority of Harris County, Houston, Tex.; B. Bolyard, Cox North Hospital, Springfield, Mo.; A. Buffenstein, Queen's Medical Center, Honolulu, Ha.; J. Burruss, Baylor College of Medicine, Houston, Tex.; M. Byerly, University of Texas Southwestern Medical Center at Dallas, Dallas; J. Canive, Albuquerque Veterans Affairs Medical Center, Albuquerque, N.M.; S. Caroff, University of Pennsylvania and Philadelphia VA; C. Casat, Behavioral Health Center, Charlotte, N.C.; E. Chavez-Rice, El Paso Community Mental Health and Mental Retardation Center, El Paso, Tex.; J. Csernansky, Washington University School of Medicine, St. Louis, Mo.; P. Delgado, University Hospitals of Cleveland, Cleveland, Oh.; R. Douyon, Veterans Affairs Medical Center, Miami, Fla.; C. D'Souza, Connecticut Mental Health Center, New Haven; I. Glick, Stanford University School of Medicine, Stanford, Calif.; D. Goff, Massachusetts General Hospital, Boston; S. Gratz, Eastern Pennsylvania Psychiatric Institute, Philadelphia; G.T. Grossberg, Saint Louis University School of Medicine–Wohl Institute, St. Louis, Mo.; M. Hale, New Britain General Hospital, New Britain, Conn.; M. Hamner, Medical University of South Carolina and Veterans Affairs Medical Center, Charleston; R. Jaffe, Belmont Center for Comprehensive Treatment, Philadelphia, Pa.; D. Jeste, University of California, San Diego, Veterans Affairs Medical Center, San Diego; A. Kablinger, Louisiana State University Health Sciences Center, Shreveport; A. Khan, Psychiatric Research Institute, Wichita, Kans.; S. Lamberti, University of Rochester Medical Center, Rochester, N.Y.; M.T. Levy, Staten Island University Hospital, Staten Island, N.Y.; J.A. Lieberman, University of North Carolina School of Medicine, Chapel Hill; G. Maguire, University of California Irvine, Orange; T. Manschreck, Corrigan Mental Health Center, Fall River, Mass.; J. McEvoy, Duke University Medical Center, Durham, N.C.; M. McGee, Appalachian Psychiatric Healthcare System, Athens, Ohio; H. Meltzer, Vanderbilt University Medical Center, Nashville, Tenn.; A. Miller, University of Texas Health Science Center at San Antonio, San Antonio; D.D. Miller, University of Iowa, Iowa City; H. Nasrallah, University of Cincinnati Medical Center, Cincinnati; C. Nemeroff, Emory University School of

Medicine, Atlanta; S. Olson, University of Minnesota Medical School, Minneapolis; G.F. Oxenkrug, St. Elizabeth's Medical Center, Boston; J. Patel, University of Massachusetts Health Care, Worcester; F. Reimherr, University of Utah Medical Center, Salt Lake City; S. Riggio, Mount Sinai Medical Center–Bronx Veterans Affairs Medical Center, Bronx, N.Y.; S. Risch, University of California, San Francisco, San Francisco; B. Saltz, Mental Health Advocates, Boca Raton, Fla.; G. Simpson, University of Southern California Medical Center, Los Angeles; M. Smith, Harbor–UCLA Medical Center, Torrance, Calif.; R. Sommi, University of Missouri, Kansas City; R.M. Steinbook, University of Miami School of Medicine, Miami; M. Stevens, Valley Mental Health, Salt Lake City, Utah; A. Tapp, Veterans Affairs Puget Sound Health Care System, Tacoma, Wash.; R. Torres, University of Mississippi, Jackson; P. Weiden, SUNY Downstate Medical Center, Brooklyn, N.Y.; J. Wolberg, Mount Sinai Medical Center, New York, N.Y.

Introduction

The history of the CATIE study

The approval of clozapine in the United States in 1989 by the Food and Drug Administration (FDA), and its marketing for clinical use in 1990, heralded the era of a "second-generation" of antipsychotic medications (SGAs) with "atypical" characteristics. Over the ensuing decade, five additional putative SGAs would move through clinical development and be approved for marketing and clinical use. The excitement and anticipation around these events was palpable, and the fields of psychiatry and mental health care genuinely believed that they were on the threshold of a great step forward in the treatment of mental illness. Clinicians and patients, urged on by pervasive and sophisticated marketing campaigns, embraced the new medications so fully that they were preferentially used when patients with new-onset psychosis began treatment or when patients with chronic illness changed their medications. The market share of the new medications increased rapidly, and with it the amount of health care dollars spent on pharmaceuticals.

At first this did not attract attention or cause concern. This was because it was fervently anticipated that the SGA medications would produce better treatment outcomes, prevent relapses, reduce the need for health care services, and prove to be cost effective over time. Moreover, patients, their families, and advocates clamored for new, better, and safer medications, confident in their belief that the long wait for a therapeutic breakthrough, if not panacea, had finally arrived. For their part, many clinicians willingly complied, firmly believing that prescribing the new medications was the right thing to do and that they were at the leading edge of a new standard of care.

All constituencies were encouraged by a burgeoning army of marketing personnel conscripted by the pharmaceutical companies to spread the gospel of atypicality in antipsychotic drug treatment. At the same time, a meta-psychopharmacology of novel neuro-receptor profiles evolved to explain the unique and superior effects of the SGAs as a class and as each successive agent was introduced. Enthusiasm for the new medications was so high that few questioned the concept of atypicality or the expected clinical advantages of drugs with novel mechanisms of action.

As the second millennium drew to a close, the US Congress had resolved to double the NIH budget. The NIMH, sensitive to criticism that it had not supported a sufficient amount of treatment research, decided that the time was right to employ the strategy that the National Heart, Lung and Blood Institute (NHLBI) and the National Cancer Institute (NCI) had previously pursued with considerable success by conducting large scale practical clinical trials designed to assess the effectiveness of treatments. This was a novel concept for the NIMH, which had not supported, much less orchestrated, the kind of large scale practical clinical trials as had some of its sibling institutes. Indeed one had to go back to the initial trials of the original antipsychotic and antidepressant drugs by the NIMH in the 1960s and 1970s to find large treatment trials in the NIMH portfolio. Since then, effectiveness research and practical trials had gained importance in the medical research community and found favor with the government, policy makers, and health care administrators as they addressed key questions that would influence resource allocation. They also provided a bridge from rarefied basic and translational science to clinical care and health services, and a means to determine how well new treatments worked in the real world and their cost-effectiveness.

Ever since the Clinton Administration's well intentioned but failed effort to reform the health care system, concern about the rising cost of health care had been mounting. It had not gone unnoticed that the cost of pharmaceuticals was one of the fastest growing components of the health care budget. In this context, the NIMH initiative to pursue effectiveness research was seen as a timely and much needed initiative.

The CATIE project was conceived by the NIMH officers and staff (Steve Hyman, Richard Nakamura, Grayson Norquist, Barry Lebowitz, John Hsiao, and Joanne Severe) and orchestrated by the Division of Services and Intervention Research to evaluate the effectiveness of antipsychotic medications for the psychiatric illnesses in which they were indicated [1]. Originally, it was conceived as three projects in one contract: one trial each in schizophrenia, Alzheimer's disease (AD), and psychotic depression. In the course of the application process, psychotic depression was dropped largely for budgetary reasons, but also because the level of existing knowledge about the use of antipsychotic drugs for this condition was less extensive and it was believed that a practical clinical trial was premature.

A Request for Information was issued in August of 1998 in which comments on the concept of the CATIE project (such as it was at that time) were invited from the field. A Request for Proposals was issued in November 1998 and groups of academic investigators began forming teams to respond with applications. Our team involved investigators from a consortium of universities (UNC, Duke, Yale, USC, Rochester). Brown and Stanford were also part of the team but dropped off when the psychotic depression component of the project was abandoned. We also subsequently invited Quintiles, the contract research organization founded and operated by former members of the UNC School of Public Health, to join our team to assume the functions of study and data management. Ultimately, we also recruited a network of 84 clinical sites (57 for schizophrenia and 27 for AD) from various systems of care throughout the United States.

Our application was submitted to the NIMH by 25 January 1999, deadline. Responses to queries and negotiations were conducted between the NIMH and our team over the ensuing spring and summer. The award was made at the end of September 1999.

The first phase of the project involved designing and vetting the protocol. To do this, we divided the CATIE investigators into two teams: those involved in the schizophrenia study and those with the Alzheimer's disease study. A small number of investigators and support staff were involved with both, and the staff of Quintiles supported both studies. The CATIE schizophrenia investigators revised the protocol that had been proposed in the original application and then invited experts in schizophrenia interventions, including many who had been members of other applicant groups for the CATIE contract, to meet and review and comment on it. We also solicited input from other stakeholder groups, including mental health advocates, consumers, and mental health care administrators. This resulted in significant modifications to the protocol. For example, the long-acting injectable antipsychotic treatment arm that we had wanted to include was dropped due to feedback from research experts, and input from advocates and consumers resulted in patient preference being incorporated into the process by which it was decided into which pathway patients were re-randomized in Phase 2 of the study.

The FDA had been considering the New Drug Application for ziprasidone during the period in which the CATIE protocols were being designed and revised. Knowing this and wanting the results of the CATIE studies to be as relevant and informative as possible at the time of their conclusion, NIMH asked us to design the study to be able to add ziprasidone to all phases of the schizophrenia study. Because of concern about the potential for ziprasidone to cause prolongation of the QT interval, the NIMH required us to wait for some 9 months following its approval by the FDA before activating the ziprasidone arm in the randomization scheme of CATIE.

Almost 1500 patients enrolled in CATIE between early 2001 and mid-2003. The last patient completed the study in December 2004, the database was locked in March 2005, and data analyses started immediately. We began to draft the first paper to report the primary outcome results of Phase 1 of the study while analyses were being carried out and added the results and discussion as they were completed. The first paper was submitted to the *New England Journal of Medicine* (*NEJM*) in April 2005 and underwent a process of review and revision over the course of the summer before being published in September 2005 [2]. When the embargo was lifted by the *NEJM,* the first results were eagerly anticipated. Over the entire trial, but particularly in the period during data analysis and following submission of the manuscript, there was intense interest and tremendous pressure to reveal the findings. However, we had made the decision along with NIMH not to present the results at a scientific meeting or any other forum before the first article describing the primary results was published. Rumors of the results abounded, and reports of pirated copies of the manuscript permeated the field. We are proud that strict confidentiality was maintained until the very end and that, until the time when the embargo was lifted and the paper released to the press electronically, no one but the CATIE investigators and our NIMH collaborators had any knowledge of the results. (The only exception being the *NEJM* editors and reviewers.)

The main results of the first paper were that all treatments were associated with high discontinuation or switch rates, indicating the limitations of effectiveness of antipsychotic medications as a class. The drug that did best was olanzapine, an SGA, but perphenazine, the first-generation older drug, was not much less effective than olanzapine and was comparable to the other SGAs. The latter finding was the most shocking result. Most people, ourselves included, had expected the new medications to be vastly superior to the proxy for the older drugs, but clearly they were not. In addition, there was no superiority in the effectiveness of the new medications on symptoms (and, as we learned in subsequent analyses, on cognitive impairment). Finally, perphenazine, at the doses used, did not cause more extrapyramidal side effects, as was expected, while the newer medications, with the exception of ziprasidone, caused more weight gain and adverse metabolic effects.

A press briefing at the time of the *NEJM* publication was held with members of the NIMH and CATIE investigators participating. The lay media reported the story extensively over the ensuing days and the *New York Times* ran an editorial on the study [3]. The story line was "government study finds new drugs no better than older less costly drug." The study immediately became a topic of even greater controversy in the psychiatric research community than it had already been, and other stakeholder groups were drawn into the debate. Although people expressed a myriad of different interpretations and opinions of the results, three main themes emerged from the cacophony of comments about CATIE. One point of view held that the results were accurate, confirming what many suspected but lacked evidence to verify, that the "emperor had no clothes." The second common reaction was that of the stakeholders (clinicians, consumers and advocates, administrators). They did not question the results of the study *per se* but were concerned that the study would be used to restrict access to the newer medications and further limit resources allocated to mental health care through tiered formularies, prior approval mechanisms, and treatment algorithms. The third set of responses came from the chorus of critics of the methodology of the CATIE study. These were largely due to people not having understood the study design and statistical analyses adequately or because of the unconventional "pragmatic" or "effectiveness" trial design, which was hard for clinical trial purists to accept as methodologically valid. Based on these criticisms, these persons questioned the accuracy of the CATIE results.

Despite the chorus of comments and criticisms, we never doubted the soundness of the methodology or the accuracy of the results of the CATIE study. Of course the proof of any study's findings are in their replication. In the time since the CATIE results have been published, there have been several studies and meta-analyses which pretty much bear out the CATIE findings. These include the CUtLASS study [4,5], the TEOSS study [6], the EUFEST study [7], and two meta-analyses by Leucht *et al.* [8,9].

By the middle of 2009, more than 40 original research articles based on CATIE data had been published. A public access database of the study has been made available to any interested party through the NIMH, and the DNA collected from subjects in the study and stored at the NIMH Genetics Repository at Rutgers, has been made available to investigators through the NIMH genetics policy.

One of the most common questions asked about the CATIE study is what impact it has had on clinical practice. This is a difficult question to answer as the data needed to assess this are not readily available and the process of changing practice is usually slow. Nevertheless, it is our impression that it has not changed prescribing patterns or the market shares of individual drugs dramatically. However, what has definitely changed since CATIE is the debate about the relative value and selection of treatments. It is no longer accepted that the new antipsychotic medications are a tremendous therapeutic breakthrough but rather an incremental advance and pharmacologic refinement of the dopamine 2 receptor mediated therapeutic mechanism of antipsychotics. It is no longer considered substandard practice to use first-generation antipsychotic drugs, particularly intermediate potency drugs, at moderate doses. And since we have come to realize the limits of the effectiveness of antipsychotic drugs as a class, and their lack of efficacy on negative and cognitive symptoms, the process of pursuing targets and drug development for new treatments for these pathologic dimensions of schizophrenia has resumed in earnest and with greater emphasis.

The major reason we believe that the CATIE study has become so controversial and such a lightning rod for criticism is because it essentially delivered the unwelcome news that the new drugs were not as great as they had been made out to be and we had thought [10]. How had an entire field of professionals and researchers become so enthralled with an exaggerated if not false belief? Our British colleague Peter Jones, Professor of Psychiatry at Cambridge University, may have put it best by saying that "we had allowed ourselves to be beguiled into believing that these drugs were so much better than they were because we all had so badly wanted our treatments to be better." If nothing else this book, which provides the most complete collection of the results of the NIMH CATIE schizophrenia study, should serve to help prevent ourselves from being beguiled again and spur us on to even greater efforts to develop and test truly novel and superior treatments.

References

1. Lebowitz BD, Vitiello B and Norquist GS. Approaches to multisite clinical trials: The National Institute of Mental Health perspective. *Schizophrenia Bulletin* 2003;**29**:7–13.

2. Lieberman JA, Stroup TS, McEvoy JP, *et al*; for the Clinical Antipsychotic Trials of Intervention Effectiveness (CATIE) investigators. Effectiveness of antipsychotic drugs in patients with chronic schizophrenia. *New England Journal of Medicine* 2005;**353**:1209–23.

3. New York Times. *Editorial: Comparing Schizophrenia Drugs*. The New York Times September 21, 2005.

4. Jones PB, Barnes TR, Davies L, *et al*. Randomized controlled trial of the effect on quality of life of second- vs first-generation antipsychotic drugs in schizophrenia: Cost Utility of the Latest Antipsychotic Drugs in Schizophrenia Study (CUtLASS 1). *Archives of General Psychiatry* 2006;**63**:1079–87.

5. Lewis SW, Barnes TR, Davies L, *et al*. Randomized controlled trial of effect of prescription of clozapine versus other second-generation antipsychotic drugs in resistant schizophrenia. *Schizophrenia Bulletin* 2006;**32**:715–23.

6. Sikich L, Frazier JA, McClellan J, *et al*. Double-blind comparison of first- and second-generation antipsychotics in early onset schizophrenia and schizoaffective disorder: Findings from the Treatment of Early-Onset Schizophrenia Spectrum Disorders (TEOSS) study. *American Journal of Psychiatry* 2008;**165**:1420–31. Erratum in *American Journal of Psychiatry* 2008;**165**:1495.

7. Kahn RS, Fleischhacker WW, Boter H *et al*; for the EUFEST study group. Effectiveness of antipsychotic drugs in first-episode schizophrenia and schizophreniform disorder: An open randomized clinical trial. *Lancet* 2008;**371**:1085–97.

8. Leucht S, Corves, C, Arbter D, Engel RR, Li C, Davis JM. Second-generation versus first-generation antipsychotic drugs for schizophrenia: A meta-analysis. *Lancet* 2009;**737**:31–41.

9. Leucht S, Komossa K, Rummel-Kluge C, *et al*. A meta-analysis of head-to-head comparisons of second-generation antipsychotics in the treatment of schizophrenia. *American Journal of Psychiatry* 2009;**166**:152–63.

10. Lewis SW and Lieberman JA. CATIE and CUTLASS: can we handle the truth? *British Journal of Psychiatry* 2008;**192**:161–3.

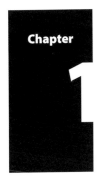

Chapter

1

Study design and protocol development process

T. Scott Stroup, Joseph P. McEvoy, and Jeffrey A. Lieberman

As part of its public mental health care treatment initiative the US National Institute of Mental Health (NIMH) in 1998 issued a request for proposals (RFP) for a research program to evaluate the comparative effectiveness of antipsychotic drugs in schizophrenia, Alzheimer's disease, and depression with psychotic features [1]. The RFP specified that the research protocols should focus on the newer (atypical or second-generation) antipsychotic drugs and should follow a public health model. In particular, the RFP stated that the trials should include the following features: focus on effectiveness and other outcome measures broader than efficacy alone; examine cost-effectiveness and the impact of external factors on treatment delivery, adherence, and outcomes; enhance generalizability by being as inclusive as possible, without exclusions for co-morbid psychiatric disorder, drug abuse, or medical illness; place a premium on demographic and geographic diversity; use multiple types of treatment settings that generally represent the systems of care in which patients with schizophrenia are treated; and generate results that inform community clinical practice. In addition, the RFP called for the program to develop a network of sites and investigators able to respond to future needs for effectiveness research and to serve as a platform for ancillary clinical investigations. Because additional new antipsychotics were expected to be introduced soon, the RFP also specified that proposals should include a mechanism for adding new medications. After an extended competitive bidding process, the Clinical Antipsychotic Trials of Intervention Effectiveness (CATIE) program was funded through a contract with the University of North Carolina (UNC).

In this chapter, we describe the development of the study designed to assess the effectiveness of antipsychotic drugs for persons with chronic schizophrenia. The protocol was developed by a team of academic investigators through an inclusive, iterative, and systematic process. The group of investigators at UNC, Duke University, and Yale University who drafted an original study design during the contract application process formed a protocol development committee that included other schizophrenia researchers who were not part of the original team. The trial designs submitted in the application process were a starting point for the protocol development process. An initial in-person meeting of the protocol development committee was followed by weekly teleconference meetings over 4 months. Additional input was sought from various stakeholder groups, including consumer representatives, mental health care administrators, and policy makers.

In January 2000, a draft study design was presented to consumer representatives at an NIMH-convened workshop entitled "Clinical Trials Recruitment: What Motivates People to Participate?" Feedback from this meeting led to additional protocol modifications, including the introduction of consumer choices in the protocol. In March 2000, a draft protocol

Antipsychotic Trials in Schizophrenia, ed. T. Scott Stroup and Jeffrey A. Lieberman. Published by Cambridge University Press. © Cambridge University Press 2010.

was submitted to the NIMH for review by a newly formed External Scientific Advisory Committee for the CATIE program. This committee made further recommendations that were incorporated into the final protocol.

Rationale for trial design

The CATIE schizophrenia trial was designed to address a discrepancy between research demonstrating the efficacy of antipsychotic drugs (i.e., how well they can work under ideal circumstances) and disappointing findings regarding their effectiveness (i.e., how they work in typical, less-than-ideal circumstances) and the ostensible superiority of second-generation antipsychotic (SGA) medications relative to first-generation antipsychotic drugs (FGA) medications. To address this so-called efficacy-effectiveness gap, the study designers adapted many of the characteristics of practical (or pragmatic) randomized controlled trials (RCTs). Pragmatic RCTs aim to answer questions of practical significance to clinicians and patients in typical clinical settings, which have varied levels of ancillary services and serve patients with co-morbid psychiatric illnesses, general medical problems, and substance use disorders [2,3]. Practical trials are intended to inform decision makers about the "real-world" impact of various treatment options [4]. Importantly, practical trials randomize interventions and ensure that treatments and the assessment of outcomes are blinded, where possible, to guard against ascertainment and performance biases [5].

The primary aim of the CATIE schizophrenia trial was to determine the comparative effectiveness of a representative FGA and the different SGA medications for patients with chronic schizophrenia. Treatment discontinuation for any reason, meant to reflect patient and physician judgments about both efficacy and tolerability, was selected as the primary outcome measure of effectiveness. Because rating-scale measures of efficacy were considered undesirable due to questionable clinical significance and reliability, and due to problems with missing data, we selected treatment discontinuation as an unambiguous, clinically meaningful outcome measure that would not be missing. Discontinuation was considered clinically important because of the distress of adverse effects or continued symptoms, and because of the increases in service use, often including hospitalization or an increased frequency of outpatient visits, associated with medication changes.

Some of the key study design decisions made by the Schizophrenia Protocol Development Committee, with input from various "stakeholder" groups, and their rationales are reviewed below.

Patient sample

Patients who entered the study were those with chronic schizophrenia for whom a new medication was needed or for whom a change in medications was an appropriate option due to incomplete symptom remission or adverse effects. In order to make the results of the trial generalizable and representative of the broad group of patients with chronic schizophrenia, inclusion criteria were broad and there were few exclusion criteria (Table 1.1). Patients with medical or psychiatric co-morbidities and those who required concomitant medications were included. First-episode patients and patients with refractory illness were excluded. First-episode patients were excluded because of their high rates of response to antipsychotic medications at relatively low doses. Patients with refractory illness were excluded because it was thought that their severe illness could preclude detection of differential effectiveness that would be apparent in treatment-responsive patients.

Table 1.1. Inclusion and exclusion criteria

Inclusion:

1. 18–65 years of age.

2. Diagnosis of schizophrenia by DSM-IV criteria.

3. Appropriate for treatment with an oral medication.

4. Adequate decisional capacity to make a choice about participating in this research study.

Exclusion:

1. Patients with schizoaffective disorder, mental retardation, pervasive developmental disorder, delirium, dementia, amnesia, or other cognitive disorders.

2. Patients with well-documented, drug-related, serious adverse reactions to even one of the proposed treatment arms.

3. Patients in their first episode of schizophrenia (first began antipsychotic drug treatment for psychosis within the previous 12 months and had psychotic symptoms for less than 3 years).

4. Patients with well-documented histories of failure to respond to even one of the proposed treatment arms. Treatment failure has occurred if the patient continued to demonstrate *severe* psychopathology in spite of fully adhering to treatment at an adequate dose of the medication for 6 consecutive weeks. Specific dose criteria are as follows:

    Olanzapine at dosages $\geq$ 30 mg/day

    Quetiapine at dosages $\geq$ 800 mg/day

    Perphenazine at dosages $\geq$ 32 mg/day

    Risperidone at dosages $\geq$ 6 mg/day

    Ziprasidone at dosages $\geq$ 160 mg/day

5. Patients currently, or in the past, treated with clozapine *for treatment resistance* are excluded. Patients who have taken clozapine for reasons other than treatment resistance may be eligible.

6. Patients currently stabilized on haloperidol decanoate or fluphenazine decanoate and who require long-acting injectable medication to maintain treatment adherence are excluded.

7. Women who are pregnant or currently breast-feeding (Women of child-bearing potential must agree to use appropriate contraception in order to enroll).

8. Patients with a contraindication to any of the drugs to which they might be assigned.

9. Patients with a medical condition that is serious and acutely unstable.

10. Patients with the following cardiac conditions are excluded:

    Recent myocardial infarction (<6 months)

    QTc prolongation (screening ECG with QTc > 450 msec for men, QTc > 470 msec for women)

    History of congenital QTc prolongation

    Sustained cardiac arrhythmia or history of sustained cardiac arrhythmia

    Uncompensated congestive heart failure

    Complete Left Bundle Branch Block (LBBB)

    First-degree heart block with PR interval $\geq$ .22 seconds

Table 1.1. (*cont.*)

11. Patients treated with dofetilide, sotalol, quinidine, other Class Ia and III anti-arrhythmics, mesoridazine, thioridazine, chlorpromazine, droperidol, pimozide, sparfloxacin, gatifloxacin, moxifloxacin, halofantrine, mefloquine, pentamidine, arsenic trioxide, levomethadyl acetate, dolasetron mesylate, probucol, or tacrolimus.

12. Patients who have taken any investigational drug within 30 days of the baseline visit.

Note: Patients with tardive dyskinesia are excluded from assignment to conventional antipsychotic treatment arms.

A summary of the demographic and clinical characteristics of the study participants is given in Table 1.2 Some patients who enrolled in the CATIE study were experiencing an acute exacerbation of symptoms while others were taking an antipsychotic that had provided benefit but who remained symptomatic (due to lack of efficacy or inability to tolerate an efficacious dose) or who experienced significant side effects, commonly consider a change in medications. Some patients who were seemingly doing well on their current medication but who wished to consider a change for a chance at greater improvement or better tolerability also enrolled.

Inclusion of FGA medications

The CATIE trial provided an important opportunity to compare definitively the effectiveness of SGAs to FGAs. Although the newer drugs had gained marketplace dominance, clear evidence of superior effectiveness was lacking. Perphenazine was selected as the FGA because it was a mid-potency medication associated with only a moderate incidence of extrapyramidal side effects (EPS) (relative to high-potency medications and other mid-potency medications) and sedation (relative to low-potency medications).

Exclusion of individuals with tardive dyskinesia from assignment to the FGA perphenazine

With input from NIMH and scientific advisors, we decided based on available evidence and current clinical consensus that tardive dyskinesia (TD) should be a contraindication for treatment with perphenazine because of evidence suggesting that FGAs posed greater risk for TD than SGAs. Therefore, the randomization scheme was stratified so that patients with TD at study entry were excluded from assignment to perphenazine and could only receive treatment with olanzapine, quetiapine, risperidone, or ziprasidone. We called this Phase 1A of the study.

Double-blinded treatment conditions in Phases 1 and 2

The treatments in Phases 1 and 2 were blinded to enable wholly objective comparisons of treatment effectiveness between drugs. The rationale for blinding to minimize biases was considered sufficiently compelling despite the complications it introduced to the study's implementation and its ecological validity. Blinding was deemed necessary because the oral medications used in Phases 1 and 2 had been marketed for several years so that clinicians and patients were expected to have preconceived notions about the efficacy and side effect profiles of the medications that could have introduced considerable biases to ratings and decisions about treatment discontinuation. However, because of the logistical complexities

Table 1.2. [12] Baseline demographic and clinical characteristics of randomized patients.*

Characteristic	Olanzapine (N=336)	Quetiapine (N=337)	Risperidone (N=341)	Perphenazine (N=261)†	Ziprasidone (N=185)	Total (N=1460)
Demographic characteristics						
Age—yr	40.8±10.8	40.9±11.2	40.6±11.3	40.0±11.1	40.1±11.0	40.6±11.1
Sex—no. (%)						
Male	244 (73)	255 (76)	253 (74)	199 (76)	129 (70)	1080 (74)
Female	92 (27)	82 (24)	88 (26)	62 (24)	56 (30)	380 (26)
Race—no. (%)‡						
White	196 (58)	213 (63)	204 (60)	152 (58)	109 (60)	874 (60)
Black	119 (35)	114 (34)	122 (36)	93 (36)	65 (36)	513 (35)
Other	21 (6)	10 (3)	15 (4)	16 (6)	9 (5)	71 (5)
Spanish, Hispanic, or Latino ethnicity—no. (%)	42 (12)	48 (14)	38 (11)	24 (9)	18 (10)	170 (12)
Education—yr	12.2±2.2	12.1±2.4	12.0±2.2	12.1±2.1	12.0±2.5	12.1±2.3
Marital status—no. (%)						
Married	36 (11)	34 (10)	37 (11)	43 (16)	17 (9)	167 (11)
Previously married§	105 (31)	90 (27)	101 (30)	68 (26)	61 (33)	425 (29)
Never married	195 (58)	213 (63)	203 (60)	150 (57)	107 (58)	868 (59)
Unemployed—no. (%)¶	281 (85)	274 (84)	288 (86)	219 (85)	155 (85)	1217 (85)
Exacerbation in previous 3 mo—no. (%)	90 (27)	89 (26)	95 (28)	68 (26)	60 (32)	402 (28)
PANSS total score‖	76.1±18.2	75.7±16.9	76.4±16.6	74.3±18.1	75.4±18.6	75.7±17.6
Clinician-rated CGI severity score**	4.0±1.0	3.9±0.9	4.0±0.9	3.9±1.0	3.9±0.9	4.0±0.9

5

Table 1.2. (cont.)

Characteristic	Olanzapine (N=336)	Quetiapine (N=337)	Risperidone (N=341)	Perphenazine (N=261)†	Ziprasidone (N=185)	Total (N=1460)
Psychiatric history						
Age at 1st treatment for any behavioral or emotional problem—yr	24.1±9.0	23.6±8.1	23.7±9.3	24.5±8.6	24.1±9.7	24.0±8.9
Years since 1st antipsychotic medication prescribed	14.5±11.0	14.6±10.3	14.8±10.7	13.8±11.0	14.0±10.5	14.4±10.7
SCID diagnosis in past 5 yr—no. (%)						
Depression	85 (26)	84 (25)	104 (30)	71 (27)	60 (32)	405 (28)
Alcohol dependence or alcohol abuse	74 (22)	81 (24)	92 (27)	74 (28)	37 (20)	358 (25)
Drug dependence or drug abuse	86 (26)	95 (28)	110 (32)	74 (28)	57 (31)	422 (29)
Obsessive-compulsive disorder	10 (3)	22 (7)	21 (6)	12 (5)	8 (4)	73 (5)
Other anxiety disorder	44 (13)	46 (14)	52 (15)	29 (11)	28 (15)	199 (14)
Baseline antipsychotic medications—no. (%)††						
Olanzapine alone	78 (23)	69 (20)	76 (22)	58 (22)	41 (22)	322 (22)
Quetiapine alone	24 (7)	17 (5)	22 (6)	15 (6)	17 (9)	95 (7)
Risperidone alone	57 (17)	59 (18)	63 (18)	64 (25)	32 (17)	275 (19)
Any combination including olanzapine, quetiapine, or risperidone	31 (9)	32 (10)	33 (10)	21 (8)	8 (4)	95 (7)
All others	52 (15)	58 (17)	60 (18)	30 (11)	29 (16)	229 (16)
None	94 (28)	102 (30)	87 (26)	73 (28)	58 (31)	414 (28)

Baseline medical diagnoses—no. (%)

Diabetes (type 1 or 2)	36 (11)	40 (12)	32 (9)	29 (11)	17 (9)	154 (11)
Hyperlipidemia	56 (17)	44 (13)	42 (12)	36 (14)	26 (14)	204 (14)
Hypertension	68 (20)	67 (20)	63 (18)	60 (23)	31 (17)	289 (20)

Notes: *Plus-minus values are means ±SD. Because of rounding, percentages may not sum to 100. SCID denotes Structured Clinical nterview for DSM-IV.

†Patients with tardive dyskinesia were excluded from the perphenazine group.

‡Race was self-reported. "Other" includes American Indian or Alaska Native (less than 1 percent of patients), Asian (2 percent), Native Hawallan or other Pacific Islander (less than 1 percent), and two or more races (2 percent). Percentages are based on the number of patients with data available: 336 in the olanzapine group, 337 in the quetiapine group, 341 in the risperidone group, 261 in the perphenazine group, and 183 in the ziprasidone group.

§This category includes patients who were widowed, divorced, or separated.

•Percentages are based on the number of patients with data available: 330 in the olanzapine group, 328 in the quetiapine group, 336 in the risperidone group, 259 in the perphenazine group, and 182 in the ziprasidone group.

‖Scores on the Positive and Negative Syndrome Scale (PANSS) for schizophrenia can range from 30 to 210, with higher scores indicating more severe psychopathology.

**The CGI severity score can range from 1 to 7, with higher scores indicating greater severity of illness.

††Percentages for baseline medications are based on the number of patients with data on concomitant medications: 333 in the olanzapine group, 333 in the quetiapine group, 340 in the risperidone group, 259 in the perphenazine group, and 184 in the ziprasidone group.

Copyright ©2005 Massachusetts Medical Society. All right reserved.

that blinding it would have created given the need for white blood count monitoring, clozapine was used open-label.

Patient and clinician involvement in decision making

In response to feedback from consumer and advocacy groups to a draft protocol, it was decided to include participant input when determining possible treatment options. Consumer advocates suggested that this feature would make the study more appealing to consumers and their family members and thus would improve enrollment and retention rates. As a result, when participants entered Phase 2, they were referred to the appropriate Phase 2 protocol but given the option of exercising their own choice between the two Phase 2 studies. In addition, subjects and their clinicians made a shared decision about which open-label treatment to choose in Phase 3.

Determination of drug doses

The decision to encapsulate study medications so that study personnel and participants would be blinded to the treatment assignment meant that a decision had to be made regarding the dosage strength in each capsule. For simplicity, we chose to have only one dosage strength for each medication and to allow flexible dosing between one and four capsules per day. Because NIMH wanted the makers of the drug to provide study medication for free and to have some input about the use of their drug, we met with representatives of each company to describe the protocol and to present proposed dosage ranges for the study drugs. The original recommendations were based on dosage data from national pharmacy databases, FDA labeling, and the input of expert clinicians. We did not necessarily restrict the doses according to the approved dose if practice patterns or practical considerations suggested otherwise; for both olanzapine and quetiapine the maximum dose allowed in the study exceeded the upper limit of the FDA-approved range. Company representatives made recommendations for dosing of the company's drug only. For risperidone, although we proposed a dosage far lower than the FDA maximum of 16 mg/day (2–8 mg/day), company representatives chose to support an even lower dose range of 1.5–6 mg/day. Because ziprasidone had only recently been approved by the FDA and because of concern about its effect on cardiac repolarization, we and its makers strictly adhered to the FDA-approved dose range. Because perphenazine was generic, we did not meet with any company representatives but selected a moderate dose range that we thought would optimize efficacy while minimizing its risk of causing EPS.

Primary outcome

Time to all-cause treatment discontinuation was selected as the primary outcome variable because it is a discrete, clinically meaningful measure that reflects efficacy and tolerability as well as the input of both the patient and clinician. The need to change medications reflects the possibilities that the treatment was not sufficiently effective or tolerable, or the belief that another treatment would be superior. Because such changes are commonly associated with the increased need for health services they have significant cost implications.

Study physicians were provided with training and ongoing support from the principal medical officer to ensure that physician-initiated treatment changes were made only for clinically justifiable reasons, so that each treatment to which patients were assigned was given every chance to be effective before discontinuation. Clinicians were encouraged to optimize dosing and use adjunctive medications before determining that the assigned study drug was not efficacious or tolerable.

Inclusion of newly approved antipsychotics

To make the study maximally informative regarding clinical practice when completed, and because this was specified in the RFP, we made contingency plans to allow the inclusion of new antipsychotic drugs that gained FDA approval during the study's enrollment period. In February 2001, ziprasidone was approved by the FDA and was then added to Phases 1, 2, and 3 of the study. In November 2002, aripiprazole was approved by the FDA and was then added only to Phase 3 as an open-label treatment because it was considered too late to obtain meaningful information about it in the randomized, double-blinded phases of the study. Thus, we obtained information from randomized, blinded portions of the trial about ziprasidone, but only open-label, descriptive data about aripiprazole.

Methods

The overarching goal of the study was to obtain objective data about the comparative effects of antipsychotic drugs for the treatment of schizophrenia. While the initial impetus for the study was to examine the comparative effectiveness of the newer drugs that had become the dominant choices in the marketplace, a comparison between the newer drugs and an older drug became a major goal as the trial was designed.

The Specific Aims and Hypotheses, along with the statistical methods used to test hypotheses and present other results, are presented in detail in Chapter 2.

Study design

The CATIE schizophrenia trial was a multi-site, multi-phase randomized controlled trial of antipsychotic medications that enrolled almost 1500 persons with schizophrenia. Figure 1.1 represents a schematic diagram of the trial design. Participants were broadly representative of persons with the chronic and recurrent forms of schizophrenia. Patients were followed for at least 18 months. The study included three treatment phases and a naturalistic follow-up phase for those who discontinued study medication in all three treatment phases or who did not want to continue receiving protocol-driven treatment. Those who did well on an assigned treatment remained on that treatment for the duration of the 18-month treatment period. If an assigned treatment was discontinued, the patient moved to the next phase of the study to receive a new treatment.

We collected a broad array of outcome measures intended to capture meaningful information about the lives of the participants, their quality of life, cognitive functioning, and their use of general, mental health, substance abuse, and rehabilitative services. The study sought to include a sample of subjects that would be representative of those seen in typical clinical settings by recruiting "real-world" patients, including those with co-morbid conditions (e.g., substance use disorders or medical problems) that would exclude them from most clinical trials. The study was conducted at sites selected to represent a broad array of clinical settings (i.e., state mental health hospitals, community mental health centers, university hospitals and clinics, Veterans' Affairs Medical Centers, and private practices) to produce generalizable and practically relevant study findings.

In Phase 1 of the trial, patients were randomly assigned to double-blinded treatment with oral perphenazine, olanzapine, quetiapine, risperidone, or ziprasidone. Patients with

CATIE Schizophrenia Trial Design

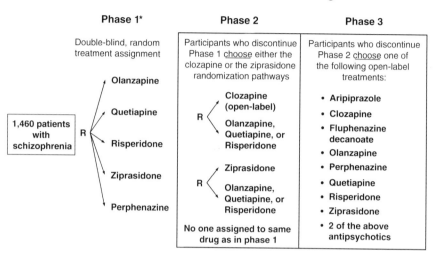

*Phase 1A: participants with Tardive Dyskinesia (TD) (N = 231) not randomized to perphenazine; Phase 1B: participants who discontinue perphenazine randomized to an atypical (olanzapine, quetiapine, or risperidone) before eligibility for Phase 2. R = randomized.

Figure 1.1. The CATIE schizophrenia trial design. From Stroup *et al.* The National Institute of Mental Health Clinical Antipsychotic Trials of Intervention Effectiveness (CATIE) Project: Schizophrenia Trial Design and Development, Schizophrenia Bulletin, 2003, volume 29, Issue 1, p. 19. Reused with permission of Oxford University Press.

tardive dyskinesia (TD) did not enter Phase 1 (and the possibility of assignment to perphenazine) but entered Phase 1A and were randomly assigned to treatment with oral olanzapine, quetiapine, risperidone, or ziprasidone. Ziprasidone was added to the study after 40% of participants had enrolled.

Participants who discontinued treatment with the conventional antipsychotic (oral perphenazine) in Phase 1 were randomly assigned to double-blinded treatment with olanzapine, quetiapine, or risperidone (Phase 1B). Phase 1B was intended to ensure that all study participants had discontinued a newer (second-generation) antipsychotic prior to entering Phase 2.

In Phase 2, participants who discontinued their assigned treatment with an SGA in Phase 1, 1A, or 1B were recommended to one of two randomized pathways based on their reason for discontinuation. The Tolerability pathway (Phase 2T) offered randomization to ziprasidone or one of the other atypical antipsychotics (olanzapine, quetiapine, or risperidone) not previously received by the patient in the study. Patients who discontinued their previous treatment with an SGA because of intolerance (e.g., weight gain or EPS) were recommended to enter Phase 2T. The Efficacy pathway (Phase 2E) offered randomization to clozapine or an SGA (olanzapine, quetiapine, or risperidone) not previously received by the patient in the study. Patients who discontinued their previous treatment because of inadequate efficacy were encouraged but not required to enter Phase 2E.

Phase 3 was for persons who discontinued the treatment assigned in Phase 2. Research and clinical personnel examined reasons for failure of the treatments assigned in Phases 1 and 2. Based upon this review, and upon partially blinded information regarding previous treatments, the clinician and patient selected an open-label treatment for Phase 3.

Table 1.3. Dosing for blinded medications

Blinded medications	Dose per standard study capsule	Dose range
Olanzapine	7.5 mg	7.5–30 mg/day
Perphenazine	8 mg	8–32 mg/day
Quetiapine	200 mg	200–800 mg/day
Risperidone	1.5 mg	1.5–6 mg/day
Ziprasidone	40 mg	40–160 mg/day

From Stroup *et al.* 2003, p. 22. Reused with permission of Oxford University Press.

The Follow-up Phase was for persons who are no longer willing to continue taking study medication or who discontinued their Phase 3 medication before 18 months from the time of initial randomization have elapsed. Follow-up Phase participants were not provided with study medication but were followed naturalistically and attended quarterly visits to provide basic outcome data through 18 months from the time of initial randomization.

Subjects

A sample of 1,460 men and women, 18–65 years of age, who met DSM-IV diagnostic criteria for schizophrenia, based upon the Structured Clinical Interview for DSM-IV (SCID), review of their clinical records, and input from available informants, enrolled in the study. Inclusion and exclusion criteria are listed in Table 1.2. Patients who entered the study were those with chronic schizophrenia for whom a new medication was needed or for whom a change in medications was an appropriate option.

Treatments
Pharmacologic treatments
Dosing of study medications

Standard study capsules contained olanzapine 7.5 mg, quetiapine 200 mg, risperidone 1.5 mg, ziprasidone 40 mg, or perphenazine 8 mg (Table 1.3). Clinicians prescribed one to four capsules daily, based upon individual patients' therapeutic response and side effect burden.

Once and twice daily medication schedules

Quetiapine and ziprasidone required twice daily (BID) dosing, whereas perphenazine, olanzapine, and risperidone could be taken once daily (QD). Because it would deviate from clinical practice patterns to insist on BID dosing in all cases, we sought to minimize the number of patients required to take their medication BID, and still maintain blinding to the extent possible. Throughout the study, half of the patients randomized to perphenazine, olanzapine, and risperidone were assigned to BID dosing, and half were assigned to QD dosing. All quetiapine and ziprasidone patients were assigned to receive BID dosing unless determined to need only one capsule per day.

Because of quetiapine's relatively slow recommended initial titration schedule, patients assigned to a BID dosing schedule began their treatment using an initial dose strength of

100 mg and titrate up to 200 mg BID over 4 days. After the initial titration period using a starter pack of five capsules, the total BID dose of all blinded study medications was identical to the QD dosing schedule for each drug.

Dosing for open-label medications

The recommended dose range for open-label clozapine in Phases 2 and 3 was 200–600 mg QD. The recommended dose range for fluphenazine decanoate injections available in Phase 3 was 12.5–50 mg IM every 2 weeks. The recommended dose range for aripiprazole in Phase 3 was 10–30 mg QD.

Transition to study medications

A cross-titration period of up to 28 days was permitted for patients who were already taking an antipsychotic at the time of study enrollment. Because the study addressed long-term effectiveness and tolerability rather than acute efficacy, the cross-titration period was used to facilitate the transition of patients onto their study medications and to minimize the risk of destabilization by this process. Clinicians were given substantial leeway in implementing these transitions according to clinical judgment.

Summary of pharmacologic treatments

The methods allowed double-blind comparisons across commonly prescribed dose ranges of the study drugs (olanzapine 7.5–30 mg daily, quetiapine 200–800 mg daily, risperidone 1.5–6 mg daily, ziprasidone 40–160 mg daily, and perphenazine 8–32 mg daily) with equivalent numbers of capsules, i.e., 1–4 daily.

Clinicians could adjust the dose of the assigned antipsychotic as clinically indicated within the range of 1–4 standard study capsules. Clinicians were allowed to prescribe adjunctive and concomitant medications whenever indicated, but antipsychotics other than the assigned study medicines were not allowed on an ongoing basis. Continuing need for an additional antipsychotic was considered a criterion for discontinuation of the study treatment.

Psychosocial interventions

Research participants were offered psychosocial interventions directed at improving patient and family understanding of the illness, decreasing the burden of illness on the family, maximizing treatment adherence, minimizing relapse, enhancing access to a range of community-based rehabilitative services, and improving study retention. Interventions included:

- patient and family education,
- opportunities for family support,
- adherence enhancement,
- broker/linking style case management or liaison with existing case management services.

Patient and family education

All participants were offered an individually tailored educational plan adapted from the Texas Medication Algorithm Project (TMAP). The TMAP education plan was conducted in several phases and invited family participation if desired by the patient. Each phase involved one or more individual sessions, with patients moving to the next phase as appropriate. All sessions were presented orally, with supplementary print materials offered. Videotape educational presentations were also available. In order to assess the intensity of educational efforts, research staff kept a record of the educational sessions provided to each subject.

The phases of the educational plan included the following:

- Individual introductory education. Content included diagnosis, medications, and symptom self-monitoring.
- Individual follow-up. Content included self-assessment of symptoms and side effects, assessing changes in symptoms, etc.
- Ongoing education. Content included more extensive information about the illness and treatment and reinforcement of earlier content.
- Group education/support. This phase offered opportunities for patients to discuss the illness with each other and provided referrals to other support groups.

Family support

Study sites were encouraged to work with the National Alliance for the Mentally Ill (NAMI) to facilitate offerings of family support groups at study sites or in the local community.

Adherence enhancement

Kemp's Compliance Therapy intervention was adapted for CATIE to guide and enhance patient and family education on medication adherence [6]. This intervention uses techniques from cognitive behavioral therapy and motivational interviewing to equip therapists to address common problems of denial of illness and resistance to treatment. In the initial phase, the patient's stance toward treatment is elicited. In the second phase, ambivalence to treatment is explored, common misgivings are addressed, misconceptions are corrected, and indirect benefits of medications are emphasized. The third phase of Compliance Therapy focuses on treatment maintenance.

Case management

Although sites varied in the availability of case management, all participants could access locally available community-based treatment and rehabilitative services. For subjects with active case management, study sites did not duplicate these services. Where subjects did not have case management, site personnel served as broker/linking style case managers, attempting to gain entry for subjects to community services.

Measures and assessment of outcomes

Subjects attended monthly study visits for clinical examinations and to participate in assessments following the study's Schedule of Events (Table 1.4). Outcome measures were obtained from a variety of sources, including patient self-report and ratings by trained study personnel.

Table 1.4. Schedule of outcome measures

Months	Screening	Baseline	1	2	3	4	5	6	7	8	9	10	11	12	13	14	15	16	17	18	Unscheduled end of phase
Eligibility assessments:																					
Demographics, SCID, physical exam, vital signs	X																				
MacCAT-CR[1]	X																			X	X
Ophthalmoscopic exam	X							X						X						X	X
Weight, waist, hip measurement, blood pressure & pulse		X			X			X			X			X			X			X	X
Medical diagnoses		X						X						X						X	X
Concomitant/adjunctive medications		X	X	X	X	X	X	X	X	X	X	X	X	X	X	X	X	X	X	X	X
Medication adherence			X	X	X	X	X	X	X	X	X	X	X	X	X	X	X	X	X	X	X
General status (CGI-S,[2] self-reported CGI, AUS/DUS,[3] habits, global satisfaction)		X	X		X			X			X			X			X			X	X
PANSS[4]		X	X	X	X			X			X			X			X			X	X
Calgary Depression Rating Scale (CDRS)		X	X		X			X			X			X			X			X	X
Adverse events/side effects																					
EPS rating scales: Barnes akathisia, Simpson-Angus, AIMS[5]		X	X		X			X			X			X			X			X	X

Side effect inquiry	X	X	X	X	X	X	X	X		X	X	X
Psychosocial measures												
Quality of life			X		X					X	X	X
MacArthur Risk Assessment Instrument			X		X						X	X
SF-12[6]			X		X					X	X	X
Insight (ITAQ)			X		X					X	X	X
Drug Attitude Inventory (DAI)		X	X		X	X	X	X	X	X	X	X
SURF-monthly[7]	X	X	X	X	X	X	X	X	X	X	X	
SURF-quarterly	X	X		X	X		X			X	X	X
Family Experiences Interview	X			X	X					X	X	X
Laboratory measurements												
Pregnancy test (serum B-hCG)	X											
Thyroid stimulating hormone (TSH)	X											
Prolactin	X		X		X						X	X
Chemistries, CBC, liver function tests, hemoglobin A1C	X		X		X						X	X
Antipsychotic drug level		X	X		X		X				X	X
Urine drug screen	X	X	X		X		X				X	X
Radioimmunoassay test of hair for drugs	X				X		X				X	X

Table 1.4. (cont.)

Months	Screening	Baseline	1	2	3	4	5	6	7	8	9	10	11	12	13	14	15	16	17	18	Unscheduled end of phase
ECG	X	X																		X	X
Neurocognitive battery		X						X												X	
WRAT-III Reading Test		X																			

Notes: [1]MacArthur Competence Assessment Tool for Clinical Research.
[2]Clinical Global Impressions Scale-Severity.
[3]Clinician's Alcohol Use Scale, Drug Use Scale.
[4]Positive and Negative Syndrome Scale.
[5]Abnormal Involuntary Movement Scale.
[6]Medical Outcomes Survey Short Form-12 Items.
[7]Service Utilization and Resources Form.
From Stroup *et al.* 2003, pp 24–25. Reused with permission of Oxford University Press.

Table 1.5. Clinical and functional outcome measures

Psychopathology	Positive and Negative Syndromes Scale (PANSS)
	The Clinical Global Impressions Scale (CGI)
	Calgary Depression Rating Scale (CDRS)
Quality of life, health status and functioning	Heinrichs-Carpenter Quality of Life Scale (QLS)
	Medical Outcomes Study Short Form-12 (SF-12)
	Lehman Quality of Life Interview (QOLI)
	MacArthur Community Violence Instrument
Side effects and adverse effects measures	Abnormal Involuntary Movement Rating Scale (AIMS)
	Simpson Angus Extrapyramidal Side Effect Scale (SAEPS)
	Barnes Akathisia Scale (BAS)
	Systematic Inquiry of Adverse Effects/Side Effects
Family experiences	Family Experiences Interview Schedule (adapted)
Measures of attitude toward treatment	Drug Attitude Inventory (DAI)
	Insight into Treatment Attitude Questionnaire (ITAQ)

From Stroup *et al.* 2003, p. 26. Reused with permission of Oxford University Press.

Clinical and functional assessments
Primary outcome
Time to all-cause treatment discontinuation, reflecting the decision to discontinue and change medications, was the primary outcome in the study. Non-adherence, exacerbation of psychopathology, or hospitalization did not necessarily require discontinuation of the study antipsychotic. (For example, if a recurrence of symptoms resulted from a trip during which the patient forgot to bring his or her medication and therefore did not take it.) Similarly, only side effects that produced significant subjective distress or objective dysfunction that could not be resolved by dose adjustment or adjunctive medications was expected to lead to clinician-initiated treatment discontinuation. The well-being of patients was the primary consideration in all clinical decision making.

In addition to the primary outcome measure, the clinical and functional outcome measures listed in Table 1.5 were used to assess psychopathology, recovery, relapse, and severity of illness over the course of the study.

Side effects and adverse effects measures
Vital signs, weight, waist circumference, and laboratory tests including lipid profiles, glycosolated hemoglobin, and fasting glucose levels were monitored regularly according to the Schedule of Events (Table 1.4).

Adverse effects

Given the substantial clinical experience already available with these drugs, we elected to focus monitoring on 18 well-known adverse effects that had been commonly reported with one or more of the study antipsychotics to determine the relative frequencies and severities of these common and important adverse effects. However, a general inquiry section was used to record information about additional treatment-emergent adverse effects. Serious adverse effects, including hospitalizations due to exacerbation of schizophrenia, were recorded according to the guidelines of the US Food and Drug Administration.

Family/caregiver experiences

Family experiences were measured to assess the impact of schizophrenia on patients' families using a revised version of the Family Experiences Interview Schedule [7]. Families and caregivers were asked about any instrumental support, limit setting for disturbing behavior, time spent directly related to care for the patient, lost productivity, and financial contributions to the patient's care. The interview also included questions about the positive aspects of caregiving and positive contributions of patients to family functioning.

Medication adherence

Medication adherence was measured at each monthly visit using pill counts. In addition, at each visit study personnel synthesized information from the pill count and any other relevant information into a Global Judgment of Medication Adherence. In order to enhance understanding of the relationship between patient attitudes toward medications, insight into illness, and medication adherence, we administered the Drug Attitude Inventory (DAI) [8] and the Insight into Treatment Attitude Questionnaire (ITAQ) [9] at specified intervals according to the Schedule of Events (Table 1.4).

Substance use

Substance use was examined in multiple ways. Subjects were asked quarterly about drug and alcohol use. Urine drug screens and radioimmunoassay (RIA) of hair samples were used to detect substances of abuse. The Clinician Alcohol Use Scale and Drug Use Scale were used to rate substance use on a 5-point scale, with anchors ranging from abstinence to dependence requiring institutionalization. More information on these methods is described in Chapter 11.

Neurocognitive assessments

As described in Chapter 8, a Neurocognitive Advisory Group was selected in concert with the NIMH project officer and the External Scientific Advisory Board. Selection of members was designed to ensure maximum consensus and integration of personnel across committees.

The neurocognitive battery was completed according to the Schedule of Events in Table 1.4. The tests are listed below.

- Controlled Oral Word Association Test
- WISC-R Mazes
- Letter-Number Test

- Hopkins Verbal Learning Test
- Face Emotion Discrimination Task
- Revised WAIS-R Digit Symbol Test
- Grooved Pegboard
- Computerized Continuous Performance Test
- Computerized Spatial Working Memory test
- Computerized Wisconsin Card Sorting Test

These tests and the neurocognitive functions measured by them are described in Chapter 8.

Health services and cost-effectiveness

External factors such as the contacts between the patient and his or her health care setting and psychosocial support system (including family interactions, living situation, environmental safety, and financial resources) may affect outcomes and also reflect the effectiveness of treatments. The methods used to examine the organizational context of care, subject service utilization, and the basis for the study's cost-effectiveness and cost-benefit analyses in CATIE are described in detail in Chapter 4.

Safety

Serious Adverse Events, as defined by the Food and Drug Administration, were assessed according to FDA guidelines, and included all events that resulted in death, initial or prolonged hospitalization, a congenital anomaly, were severely or permanently disabling, or were life threatening or medically significant. Treatment-emergent adverse effects were monitored using the Adverse Events/Side Effects measure described above.

Clinical monitoring and laboratory tests

The schedule for clinical monitoring and laboratory testing appears in the Schedule of Events (Table 1.4). Screening evaluations were intended to identify medical abnormalities and to establish baseline levels. Laboratory Assessments are collected and processed via a central laboratory, while ECGs are processed through a central ECG laboratory.

Vital signs and weight were recorded at screening, month 1, month 3, and quarterly thereafter. Height was recorded at screening. In addition to a screening ECG, an ECG was conducted at the month 18 visit, at each End of Phase visit, and 1 month after a participant started on a new study medication.

A simple ophthalmoscopic exam to evaluate for the presence of cataracts was conducted as part of the screening physical exam. Follow-up ophthalmoscopic exams were conducted every 6 months and at End of Phase visits.

Statistical methods and analytic plan

The statistical methods and analytic plan of the CATIE schizophrenia trial are described in detail in Chapter 2.

Human subjects considerations

Given the heightened public and scientific concern about the participation of mentally ill subjects in research, a CATIE Ethics Committee was established to review all human subjects considerations. This committee recommended the procedures that are described in detail in Chapter 14. Briefly, all prospective research participants were screened for decision-making capacity using the MacArthur Competence Assessment Tool-Research (MacCAT-CR) [10]. Only individuals who demonstrated adequate capacity to consent in this study and who chose to participate enrolled.

Persons who were initially assessed not to have the capacity to provide informed consent but who wanted to participate were offered a brief educational program based on the one used by Carpenter *et al.* [11]. After the program was completed, decision-making capacity was again assessed using the MacCAT-CR. Persons who demonstrated adequate decision-making capacity after completing the educational program could then enter the study. In order to assess decision-making capacity longitudinally, and to examine the effects of the study medications on decisional capacity, the MacCAT-CR is administered to participants at screening, month 6, month 18, and at each End of Phase visit.

Summary

This chapter has summarized the rationale, aims, and design of the CATIE schizophrenia trial, its procedures, and its proposed method of evaluating the effectiveness of antipsychotic medications[12]. The study design was that of a practical clinical trial intended to evaluate the effectiveness of treatments in everyday settings to generate results intended to inform clinicians, administrators, policy makers, and patients. In the context of clinical therapeutics and interventions research, practical trials provide an important bridge for the verification and translation of findings from traditional randomized controlled trials to clinical practice and public mental health care.

References

1. Lebowitz BD, Vitiello B and Norquist GS. Approaches to multisite clinical trials: The National Institute of Mental Health perspective. *Schizophrenia Bulletin* 2003;**29**:7–13.

2. Hotopf M, Churchill R and Lewis G. Pragmatic randomised controlled trials in psychiatry. *British Journal of Psychiatry* 1999;**175**:217–23.

3. March JS, Silva SG, Compton S, *et al.* The case for practical clinical trials in psychiatry. *American Journal of Psychiatry* 2005;**162**:836–46.

4. Tunis SR, Stryer DB and Clancy CM. Practical clinical trials: Increasing the value of clinical research for decision making in clinical and health policy. *Journal of the American Medical Association* 2003;**290**:1624–32.

5. Stroup TS and Geddes JR. Randomized controlled trials for schizophrenia: Study designs targeted to distinct goals. *Schizophrenia Bulletin* 2008;**34**:266–74.

6. Kemp R, Hayward P, Applewhaite G, *et al.* Compliance therapy in psychotic patients: Randomised controlled trial. *British Medical Journal* 1996;**312**:345–9.

7. Tessler RGG. *Family Experiences Interview Schedule Toolkit.* Cambridge, MA: Human Services Research Institute; 1995.

8. Awad AG. Subjective response to neuroleptics in schizophrenia. *Schizophrenia Bulletin* 1993;**19**:609–18.

9. McEvoy JP, Apperson LJ, Appelbaum PS, *et al.* Insight in schizophrenia. Its relationship to acute psychopathology. *The Journal of Nervous and Mental Disease* 1989;**177**:43 7.

10. Appelbaum PS, Grisso T. *MacArthur Competence Assessment Tool for Clinical Research*. Sarasota, FL: Professional Resource Press; 2001.

11. Carpenter WT Jr, Gold JM, Lahti AC, *et al.* Decisional capacity for informed consent in schizophrenia research. *Archives of General Psychiatry* 2000;**57**:533–8.

12. Lieberman JA, Stroup TS, McEvoy JP, *et al.* Effectiveness of antipsychotic drugs in patients with schizophrenia. *New England Journal of Medicine* 2005;**353**:1209–23.

Chapter

2

Statistical considerations

Sonia M. Davis, Gary G. Koch, Robert A. Rosenheck, and Vicki G. Davis

Introduction

The CATIE (Clinical Antipsychotic Trials of Intervention Effectiveness) schizophrenia study sought to compare the effectiveness and cost-effectiveness of four second-generation antipsychotics and one first-generation antipsychotic in the treatment of schizophrenia. The study design was a multi-phase double-blind randomized clinical trial. CATIE was uniquely complex in that 1) it included five medications, which were intended to be compared in a pair-wise fashion; 2) multiple treatment phases involved re-randomizing subjects to a unique subset of the study drugs; 3) in the first phase, different exclusion criteria were applied to different treatments: subjects with tardive dyskinesia (TD) were not included in the randomization to perphenazine, resulting in a stratified randomization design; and 4) one drug became available after 40% of the sample had been recruited, further extending the stratified randomization design. These complicating factors required a unique and complex set of analytic strategies.

In the first phase of the CATIE study, subjects were randomized to perphenazine, a "typical" antipsychotic, or one of four "atypical" antipsychotic medications. The study originally started with three atypicals: olanzapine, quetiapine, and risperidone. The fourth, ziprasidone, was not yet approved by the FDA at the beginning of the trial, and was added after 40% of subjects had been enrolled. In addition, due to side effect concerns, subjects with TD were stratified into a subgroup labeled Phase 1A, in which the randomization schedule excluded perphenazine.

If the Phase 1/1A treatment was found to be unsatisfactory for any reason including subject decision, subjects could discontinue the first treatment phase and be re-randomized to a new double-blind treatment in Phase 2. The second phase was designed for subjects who discontinued from an atypical antipsychotic. Therefore, subjects who received perphenazine in Phase 1 first entered Phase 1B and were randomized to one of the three original study atypicals. They could subsequently enter Phase 2 if they discontinued from Phase 1B. At the second phase, subjects chose either a tolerability pathway that randomized them to ziprasidone versus one of the three original study atypicals, or an efficacy pathway that randomized them to open-label clozapine versus one of the three original atypicals. Before ziprasidone was added to the study, the tolerability arm simply contained the other three atypicals. Subjects could subsequently choose to discontinue the second treatment phase and enter an unrandomized open-label phase (Phase 3).

Subjects were to be followed in the study for 18 months. Double-blind medication was over-encapsulated and distributed in bottles. Investigators prescribed dosing between one

Antipsychotic Trials in Schizophrenia, ed. T. Scott Stroup and Jeffrey A. Lieberman. Published by Cambridge University Press. © Cambridge University Press 2010.

and four capsules daily, depending on individual patient response. The primary outcome in each phase was the time until stopping the phase for any reason, referred to as all-cause treatment discontinuation.

This study design posed several challenges for statistical analysis. We first describe the stratified Phase 1/1A randomization, and explain the steps for comparing treatment groups within the stratified randomization structure. Second, we describe strategies to perform treatment group comparisons that control the inflation of Type 1 error due to multiple pair-wise testing. Third, we focus on the evaluation of multiple outcomes. Fourth, we examine the advantages of using all-cause treatment discontinuation as the primary effectiveness outcome and the specific statistical issues for its analysis. Fifth, we address the impact of missing data due to phase discontinuation on analysis of the secondary outcomes. We contrast the statistical methods we employed to address this issue, and consider further methods. Several analysis options that combine data from multiple phases are also described.

Stratified randomization and its impact on statistical analysis

The treatment group randomization scheme for all phases is displayed in Table 2.1.

Randomization scheme for the first phase

The randomization for the first phase in the CATIE study was stratified by whether subjects had tardive dyskinesia (TD), by the cohort defined by the addition of ziprasidone to the protocol, and also by investigator site, for non-TD subjects only. The TD stratum was not stratified by site due to its small size.

Operationally, each of the strata in the first phase defined by the cross-classification of TD status and the ziprasidone cohort had a separate randomization schedule. There were four strata: (A) no TD, pre-ziprasidone; (B) no-TD, post-ziprasidone, (C) TD, pre-ziprasidone; and (D) TD, post-ziprasidone. Within each stratum, subjects were allocated to treatments in equal ratios. The set of treatments to which subjects were randomized differed across the four strata. Olanzapine, quetiapine, and risperidone were included in all strata. Perphenazine was in strata A and B, and ziprasidone was in strata B and D. The number of subjects randomized to each treatment group within each stratum is displayed in Table 2.2. Patients randomized to one site with concerns regarding data quality were excluded from analyses prior to unblinding, and are not included in these counts.

Independently of the treatment group randomization, some subjects were also randomized to once a day or twice a day dosing. Those assigned to receive twice a day dosing were to split their daily dose equally between a morning and an evening dose. Once a day subjects took their entire daily dose in the morning. Quetiapine (Q) and ziprasidone (Z) were administered twice a day to all subjects, as required by the prescription labeling for these drugs. Subjects who were randomized to olanzapine (O), perphenazine (P), or risperidone (R), which are to be taken once per day per the prescription labeling, were randomized to either once a day or twice a day dosing in a 1:1 ratio. The randomization to daily dosing frequency was applied independently of treatment randomization. The purpose of this randomization was to mask the treatment assignment for people who received twice a day dosing, yet also minimize the number of subjects taking medication in a way different from the prescription labeling instructions. It should

Table 2.1. CATIE schizophrenia trial randomization scheme

Phase	Pre-ziprasidone cohort	Ziprasidone cohort
Phase 1 For subjects without TD	Stratum A Site stratified, 4 groups O:Q:R:P – 1:1:1:1 Blocks of size 8	Stratum B Site stratified, 5 groups O:Q:R:P:Z – 1:1:1:1:1 Blocks of size 5
Phase 1A Subgroup of Ph. 1 for subjects with TD not eligible for treatment with perphenazine	Stratum C Central, 3 groups O:Q:R – 1:1:1 Blocks of size 3	Stratum D Central, 4 groups O:Q:R:Z – 1:1:1:1 Blocks of size 4
Phase 1B For subjects randomized to perphenazine in Phase 1	Central, 3 groups O:Q:R – 1:1:1 Blocks of size 3	Z was not added
Phase 2 Clozapine pathway Subjects were not eligible for treatments received in prior phases	Central, 4 groups C:O:Q:R – overall 3:1:1:1 Blocks of size 4 or 6 Stratified by Phase 1/1A/1B treatment: Ph. 1/1A/1B Trt: Blocks: O C:Q:R 2:1:1 Q C:O:R 2:1:1 R C:O:Q 2:1:1 Z C:O:Q:R 3:1:1:1	Z was not added
Phase 2 Ziprasidone pathway Subjects were not eligible for treatments received in prior phases	Central, 3 groups O:Q:R – overall 1:1:1 Blocks of size 4 Stratified by Phase 1/1A/1B treatment: Ph. 1/1A/1B Trt: Blocks: O Q:R 2:2 Q O:R 2:2 R O:Q 2:2	Central, 4 groups Z:O:Q:R – overall 3:1:1:1 Blocks of size 3 or 4 Stratified by Phase 1/1A/1B treatment: Ph. 1/1A/1B Trt: Blocks: O Z:Q:R 2:1:1 Q Z:O:R 2:1:1 R Z:O:Q 2:1:1 Z O:Q:R 1:1:1
Phase 3	Non-randomized Open-label choice	Non-randomized Open-label choice

Abbreviations: O = olanzapine; Q = quetiapine; R = risperidone; P = perphenazine; Z = ziprasidone;
C = open-label clozapine.
Pre-ziprasidone randomizations occurred before ziprasidone was added to the study.
Subjects discontinuing Phase 1 or 1A were eligible for Phase 2, except for subjects who received perphenazine
in Phase 1, who were first eligible for Phase 1B, and were subsequently eligible for Phase 2 upon discontinuation
of Phase 1B.
Note: Block sizes were unknown to CATIE investigators.

be noted that this strategy partially unmasked treatment assignments, since only three of
the five drugs were eligible for once a day dosing. An alternate strategy, such as study
drug administration with blister cards using dummy placebo capsules, would have been
prohibitively expensive. The comparison of daily dosing frequencies was not an *a priori*

Table 2.2. Randomized subjects in Phase 1/1A by randomization stratum

Randomization strata	OLZ (O)	PERP (P)	QUET (Q)	RISP (R)	ZIPR (Z)	Total
Stratum A Phase 1: no TD, pre-ziprasidone	118	110	116	127	–	471
Stratum B Phase 1: no TD, ziprasidone cohort	152	151	154	148	153	758
Stratum C Phase 1A: TD subjects, pre-ziprasidone	33	–	34	33	–	100
Stratum D Phase 1A: TD subjects, ziprasidone cohort	33	–	33	33	32	131
Total	336	261	337	341	185	1460

research question, and since it was not applicable to all treatments, it was not included as a factor in the statistical comparison of treatment groups.

Exacerbation status, defined as whether the subject had been hospitalized for crisis stabilization in the past 3 months, was expected to be a key predictor of outcome. It was considered during sample size and power calculations at study planning, and was included *a priori* as a covariate in statistical comparisons of treatment groups, but was not a randomization stratum.

Subject groupings for analysis of the first phase

Because the treatment group options for perphenazine and ziprasidone differed across the four randomization strata in the first phase, statistical comparisons involving perphenazine and ziprasidone might have been biased if not limited to subjects from these strata. For example, a comparison of the perphenazine treatment group, which contained no TD subjects, versus *all* subjects randomized to another treatment group would likely find that the perphenazine group had lower mean abnormal movement scale scores at baseline. On the other hand, for treatment groups whose membership did not vary across strata (olanzapine, quetiapine, and risperidone), an optimal and unbiased analysis combines all subjects from the stratification groups.

Therefore, to both avoid bias and maximize efficiency, treatment group comparisons for key outcomes were conducted on four analytic data sets with overlapping membership based on the TD and ziprasidone cohort stratification. As shown in Table 2.3, each data set only included subjects who had an equal chance of randomization to the treatments under comparison. Perphenazine subjects, in particular, were only compared to equivalent subjects who did not have TD at baseline, and ziprasidone subjects were only compared to subjects who were enrolled after ziprasidone was added.

Analytic Set 1 was used specifically for comparisons of perphenazine with the other antipsychotics available at the start of the study, and was limited to subjects in Phase 1, i.e., those without TD. Ziprasidone was excluded from this primary analysis because it was added to the trial late. However, subjects not randomized to ziprasidone in the Phase 1

Table 2.3. Randomized subjects in Phase 1/1A by analytic dataset

Analytic data set	OLZ (O)	PERP (P)	QUET (Q)	RISP (R)	ZIPR (Z)	Total
Analytic Set 1: P vs. O vs. Q vs. R Excluding subjects on Z and Phase 1A:TD subjects	270	261	270	275	–	1076
Analytic Set 2: O vs. Q vs. R Excluding subjects on P or Z	336	–	337	341	–	1014
Analytic Set 3: Z vs. O, Q, R Limited to ziprasidone cohort, Excluding subjects on P	185	–	187	181	185	738
Analytic Set 4: Z vs. P Limited to ziprasidone cohort, Excluding Phase 1A:TD subjects	–	151	–	–	153	304

ziprasidone cohort were included in this analytic set, as these subjects all had an equal chance of being randomized to one of the other four treatments. Therefore, Analytic Set 1 contains all subjects from Stratum A, as well as all subjects in Stratum B, except those who were randomized to ziprasidone.

Analytic Set 2 was used specifically for comparisons of olanzapine, quetiapine, and risperidone. Since each of these three treatments was included in all four randomization strata, all four strata were combined together for comparisons of these treatments.

All ziprasidone comparisons were limited to subjects in the ziprasidone cohort. Therefore, Analytic Set 3, used for comparison of Z vs. O, Q, and R, includes all subjects from stratification group D as well as all subjects in Stratum B, except those who had been randomized to perphenazine. Analytic Set 4, used for comparisons of Z vs. P, is limited to subjects randomized to Z or P in Stratum B, i.e., subjects without TD randomized after ziprasidone was added.

Strategies for pair-wise treatment group comparisons

The previous section described the analysis data sets used for key treatment group comparisons. This section describes null hypotheses, step-down testing, and adjustment for multiple comparisons that comprise the primary analysis steps. Outcome measures upon which these steps were applied are described in later sections.

Primary strategy for treatment group comparisons in the first phase

The primary CATIE objective compared olanzapine, quetiapine, and risperidone to perphenazine and was updated during the course of the trial. Since ziprasidone was added partway through the study, it was not included in the primary objective. The original primary hypothesis, specified in 1999, was that the three atypical antipsychotics, pooled together, would be superior to perphenazine. The second step of the primary analysis was to compare the three atypical antipsychotics to each other, if they were together found to be superior to perphenazine.

However, analyses presented in 2003, particularly a large influential meta-analysis of 124 randomized controlled trials, suggested that the atypical antipsychotics are not a homogeneous group and found that not all of them were substantially different from typicals such as haloperidol [1]. There were virtually no studies of intermediate potency drugs like perphenazine. In addition, a large Veterans Affairs (VA) trial found no advantage of olanzapine over haloperidol on measures of effectiveness [2].

Therefore, in 2004, while the study was still ongoing, the primary hypothesis of the CATIE trial was modified to directly compare all four treatment groups. The second step comparing the three atypicals remained the same and was to be investigated only if the primary analysis found an overall difference between the four treatments. Consideration was needed to plan the testing strategy because we sought to compare multiple drugs with multiple statistical tests, rather than performing just one test for which the conventional $p \leq 0.05$ criteria for statistical significance is appropriate.

The first step of the primary analysis was an overall 3 degree of freedom (df) test comparing the four treatment groups, excluding Phase 1A TD subjects and ziprasidone, using Analytic Set 1 (see Figure 2.1). This global test acted as a gatekeeper [3], such that subsequent evaluations for statistical significance would be completed only if this global test had $p \leq 0.05$.

Assuming a significant ($p \leq 0.05$) difference was found between the four treatment groups in Phase 1, the three atypical treatment groups were then compared for Phases 1 and 1A combined using Analytic Set 2. If a significant ($p \leq 0.05$) difference was found for the 2 df test, then pair-wise comparisons were evaluated, also relative to $p \leq 0.05$. No adjustment for multiple comparisons was needed, since the 2 df test was a step-down; i.e., it was not evaluated for significance unless there was significance for the overall 3 df test. Similarly, the pair-wise tests were a step-down of the 2 df test, and the α-level for a set of

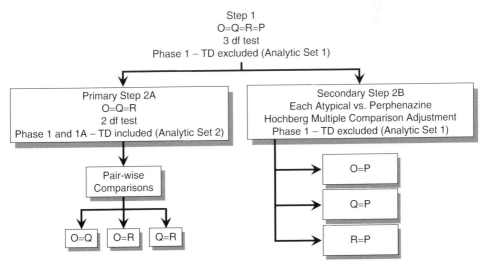

Figure 2.1. Primary Phase 1/1A treatment group comparisons.

three pair-wise step-down comparisons is protected based on closed testing procedures [4]. This testing strategy is displayed as Step 2A in Figure 2.1.

In addition, assuming a significant difference was found between the four treatment groups in Phase 1, pair-wise comparisons of the atypicals versus perphenazine were evaluated using Analytic Set 1, as displayed in Step 2B of Figure 2.1. Within Step 2B, the Type I error was maintained at 0.05 by a Hochberg modification to the Bonferroni adjustment for multiple comparisons [5,6].

The Hochberg adjustment for three multiple comparisons was conducted as follows:

- All three comparisons were considered significant if the largest p-value was ≤ 0.050.
- Otherwise, the two strongest comparisons were considered significant if the second smallest p-value was ≤ 0.025 (0.05/2).
- Otherwise, the strongest comparison was considered significant if the smallest p-value was ≤ 0.0167 (0.05/3).

Stepping down to the atypical vs. conventional comparisons was considered a secondary rather than primary test. This secondary step had an alternate focus from the primary comparison of the three atypicals, and was a separate family of comparisons. The experiment-wise Type I error rate was not strictly controlled by our method for Step 2B. However, we felt it was a reasonable strategy to address both Step 2A and 2B at the 0.05 significance level. Our strategy provided complete experiment-wise Type I error control for Step 2A, and family-wise control for Step 2B.

Ziprasidone comparisons

To avoid any potential cohort bias, whereby subjects enrolled later could be different from subjects enrolled earlier, ziprasidone was compared against the other four treatment groups only within the cohort of subjects who were enrolled after ziprasidone was added to the study. The analysis consisted of pair-wise comparisons of ziprasidone to each of the other treatment groups (O, Q, R, and P), using Analytic Set 3 for comparisons with O, Q, and R and Analytic Set 4 for comparison with perphenazine, as shown in Figure 2.2. The Type I error rate was maintained at 0.05 by a Hochberg adjustment for four multiple comparisons. The adjustment was similar to that described above for three comparisons, except that the strongest treatment comparison was considered significant if the smallest p-value was ≤ 0.0125 (0.05/4).

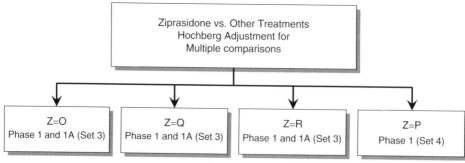

Figure 2.2. Ziprasidone Phase 1/1A treatment group comparisons for subjects enrolled after ziprasidone was added.

Secondary strategy for treatment group comparisons in the first phase

Analysis of the primary outcome, time to all-cause discontinuation, used the above primary treatment group comparison strategy (Figures 2.1 and 2.2) with each of the four overlapping analytic sets. This strategy was also used for many key secondary outcomes, such as efficacy rating scales, costs, quality of life, neurocognition, and movement disorder side effects. However, this rigorous approach was felt to be overly complex and unnecessary for other secondary outcomes in which little or no bias in treatment group comparisons was expected from the absence of TD subjects in the perphenazine arm and the late arrival of ziprasidone, such as metabolic outcomes. In the analysis of such secondary outcomes, the following secondary strategy for treatment group comparisons was implemented.

The absence of a ziprasidone cohort effect was evaluated by comparing the outcome measure for the pre- versus post-ziprasidone cohorts of the original four treatment groups. If no differences were found, then all treatment groups and all subjects were included in one analysis. A similar strategy was followed for TD patients and perphenazine. In addition, TD status at baseline was generally included as a covariate in treatment group comparisons. The first step of the treatment comparisons consisted of a 4 degree of freedom overall test of the five treatment groups. If $p \leq 0.05$, then all 10 pair-wise treatment group comparisons were conducted. The Type I error was maintained by a Bonferroni adjustment for multiple comparisons, in which a comparison was considered significant if $p \leq 0.005$ (0.05/10). Comparisons with $p \leq 0.01$ (0.10/10) were identified as noteworthy. Identifying noteworthy comparisons was a reasonable strategy for two reasons: 1) the Bonferroni correction is known to be overly conservative [6]; 2) the conservative nature was increased because we evaluated pair-wise comparisons only when the overall test had $p \leq 0.05$; a "Bonferroni-after-gatekeeper" approach. Based on closed testing, when the overall test rejects the null hypothesis, then we know there are at least some differences between treatments, and control of the Type I error would require less-stringent adjustment.

Contrasting the primary and secondary comparison strategies

The primary treatment comparison strategy is complex, but was developed *a priori* to address the stratified nature of the study design while at the same time maximizing the power for treatment comparisons. It was consistently used for all primary outcomes and major outcomes that might have been biased by the randomization design.

For secondary outcomes without a concern for bias, the secondary strategy of combining all of the treatment groups into one analysis had both advantages and disadvantages. The main advantage was that treatment comparisons were substantially simplified, usually requiring only one instead of four separate analyses. The main disadvantage was that the degree of significance level adjustment required to account for 10 pair-wise treatment group comparisons resulted in a loss of power. The primary strategy in Figure 2.1 was designed to maximize power for the primary comparisons and provides partial control of the Type I error rate since Step 2B controls family-wise error instead of experiment-wise error. Bonferroni adjustment of the 10 comparisons, on the other hand, provides full control of the Type I error, and is also overly conservative [6].

Bonferroni and its Hochberg modification can be applied to any statistical method since they are applied to the p-value, unlike some adjustment strategies that are calculated as part of the statistical test itself, and are only applicable to that particular method, such as Tukey or Dunnett. This flexibility was necessary for CATIE so that we could apply a consistent method of adjustment across all types of outcomes, regardless of statistical method.

We chose to employ Bonferroni rather than the more powerful Hochberg method in the secondary strategy for two reasons. First, Hochberg only provides full control of the Type I error rate when all comparisons are positively correlated, a condition not generally met by all pair-wise comparisons within a set of treatments [6]. Second, we noted a disadvantage of the Hochberg adjustment while interpreting the primary results. For Hochberg, the determination of statistical significance for a comparison depends on the relative ordering of the p-values within each parameter. Whether a particular numerical p-value is statistically significant depends not just on that one comparison but also on the p-values of the other comparisons within the family. Hence, it is possible to have the same numerical p-value identified as significant in the analysis of one parameter and not significant for another parameter. For the secondary strategy involving 10 pair-wise comparisons, we preferred a method with straightforward interpretation.

We found that the stratified design and the multi-tiered treatment group strategy described in Figures 2.1 and 2.2 complicated the interpretation of the results. A consequence of our plan was that the pair-wise comparisons of the treatment groups followed different rules for determining statistical significance. For example, analyses of time to all-cause discontinuation identified olanzapine as having a numerical advantage over all other treatments, with the longest median time to all-cause discontinuation [7]. Statistical significance of O versus Q and R was evaluated relative to $p = 0.05$. On the other hand, due to multiple comparison adjustment, comparisons with O were evaluated relative to $p = 0.0167$ for P and $p = 0.0125$ for Z. At the same time, comparisons for these two groups had less power because they were based on fewer subjects due to the stratified design. In summary, the comparisons that were limited to smaller sample sizes in order to obtain unbiased treatment group comparisons also had an additional decrease in power due to adjustment for multiple treatment comparisons. The trial had a statistical power of 85% to identify a difference of 12% in the rates of discontinuation between two atypical agents at $p \leq 0.05$; however, it had a statistical power of 76% for comparisons involving perphenazine and of 58% for comparisons involving ziprasidone at $p \leq 0.05$. It should be noted that these comparisons were identified *a priori* as secondary and that all samples were of substantial magnitude in comparison to most other studies.

Treatment group comparisons in subsequent phases

Treatment group comparisons in Phase 1B, the clozapine Phase 2 efficacy pathway, and the ziprasidone Phase 2 safety pathway followed strategies similar to the primary comparison strategy used in the first phase. These phases had no subject cohorts and fewer treatment groups, so methods were simpler. Specific details are described in each paper [8–10]. In Phase 3, the treatment options were numerous and non-randomized, so treatment group comparison in Phase 3 was purely descriptive [11].

Addressing multiple outcomes

Many types of outcomes were assessed in CATIE, and most were measured across each of the study phases. Without an *a priori* plan, statistical testing of all assessments would lead to an extreme inflation of the study-wise Type I error rate. Therefore, in addition to a plan for addressing multiple treatment group comparisons, we also developed a hierarchical strategy for evaluation of multiple outcomes.

Assessments were loosely grouped into domains. Overall effectiveness in the first phase was defined in the protocol as the primary domain. Secondary domains included effectiveness in the two Phase 2 pathways, cost-effectiveness, quality of life, neurocognitive functioning, efficacy, movement disorder side effects, and metabolic side effects. There were many tertiary domains, such as compliance, competency to give informed consent, family burden, violence, substance abuse, employment, use of concomitant medications, and the effect of prior antipsychotic treatments. A complete list of tertiary domains need not be specified *a priori*, as long as each domain was logically independent of others.

In general, within the primary and secondary domains, the domain-wise Type I error rate was maintained by identifying one primary analysis of one primary parameter within the domain. All other analyses of the primary parameter, as well as analyses of all other parameters within the domain, were viewed as secondary or supportive. P-values from the primary analysis were considered inferential, and p-values from all secondary analyses were considered descriptive. Descriptive p-values were presented to identify potential treatment differences without drawing conclusions about statistical significance. All p-values for the tertiary domains were descriptive, exploratory, or hypothesis-generating in nature.

For most results reported by the CATIE team, a statistical analysis plan was written prior to beginning the analysis. The plans included an identification of the primary and secondary parameters, the method for treatment group comparisons, as well as the types of statistical analyses to be applied. The CATIE executive committee took the responsibility to ensure that each statistical analysis reported by the CATIE team was focused on one domain and followed a multiple comparison strategy that addressed the multiple outcomes, multiple phases, and multiple treatment comparisons. The analysis plan for the primary effectiveness outcome was finalized prior to completion of the study.

Primary outcome: time to all-cause treatment discontinuation

The primary CATIE outcome domain was specified as overall treatment effectiveness. Although many types of overall effectiveness outcomes are possible, we chose time until all-cause treatment discontinuation because it is a discrete indicator that incorporates components of efficacy, tolerability, and compliance combined.

Treatment discontinuation was defined as withdrawal from randomized treatment or the study itself for any reason, including intolerable side effects, lack of efficacy, poor compliance, patient decision (after clinical reasoning and discussion with the patient by their clinician had taken place), or administrative reasons, which were fairly uncommon. For subjects who were lost to follow-up, the date of phase discontinuation was truncated to a maximum of 2 months plus 2 weeks following the last attended visit. Subjects who completed the study without requiring re-randomization to other study treatments were censored at the end of the study. In the statistical analysis, 1 month was defined as 28 days.

Kaplan Meier survival estimates were produced for time to treatment discontinuation. Hypothesis tests for assessing treatment differences were based on proportional hazards regression models [12] stratifying on pooled clinical site, and controlling for baseline clinical status (exacerbated, partially remitted), and TD status (Phase 1 vs. 1A), where applicable. Eight of 56 sites had 15 or fewer randomized subjects and were combined into three pooled sites based on the care setting of the site (public, university, private). Two small satellite sites were pooled with their partner, resulting in 49 sites. Once- and twice-daily dose groups were pooled for all analyses.

Discontinuation for specific reasons

The reason for discontinuation was collected, and secondary evaluations were carried out for three specific reasons for discontinuation: lack of efficacy, intolerability, and patient decision. In these analyses, subjects who discontinued due to a reason other than the one of interest were considered censored at the time of discontinuation.

This is a common method for analyzing competing risks: once a subject has discontinued for one reason, it is unknown if they might have discontinued for a different reason at a later time. The analysis provided an accurate description of the three types of events, but might not have provided an unbiased comparison of the treatment groups for each specific discontinuation reason. This is because the competing risks strategy assumes the three outcomes are independent; in other words, someone at high risk of discontinuing due to one reason is no more or less likely to discontinue due to one of the other reasons [13]. This assumption may not be valid. For instance if one treatment had both strong side effects and strong efficacy, or in the situation of patient decision, where a subject may discontinue because of side effects or lack of efficacy that the investigator did not feel warranted treatment discontinuation. Although the three reasons for discontinuation may not be completely independent, the primary evaluation of all-cause discontinuation incorporated them all together and therefore was free of bias.

Discussion of time to discontinuation

The simplicity and generality of time to discontinuation made it an excellent choice as a measurement of overall effectiveness. By including all reasons for treatment discontinuation, this outcome encompassed lack of efficacy, intolerable side effects, any combination of the two, lack of compliance, plus any other reason that led to substantial dissatisfaction with the medication, *without having to specifically identify these reasons*. In addition, it could be easily measured and understood by a general audience, without, for instance, needing to know details of specific scoring instruments. On the other hand, because of its lack of specificity, it may have limited clinical interpretation for psychiatrists and patients.

Applicable descriptive statistics for the primary outcome include median time on treatment and probability of staying on treatment for a specified duration. Because treatment group comparisons were based on hazard ratios, which could be complex for general audiences to understand, the outcome was further simplified for descriptive purposes into the proportion of subjects who discontinued the phase from each treatment group.

Time to discontinuation would not be an appropriate effectiveness outcome for acute illnesses that can be completely healed within a short time period, or intermittent illnesses with symptoms that come and go. In these cases, subjects who discontinued the drug because it was no longer required would need to be carefully separated from those for whom the drug was ineffective or intolerable. Unfortunately, this scenario is not applicable to schizophrenia, where long-term treatment is required, and where patients frequently stop taking medications for non-compliance or side effects. For schizophrenia, staying on a treatment for a longer time can in itself be considered a success in as much as it may lead to greater symptom reductions or improved quality of life.

Perhaps one of the most striking advantages of time until treatment discontinuation is the fact that the outcome was *defined by* whether a subject discontinued. This is a substantial benefit compared to many conventional outcomes which were missing, biased, or hard to interpret when a subject discontinued. Most types of outcome data in CATIE were collected in the form of repeated measurements over time, such as the PANSS, quality of life, side effect scales, cost-effectiveness, and laboratory assessments. As a subject discontinued the phase or the study, outcome data left missing for this person was not missing completely at random. For example, a subject who discontinued for lack of efficacy would likely have demonstrated high PANSS scores had they continued.

Analysis methods for outcomes measured at scheduled intervals are negatively impacted by non-ignorably missing data, and the impact increases with the amount of data that is missing. In CATIE, over a quarter of subjects had discontinued by 3 months, and 74% discontinued by 18 months. The next section of this chapter addresses several strategies for analyzing the secondary outcomes. Each strategy has a different approach to missing data caused by phase discontinuation, although none is a completely adequate way to address the large amount of data that was simply not present.

Analysis strategies for secondary outcomes

Most secondary outcomes in CATIE were assessed at repeated times, such as at months 1, 3, 6, 9, 12, 15, and 18, as well as the end of a phase. Subjects could switch from the first phase at any time, so some subjects were in a phase for 1 month or less, while others had 18 months of data. In addition, the schedule of assessments followed one plan, based on months since study baseline. Therefore, in subsequent phases, outcomes were not scheduled to be measured at the same time relative to phase switch, across subjects. We addressed this complication by combining assessments into 3-month intervals for analyses of subsequent phases.

A variety of statistical analysis methods were used to analyze the outcomes. Each is described below, along with a description of how it handles missing data due to subject discontinuations. Possible alternate strategies are also described.

Repeated measures analysis with mixed models

Change from baseline in the continuous measurements collected over the 18 months within a phase were compared across treatment groups with a mixed model including terms representing the baseline value of the dependent variable, time (treated as a classification variable), other baseline predictors in some situations, and baseline-by-time and treatment-by-time interactions. The baseline-by-time term adjusted for baseline differences in characteristics of subjects who dropped out early and thus were less well represented at later time points. A random subject effect and a spatial power covariance structure were used to adjust standard errors for the correlation of observations from the same individual. Some analyses used an autoregressive or an unstructured covariance matrix. Spatial power is an extension of the autoregressive structure that accounts for unequally spaced intervals. If the treatment-by-time interaction was not significant, it was removed from the model, in order to obtain treatment group differences averaged across all time points.

The repeated measures analysis used all available data and included all subjects with at least one post-baseline assessment. The covariance structure took into account the correlation of the repeated measurements within a person. Mixed models develop estimates under the assumption that the missing data are correlated in the same way as observed data, or in other words, that the data are missing at random. The mixed model may be fairly robust to some departure from this assumption, as has been shown by simulations of an example where the drop-out rate was 40% [14]. However, the amount of missing data in CATIE was substantial, reaching 74% by 18 months. Results from models based on such a substantial amount of missing data should be viewed with caution. In some cases, we minimized the impact of substantial missing data by excluding later months from the repeated measures model.

Assessments that were measured frequently, such as costs, PANSS, weight, and side effect scales were the best candidates for repeated measures analyses. Some assessments, such as PANSS, were measured quarterly, but also could be done at unscheduled visits or the end of the phase. In such cases, visit data were slotted into windows, and the last measure within the window was used in the model. In many papers, repeated measures results were confirmed by other secondary analyses.

Analysis at fixed time points

Some assessments, such as neurocognition, quality of life, and laboratory parameters were measured infrequently. For example, neurocognition was assessed at months 2, 6, and 18; quality of life was measured at 6, 12, and 18. For these parameters, we decided that repeated measures analysis was better as a secondary or supportive analysis, due to the small number of assessments, long duration between them, and substantial phase discontinuation over time. Instead, one of the time points was selected *a priori* as the primary time point, and the others were considered secondary. Separate treatment group comparisons were conducted at each time. For neurocognition, month 2 was selected as primary, and for quality of life, month 12 was primary. In each situation, the selection of the primary time point was driven by two competing issues: 1) selecting a meaningful time at which most of the treatment effect was expected to have been reached; and 2) selecting the earliest such meaningful time in order to include the largest number of subjects in the analysis. Treatment groups were compared with an analysis of covariance (ANCOVA) at each of the primary and secondary time points based on observed cases: subjects who had discontinued prior to reaching that time were excluded from the analysis.

The benefit of this strategy compared to the repeated measures model was that the ANCOVA was more straightforward to interpret, as it was based on data collected from just one time point. Repeated measures models, in contrast, estimate the results for all time points, but were based on sparse data for the large number of subjects who discontinued the phase.

The main disadvantage of the observed case strategy was that subjects who had discontinued before the primary time point did not contribute to the analysis. This caused both a loss of power and a limit on interpretability of the results. The effect of the treatments could only be evaluated for subjects who stayed in the phase until the primary time-point. We compared the baseline characteristics of subjects included in the primary analysis to those who were excluded to identify if the analysis sample was a selective subset. We also evaluated whether the treatment groups had balanced baseline characteristics within the primary analysis sample, since they no longer comprised a randomized sample. If a baseline imbalance was found, that parameter was included as a covariate in post-baseline comparisons.

Analysis adjusting for duration of exposure

Most of the primary analyses of key secondary parameters were analyzed with one of the two methods described above. However, for some parameters, particularly those focused on side effects, neither of these approaches was of interest. In these situations, one assessment per person was selected, such as:

- The last recorded value, collected at phase discontinuation (i.e., a last observation carried forward (LOCF) approach)
- The largest recorded laboratory value at any time during the phase
- An indicator of whether a subject ever met a certain criteria or experienced a certain event at any time during the phase

For these situations, all subjects were included in analyses. However, because subjects could discontinue the phase at any time from 1 to 18 months, subjects had different durations of exposure to the medication, and different amounts of repeated measurements. If subjects in one treatment group tended to discontinue earlier or later than other treatment groups, then treatment group comparisons of these outcomes that do not take into account the differential durations of exposure could be biased.

We sought to minimize this bias by adjusting for the duration that a subject was in the phase. One simple strategy for continuous parameters was to calculate a new outcome for each patient, such as the change in weight divided by the duration in the phase, to yield average weight change per month. We also used a more general approach via analysis of covariance in which duration of exposure was added as an independent covariate in the ANCOVA model. Treatment groups were then compared using least squares mean estimates corresponding to the average duration in the phase across all subjects. Similarly, for categorical outcomes, treatment groups were compared using Poisson regression, which took into account the duration that each subject was in the phase [15].

Advanced analysis options

The above three methods comprised most of the treatment group comparisons conducted for repeated secondary outcomes. Other more computationally advanced methods could be explored. Before fitting repeated measures models, the missing data could be estimated through a strategy of multiple imputation [16]. This was done as a supportive method for the analysis of cost effectiveness [17]. There are a number of methods available for imputation, although all should be considered cautiously when applied to large amounts of missing data, such as in CATIE.

Another promising analysis option is the joint modeling of time to discontinuation with a continuous outcome. This cutting edge strategy is currently under development [18], and is an area for future application for CATIE. At the time of writing this chapter, joint modeling of CATIE outcomes was being explored as part of a grant funded by the NIH.

Combining data from multiple phases

Most of the analyses completed by the CATIE team have been limited to the data within just one phase. However, some research questions were focused on combining data across the phases. A few methods for doing so are described in this section.

Analyses of all data based on the first randomization

One strategy that incorporates data from all phases evaluates differences in long-term outcomes as a function of the first treatment a subject received, regardless of subsequent treatment phases. It was applied in the primary CATIE cost-effectiveness analysis [16]. All collected data from each subject, including data from subsequent phases, was included in the repeated measures model. Within the model, the time classification for each measurement was defined as the number of months since initial randomization, and the treatment associated with each measurement was the initially assigned treatment. Medications assigned in the first phase were thus compared in an intent-to-treat fashion using this model.

This analysis strategy is not intended to identify acute treatment differences, but rather differences in treatment initiation strategies. Since real-world treatment often entails medication changes, this approach addresses the question, what long-term differences do we see if we start on one of five medications and apply a common algorithm to the selection of subsequent treatments? This strategy should be understood as a comparison of treatment initiation strategies and not of individual treatments, since the analysis includes data from subsequent phases without accounting for the actual subsequent treatment effects.

Analysis of treatment algorithms

Re-randomization in subsequent phases can also be viewed as a treatment algorithm. In this framework, a researcher may wish to explore whether there are treatment sequences that lead to a superior or inferior outcome. An analysis of treatment algorithms can be fit with the same repeated measures model as the intent-to-treat analysis based on the first treatment, but the single treatment assignment category for each person is expanded to account for the treatment sequence combination across the phases.

Analyses of treatment algorithms have some disadvantages. Since there are many possible treatment sequences obtained by combinations of treatments across phases in CATIE, the sample size for each sequence is fairly low, and therefore the power for identifying treatment sequence differences is low. Most importantly, in CATIE, the number of treatments that a subject received and the duration for which they took each treatment was driven by the subject's response to the treatments. The fact that a subject was re-randomized was actually part of their outcome; therefore, the treatment algorithm received by a subject in CATIE is both part treatment, and part response. To date, no analyses sponsored by the CATIE team have focused on treatment algorithms.

Combining phases within one repeated measures model

It is appealing to maximize the power available in CATIE by combining data from all of the phases within one repeated measures model that takes the phase switches into account by applying the actual treatment received at each visit, yet making one set of treatment comparisons from all phases combined. The repeated measures modeling required to fit this analysis to the CATIE design can be complex, which could hinder interpretation of treatment comparisons. However, the CATIE genetics working groups have employed this strategy to gain needed power in looking for genetic links between medications and specific outcomes [19].

Summary

This paper has addressed some of the fundamental statistical issues involved with the analysis of treatment group comparisons for the CATIE schizophrenia trial. We described the CATIE design and stratified randomization, presented a framework used to handle the multiple treatment group comparisons, motivated the primary overall effectiveness outcome of time until discontinuation from the first treatment phase, and described the advantages and limitations of several strategies used to analyze the secondary and tertiary outcomes.

Acknowledgments

The authors wish to thank C. Edward Davis for scientific input and Beth Wiener and Carolyn Deans for editorial reviews.

References

1. Davis JM, Chen N and Glick ID. A meta-analysis of the efficacy of second-generation antipsychotics. *Archives of General Psychiatry* 2003;**60**:553–64.

2. Rosenheck RA, Perlick D, Bingham S, Liu-Mares W, Collins J, Warren S and Leslie D for the Department of Veterans Affairs Cooperative Study Group on the Cost-Effectiveness of Olanzapine. Effectiveness and cost of olanzapine and haloperidol in the treatment of schizophrenia. *Journal of the American Medical Association* 2003;**290**:2693–702.

3. Dmitrienko A and Tamhane AC. Gatekeeping procedures with clinical trial applications. *Pharmaceutical Statistics* 2007;**6**:171–80.

4. Bauer P. Multiple testing in clinical trials. *Statistics in Medicine* 1991;**10**:871–90.

5. Hochberg Y. A sharper Bonferroni procedure for multiple tests of significance. *Biometrika* 1988;**75**:800–3.

6. Westfall PH, Tobias RD, Wolfinger RD and Hochberg Y. *Multiple Comparisons and Multiple Tests Using the SAS System*. Cary, NC: SAS Institute, Inc; 1999.

7. Lieberman JA, Stroup TS, McEvoy JP, et al; for the CATIE investigators. Effectiveness of antipsychotic drugs in patients with chronic schizophrenia. *New England Journal of Medicine* 2005;**353**:1209–23.

8. Stroup TS, Lieberman JA, McEvoy JP, et al; for the CATIE Investigators. Effectiveness of olanzapine, quetiapine, and risperidone in patients with chronic schizophrenia after discontinuing perphenazine: A CATIE study. *American Journal of Psychiatry* 2007;**164**:415–27.

9. McEvoy JP, Lieberman JA, Stroup TS, et al; for CATIE Investigators. Effectiveness of clozapine versus olanzapine, quetiapine and risperidone in patients with chronic schizophrenia who did not respond to prior atypical antipsychotic treatment. *American Journal of Psychiatry* 2006;**163**:600–10.

10. Stroup TS, Lieberman JA, McEvoy JP, et al; for the CATIE Investigators. Effectiveness of olanzapine, quetiapine, risperidone, and ziprasidone in patients with chronic schizophrenia after discontinuing a previous atypical antipsychotic. *American Journal of Psychiatry* 2006;**163**:611–22.

11. Stroup TS, Lieberman JA, McEvoy JP, et al; for the CATIE Investigators. Results of phase 3 of the CATIE schizophrenia trial. *Schizophrenia Research* 2009;**107**:1–12.

12. Cox D. Regression models and life tables. *Journal of the Royal Statistical Society* 1972; **B34**:187–220.

13. Alison P. *Survival Analysis Using the SAS® System: A Practical Guide*. Cary, NC: SAS Institute, Inc; 1995.

14. Mallinckrodt CH, Clark WS and David SR. Accounting for dropout bias using

mixed-effects models. *Journal of Biopharmaceutical Statistics* 2001;**11**:9–21.

15. Stokes ME, Davis CS and Koch GG. *Categorical Data Analysis using the SAS® System*. Cary, NC: SAS Institute, Inc; 2000.

16. Rubin DB. Multiple imputation after 18+ years. *Journal of the American Statistical Association* 1996;**91**:473–89.

17. Rosenheck RA, Leslie D, Sindelar J, *et al.* Cost-effectiveness of second generation antipsychotics and perphenazine in a randomized trial of treatment for chronic schizophrenia. *American Journal of Psychiatry* 2006;**163**:2080–9.

18. Henderson R, Diggle P and Dobson A. Joint modeling of longitudinal measurements and event time data. *Biostatistics* 2000;**1**:465–80.

19. van den Oord EJ, Adkins DE, McClay J, Lieberman J and Sullivan PF. A systematic method for estimating individual responses to treatment with antipsychotics in CATIE. *Schizophrenia Research* 2009;**107**:13–21.

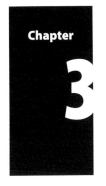

Chapter

3

Effectiveness and efficacy: staying on treatment and symptom reduction

Joseph P. McEvoy, T. Scott Stroup, and Jeffrey A. Lieberman

The goal of CATIE was to conduct a comparison of the effectiveness of the newer (atypical or second-generation) antipsychotic medications, each relative to the others, as well as to an older (conventional or first-generation) antipsychotic comparator. Efficacy studies had already demonstrated that all of these agents produced a therapeutic antipsychotic effect relative to placebo under optimal conditions. Our main goal was to determine their effectiveness relative to each other under "real-life" conditions. In this chapter, we present the rationale for the primary effectiveness outcome and results for the randomized phases of the study. In addition, we present analyses of comparative effects of the medications on symptoms in the initial phase of the study.

Efficacy studies

The primary purpose of efficacy studies is to determine if a candidate antipsychotic compound has antipsychotic efficacy. The central question around which efficacy studies are constructed is, "Does this compound reduce the manifestations of psychosis?" The optimal patients to include in efficacy studies manifest potentially treatment-responsive psychosis. In order to have the best chance of demonstrating antipsychotic efficacy, if the compound can produce such an effect, the persons conducting efficacy trials (usually sponsored by pharmaceutical companies) recruit patients who are expected to be treatment responsive, for example, patients who failed to comply with prescribed antipsychotic medication and subsequently suffered a psychotic exacerbation. If treated with an efficacious antipsychotic compound such patients' psychotic features will diminish.

For efficacy studies to be most efficient, suitable patients must take the compound reliably as prescribed, and extraneous confounds that can enhance or hamper efficacy must be avoided. Patients usually participate in efficacy studies in hospital where medication compliance can be monitored, psychosocial stressors limited, the use of other medications or substances restricted, and patient safety maintained.

For the cleanest assessment of the compound's efficacy and safety, efficacy trials avoid including patients with substantial medical problems, which may contribute to psychopathology and affect pharmacodynamics. Also excluded are patients with substance use disorders because the manifestations of substance-induced intoxications and withdrawals can confound the assessment of psychopathology, and because substance abusing patients' lifestyles predispose them to medical complications. Patients known to show little or no

Antipsychotic Trials in Schizophrenia, ed. T. Scott Stroup and Jeffrey A. Lieberman. Published by Cambridge University Press. © Cambridge University Press 2010.

therapeutic response when treated with established antipsychotic medications are also excluded from efficacy trials.

Clinician investigators implementing efficacy studies are usually experienced with the treatment of psychosis, and supported by research staff funded by trial budgets. Protocols mandate most decisions, and clinicians have little flexibility. Visits are frequent and longer than routine clinical contacts. Efficacy studies are usually 4–8 weeks in duration.

To test for antipsychotic efficacy of a new compound, the investigators contrast the compound's performance with that of a comparator that is not expected to produce antipsychotic efficacy—usually a placebo. Antipsychotic efficacy is demonstrated by differential change from the baseline on rating scales, such as the Positive and Negative Syndrome Scale (PANSS), whose items capture features of psychosis; these scales are administered at baseline and repeated at intervals after treatment is initiated. These scales have standardized interviews, item descriptors, and anchor-point descriptors, and raters are trained in their use to support consistency of rating. To avoid bias, patients, study doctors, and raters are all blinded, i.e., unaware of the treatments to which individual patients are assigned.

Efficacy trials restrict the use of adjunctive medications that may have beneficial effects on psychopathology. Such medications could interfere with the failure of placebo, making it more difficult to demonstrate efficacy advantages for the investigational compound.

After preliminary evidence of antipsychotic efficacy, extended evidence of safety, and a confident approximation of the optimal dose range for the investigational compound are obtained, drug developers conduct trials to provide convincing evidence for regulatory agencies that the new compound is safe and has substantial antipsychotic efficacy. Convincing evidence consists of at least two high-quality, clearly positive efficacy trials that are part of an overall pattern of results supporting the safety and efficacy of the new compound. As previously noted, all of the antipsychotic medications included in the CATIE trials had been proven safe and efficacious enough to achieve regulatory approval for marketing.

Efficacy studies, however, have substantial limitations in their ability to inform clinicians, patients, and policy makers regarding a medication's use in routine clinical care. The majority of patients treated in routine clinical settings are not eligible for participation in efficacy studies because they have exclusionary co-morbid medical or substance-use disorders, or are receiving excluded medications. Most patients treated in routine clinical care are outpatients who are seen infrequently, have stressful lives and co-morbid illnesses, take multiple adjunctive and concomitant medications, and are at best variably compliant with their prescribed antipsychotic medications. The majority of routine clinical care settings have fewer staff and less time to spend with patients than research teams. When a new antipsychotic medication is approved for clinical use, little or no information is available on the use of the compound in such patients at such settings. The result is that new drugs are introduced into "real-world" practice before their effectiveness is known, and before their true benefits, indications, and limitations are known [1].

Efficacy trials are almost always designed, implemented, and analyzed by pharmaceutical companies that will benefit financially if the investigational compound demonstrates antipsychotic efficacy. It is to be expected that those who bring a compound into existence will see its advantages more clearly than its disadvantages. Subtle biases in efficacy trials (e.g., the doses or titration schedules for comparator compounds) can offer advantages to the sponsors' compounds that are not replicated by independent or competing groups [2]. Until recent changes in reporting requirements for clinical trials mandated registering and reporting all trials in a compound's development, negative efficacy trials were commonly not reported.

Effectiveness studies

Effectiveness studies of any treatments for a chronic disease such as schizophrenia must incorporate a longer term view of the treatments' effects. A primary goal of such effectiveness studies is to determine the durability of the treatments, i.e., do the treatments continue to provide therapeutic benefit over the course of illness?

To ensure maximum generalizability, few patients should be excluded from effectiveness studies. In designing the CATIE schizophrenia trial, we excluded patients taking long-acting injected antipsychotic medications who had an established history of non-compliance with oral medications; such patients would be very likely to relapse because they would not take the prescribed oral study antipsychotic medications and would not test the comparisons among these medications. We excluded patients taking clozapine because of previously failed repeated trials of antipsychotic medications; such patients would be very likely to relapse because they would not be responsive to the assigned study antipsychotic medication and would not test the comparisons among the study antipsychotic medications. We also excluded patients experiencing a first episode of psychosis. Prior evidence suggested that these patients have a different pattern of treatment responsiveness, different propensities for adverse events, and are best treated at a lower dose range than is optimal with chronic schizophrenia.

We did not exclude patients with co-morbid medical disorders or co-morbid substance use disorders. The diagnostic criteria for inclusion required that patients' psychoses not be explainable entirely on the basis of co-morbid medical or substance use disorders. We accepted the reality that the manifestations of their primary psychotic illnesses could be affected by these co-morbid disorders. We included assessments to capture the manifestations of co-morbid medical and substance abuse disorders, and we documented the treatments prescribed for them.

Outcome measures in CATIE

Because schizophrenia is a persistent condition, the effectiveness of any treatment for schizophrenia should reflect the durability of that treatment over long periods of time. We sought as our primary outcome measure a summary indicator of the enduring therapeutic benefit and tolerability of the study antipsychotic medications in the judgments of both the patient and the treating clinician. We wanted to utilize an objective and clinically meaningful measure of outcome that would be comparable to those used in large simple or pragmatic trials of other fields such as cardiovascular disease and oncology. However, such outcomes as myocardial infarction, stroke, metastasis, and mortality (to name a few) that are objective, discrete, and valid are harder to define in psychiatric research. Consequently, we selected time until discontinuation of the assigned antipsychotic medication for any cause as the primary outcome measure for CATIE because it is a simple, discrete event that integrates therapeutic benefit, tolerability, and the opinions of clinician and patient, whether or not these opinions are able to fully converge solely on benefit or tolerability or some other contributing factor.

We did not dictate to site investigators what should constitute a cause for treatment discontinuation, but left the decision to patients and clinicians as is the case in usual practice. We did, however, provide guidance to minimize unnecessary switching implemented by study physicians. For example, brief exacerbations, precipitated by situational stress, temporary non-compliance, or a foray into substance abuse, which are common in routine maintenance treatment for schizophrenia, do not necessarily imply failure of the antipsychotic treatment and a need for discontinuation. If both the patient and clinician agreed that the assigned antipsychotic medication had been performing well and they wanted to continue it (even if there had been a brief interruption related to the exacerbation), then the treatment could be continued. Such exacerbations were captured in the record, and addressed via suitable interventions other than treatment discontinuation.

We gathered information about reasons for treatment discontinuation, although we are aware that these reasons are often not clear. We provided guidance to clinicians to help assign reasons for treatment discontinuation. Administrative reasons for discontinuation were those in which the patient and clinician would otherwise have continued the assigned antipsychotic medication (both were satisfied that the assigned antipsychotic medication was providing adequate therapeutic benefit and causing no intolerable side effects), but an independent, external event precluded the patient's further continued participation in the trial. An example of such an event included the patient moving to another locale.

If the clinician decided to discontinue the patient's treatment for any reason, the discontinuation was considered a "clinician's decision" even if the patient agreed with the clinician. The clinician was required to determine whether the decision to discontinue treatment was predominantly because of inadequate therapeutic effect or intolerable side effects from the assigned antipsychotic medication.

Finally, if the clinician judged that the patient would do well to continue on the assigned medication, but the patient disagreed and decided to discontinue treatment, the discontinuation was labeled a "patient decision." Although it would be valuable to understand what led to each of these patient decisions, in most cases the patient simply withdrew consent to participate or provided inadequate information to determine the primary cause of discontinuation. We accepted the reality that tolerability, efficacy, and other reasons are not mutually exclusive and could all contribute to a single decision to discontinue a drug.

Although we did not choose a measure of psychopathology as the primary outcome measure in CATIE, we obtained multiple repeated measures of the PANSS to measure psychopathology and present findings on symptom changes in Phase 1/1A here.

Long-term comparative trials such as CATIE, in which substantial discontinuation rates are expected in all arms, present problems in summarizing or encapsulating effects on psychopathology. Last observation carried forward (LOCF) measures capture patients at a single point in time in a wide variety of conditions after varying lengths of exposure to medication, and would be expected to favor a treatment that patients took for a longer period of time. An alternative approach is to examine symptom effects at specified time points including only those patients still taking the assigned medication at that time. This so-called observed cases (OC) method would be expected to reflect how well a drug might work under the favorable circumstance that the patient and doctor agree that the drug has been worth continuing. Here, we will present PANSS change scores using both LOCF and OC methods.

Treatment discontinuation results
Phase 1

The initial treatment phase of CATIE (Phase 1/1A) evaluated the relative effectiveness of olanzapine, perphenazine, quetiapine, risperidone, and ziprasidone [3]. Results are seen in Table 3.1 and Figure 3.1. The median time to treatment discontinuation for all causes was

Table 3.1. Outcome Measures of effectiveness in Phase 1/1A [3]

Outcome	Olanzapine (N=330)	Quetiapine (N=329)	Risperidone (N=333)	Perphenazine (N=257)†	p Value‡	Ziprasidone (N=183)§
Mean modal dose—mg per day/total no. of patients¶	20.1/312	543.4/309	3.9/305	20.8/245		112.8/165
Maximal dose received—no. of patients (%)	124/312 (40)	137/309 (44)	122/305 (40)	98/245 (40)	<0.001	80/165 (48)
Discontinuation of treatment for any cause						
Discontinuation—no. of patients (%)	210 (64)	269 (82)	245 (74)	192 (75)		145 (79)
Kaplan–Meier time to discontinuation—mo Median (95% CI)*	9.2 (6.9–12.1)	4.6 (3.9–5.5)	4.8 (4.0–6.1)	5.6 (4.5–6.3)		3.5 (3.1–5.4)
Cox-model treatment comparisons‖						
Olanzapine						
Hazard ratio (95% CI)		0.63 (0.52–0.76)	0.75 (0.62–0.90)	0.78 (0.63–0.96)	0.004**	0.76 (0.60–0.97)
p value		<0.001**	0.002**	0.021		0.028
Quetiapine						
Hazard ratio (95% CI)			1.19 (0.99–1.42)	1.14 (0.93–1.39)		1.01 (0.81–1.27)
p value			0.06	0.21		0.94
Risperidone						
Hazard ratio (95% CI)				1.00 (0.82–1.23)		0.89 (0.71–1.14)
p value				0.99		0.36
Perphenazine						
Hazard ratio (95% CI)						0.90 (0.70–1.16)
p value						0.43

Table 3.1. (cont.)

Outcome	Olanzapine (N=330)	Quetiapine (N=329)	Risperidone (N=333)	Perphenazine (N=257)†	p Value‡	Ziprasidone (N=183)§
Discontinuation of treatment for lack of efficacy						
Discontinuation—no. of patients (%)	48 (15)	92 (28)	91 (27)	65 (25)		44 (24)
Kaplan–Meier time to discontinuation—mo 25th percentile (95% CI)	—††	6.0 (4.5–8.0)	6.0 (4.4–9.0)	6.1 (4.5–9.1)		6.9 (3.2–12.1)
Cox-model treatment comparisons‖						
Olanzapine						
Hazard ratio (95% CI)		0.41 (0.29–0.57)	0.45 (0.32–0.64)	0.47 (0.31–0.70)	<0.001**	0.59 (0.37–0.93)
p value		<0.001**	<0.001**	<0.001**		0.026
Quetiapine						
p value			0.49	0.47		0.69
Risperidone						
p value				0.59		0.93
Perphenazine						
p value						0.44

Discontinuation of treatment owing to intolerability‡‡

Discontinuation—no. (%)	62 (19)	49 (15)	34 (10)	40 (16)	28 (15)
Cox-model treatment comparisons‖					
Risperidone					
Hazard ratio (95% CI)	0.62 (0.41–0.95)	0.65 (0.42–1.00)		0.60 (0.36–0.98)	0.79 (0.46–1.37)
p value	0.027	0.051		0.054	0.41
Olanzapine					
p value		0.84		0.49	0.28
Quetiapine					
p value				0.97	0.87
Perphenazine					
p value				0.19	

Notes: *CI denotes confidence interval.

†Patients with tardive dyskinesia were excluded from the perphenazine group.

‡ The overall *p* value is for the comparison of olanzapine, quetiapine, risperidone, and perphenazine with the use of a 3 df test from a Cox model for survival outcomes, excluding patients with tardive dyskinesia. If the difference among the groups was significant at a *p* value of less than 0.05, the three atypical agents were compared with each other by means of step-down or closed testing to identify significant differences (*p*<0.05) between groups. Each atypical agent was then compared with perphenazine by means of a Hochberg adjustment. The smallest *p* value for the perphenazine group was compared with a value of 0.017 (0.05 ÷ 3).

§Statistical analyses involving the ziprasidone group were confined to the cohort of patients who underwent randomization after ziprasidone was added to the study, with the use of a Hochberg adjustment for four pairwise comparisons. The smallest *p* value was compared with a value of 0.013 (0.05 ÷ 4).

¶The modal dose and percentages of patients taking the maximal dose are based on the number of patients with data on the dose. Information on dose was not available for some patients who dropped out early. The *p* values for the percentage of patients reaching the maximal dose were calculated with the use of a 4 df test comparing all treatment groups from a Poisson regression accounting for differential exposure times, and adjusting for whether the patient had an exacerbation in the preceding three months.

‖For pairwise comparisons of treatment groups, Cox-model hazard ratios of less than 1 indicate a greater time to the discontinuation of the first treatment listed.

**p* value is statistically significant.

†tThe Kaplan–Meier 25th percentile for discontinuation owing to lack of efficacy could not be estimated for olanzapine because of the low event rates.

‡‡The Kaplan–Meier 25th percentile for discontinuation owing to intolerability could not be estimated because of the low event rates.

Copyright © 2005 Massachusetts Medical Society. All rights reserved. With permission from Lieberman *et al.* 2005 [3].

(a)

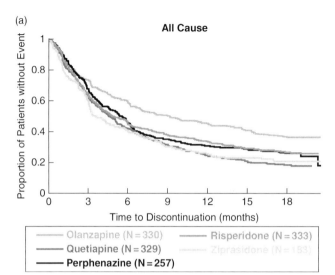

Figure 3.1. (a) Discontinuation for any reason Phases 1/1A. (b) Discontinuation due to inefficacy Phases 1/1A. (c) Discontinuation due to intolerability Phases 1/1A. (d) Switchers only. Discontinuation for any reason excluding those who were assigned to stay on the medication taken when entering the study. See plate section for color version. 3.1. a–c [3] Copyright © 2005 Massachusetts Medical Society. All rights reserved. 3.1.d. [4] Reprinted with permission from The American Journal of Psychiatry (2006), American Psychiatric Press.

(b)

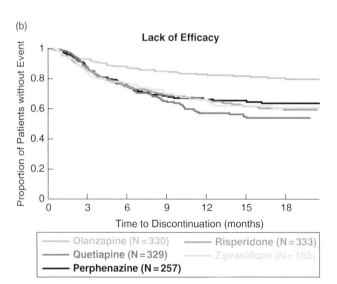

longest with olanzapine (9.2 months) compared to quetiapine (4.6 months) and risperidone (4.8 months). Perphenazine (5.8 months) and ziprasidone (3.5 months) produced similar results but did not meet the *a priori* standard of statistical significance, which adjusted for multiple comparisons. Differences in times to discontinuation because of intolerable side effects were not significant. Patients assigned to olanzapine had the longest time to discontinuation due to inadequate efficacy (although not significant compared to ziprasidone).

In a post hoc analysis, Essock and colleagues examined the impact of "staying versus switching" in Phase 1 of the trial [4]. The investigators hypothesized that the patients that

Figure 3.1. (cont.)

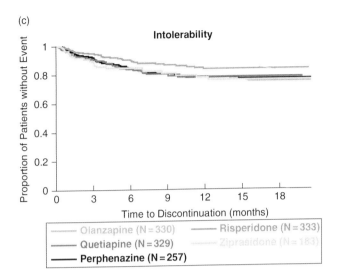

(c)

Intolerability

Olanzapine (N = 330) Risperidone (N = 333)
Quetiapine (N = 329) Ziprasidone (N = 183)
Perphenazine (N = 257)

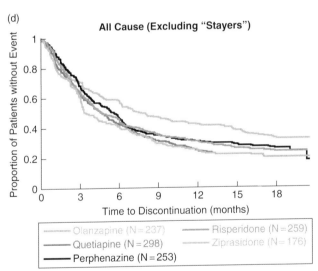

(d)

All Cause (Excluding "Stayers")

Olanzapine (N = 237) Risperidone (N = 259)
Quetiapine (N = 298) Ziprasidone (N = 176)
Perphenazine (N = 253)

were randomized to stay on the same medications that they had been on prior to entering the study would do less well as they would not have the benefit of trying a new medication. In the original report of Phase 1, however, it was found that patients randomized to olanzapine and risperidone who stayed on the antipsychotic they were taking at study entry had significantly longer times until discontinuation than did those who had switched from other antipsychotics [3]. When these "stayers" were removed, the original pattern of treatment discontinuations in Phase 1 remained, although differences seen in the original analyses were attenuated (Figure 3.1D).

Table 3.2. Phase 1B primary outcome [5]

Phase 1B Outcome	Olanzapine (N=38)	Quetiapine (N=38)	Risperidone (N=38)
Treatment discontinuation due to all causes			
Patients who discontinued			
N	23	22	32
%	61	58	84
Kaplan-Meier time to discontinuation (months)			
Median	7.1	9.9	3.6
95% CI	5.5	4.0	2.0–6.4
Cox model treatment comparisons			
Comparison with olanzapine			
Hazard ratio[a]		0.97	0.53*
95% CI		0.53–1.75	0.31–0.91
Comparison with quetiapine			
Hazard ratio[a]			0.55*
95% CI			0.32–0.95

Notes: [a]Hazard ratios less than 1 indicate greater time to discontinuation for the specified comparison treatment. *$p<0.05$.

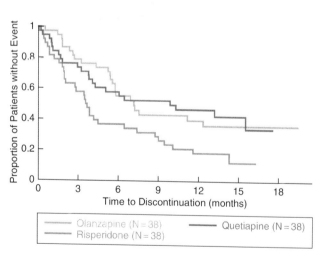

Figure 3.2. Time until all-cause discontinuation Phase 1B (patients who discontinued perphenazine). **See plate section for color version.** [5] Reprinted with permission from The American Journal of Psychiatry (Copyright 2007), American Psychiatric Association.

Phase 1B

In Phase 1B, the effectiveness of olanzapine, quetiapine, and risperidone were compared in patients who had just discontinued the older antipsychotic perphenazine [5] (see Table 3.2 and Figure 3.2). The time to treatment discontinuation was longer for patients treated with quetiapine (median, 9.9 months) and olanzapine (7.1 months) than with risperidone (3.6 months).

Table 3.3. Phase 2E primary outcome [7]

Treatment Discontinuation Measures Among Patients Randomly Assigned to Treatment with Clozapine or Another Atypical Antipsychotic							
Outcome	**Clozapine (N = 45)**		**Olanzapine (N = 17)**		**Quetiapine (N = 14)**		**Risperidone (N = 14)**	
Treatment discontinuation for any reason								
	N	%	N	%	N	%	N	%
Subjects discontinuing	25	56	12	71	13	93	12	86
	Median	95% CI	Median	95% CI	Median	95% CI	Median	95% CI
Kaplan-Meier time to discontinuation (months)	10.5	7.3–16.1	2.7	1.9–11.9	3.3	1.0–4.9	2.8	1.1–4.0
			Hazard Ratio	95% CI	Hazard Ratio	95% CI	Hazard Ratio	95% CI
Cox model treatment comparisons[a]								
Clozapine			0.57	0.29–1.16	0.39*	0.19–0.80	0.42*	0.21–0.86
Olanzapine					0.69	0.30–1.54	0.73	0.32–1.67
Quetiapine							1.07	0.48–2.37

Notes: [a]Hazard ratios less than 1 indicate greater time to discontinuation compared to the treatment listed in the first column.
*p<0.05.
Reprinted with permission from The American Journal of Psychiatry (Copyright 2006), American Psychiatric Association.

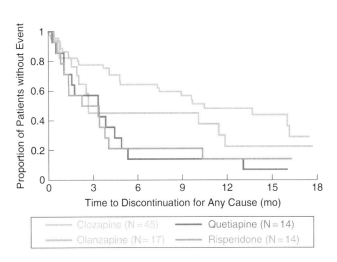

Figure 3.3. Time to all-cause discontinuation in Phase 2E. See plate section for color version. [6]
Reprinted with permission from The American Journal of Psychiatry (Copyright 2006), American Psychiatric Association.

Phase 2E

The efficacy arm of Phase 2 (Phase 2E) compared the effectiveness of clozapine versus olanzapine, quetiapine, or risperidone in patients who had discontinued treatment with olanzapine, quetiapine, risperidone, or ziprasidone in Phase 1 of the trial [6] (see Table 3.3 and Figure 3.3).

Table 3.4. Phase 2T primary outcome [7]

Treatment Discontinuation Measures Among Patients Randomly Assigned to Treatment with Olanzapine, Quetiapine, Risperidone, or Ziprasidone								
Outcome	Olanzapine (N = 66)		Risperidone (N = 69)		Quetiapine (N = 63)		Ziprasidone (N = 135)	
Treatment discontinuation for any reason								
	N	%	N	%	N	%	N	%
Subjects discontinuing	44	67	44	64	53	84	104	77
	Median	95% CI	Median	95% CI	Median	95% CI	Median	95% CI
Kaplan-Meier time to discontinuation (months)	6.3	3.5–9.7	7.0	4.1–10.0	4.0	3.1–4.8	2.8	2.4–4.4
			Hazard Ratio	95% CI	Hazard Ratio	95% CI	Hazard Ratio	95% CI
Cox model treatment comparisons[a]								
Olanzapine			1.02	0.67–1.55	0.65*	0.43–0.97	0.61**	0.43–0.87
Risperidone					0.64*	0.43–0.95	0.60**	0.42–0.85
Quetiapine							0.94	0.67–1.31

Notes: [a]Hazard ratios less than 1 indicate greater time to discontinuation compared to the treatment listed in the first column.
*$p<0.05$.
**$p<0.01$.
Reprinted with permission from The American Journal of Psychiatry (Copyright 2006), American Psychiatric Association.

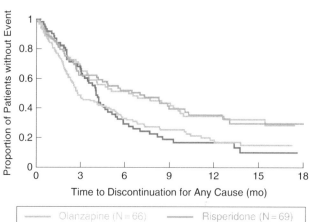

Figure 3.4. Time to discontinuation for any reason Phase 2T. **See plate section for color version.** [7] Reprinted with permission from The American Journal of Psychiatry (Copyright 2006), American Psychiatric Association.

Almost all of the 99 patients who enrolled in Phase 2E had discontinued the previous treatment due to inefficacy. No patient was assigned to a medication previously received in the trial. Time to all-cause treatment discontinuation was significantly longer for clozapine (median 10.5 months) than for quetiapine (3.3 months; $p = 0.01$) or risperidone (2.8 months; $p = 0.02$) but not olanzapine (2.7 months; $p = 0.12$). Time to discontinuation for inadequate therapeutic effect was significantly longer for clozapine than for olanzapine, quetiapine, or risperidone.

Phase 2T

In the tolerability arm of Phase 2 (Phase 2T), 444 patients who discontinued Phase 1 were randomized to a drug they had not previously received in the study, either olanzapine, quetiapine, risperidone, or ziprasidone [7] (see Table 3.4 and Figure 3.4). While the intent of this phase was to evaluate patients who discontinued Phase 1 due to intolerability, because there was a choice of which arm of Phase 2 to enter, some patients and their doctors who had stopped the previous treatment due to inadequate efficacy chose this arm, presumably to avoid possible randomization to clozapine. The time to treatment discontinuation was longer for patients treated with risperidone (median 7.0 months) and olanzapine (6.3 months) than with quetiapine (4.0 months) and ziprasidone (2.8 months). Among the patients who discontinued the previous treatment due to inefficacy, olanzapine was more effective than quetiapine and ziprasidone, and risperidone was more effective than quetiapine. There were no significant differences between treatments among those who discontinued the previous treatment due to intolerability.

Symptom outcomes

Because symptom reduction remains an important goal of antipsychotic treatment and is the typical outcome in antipsychotic drug trials, we include in this chapter results of how olanzapine, perphenazine, quetiapine, risperidone, and ziprasidone compared in their effects on the core psychopathology of schizophrenia. The PANSS, which includes positive and negative symptom subscales, was administered to all subjects at baseline, after 1 month of treatment, after 3 months of treatment, and every 3 months after that until the medication was discontinued or 18 months of treatment were completed. Table 3.5a shows symptom change scores for persons still taking the drug at specific points in time. In these "observed cases", there was no overall difference in average positive, negative, or total symptom score changes for the drugs at 3 months, while at 6 months only the change scores for the negative symptom scale met the common (though unadjusted) criterion for statistical significance. Pairwise comparisons found larger symptom reductions for olanzapine than risperidone. For the final visit in Phase 1/1A, there were overall differences in change scores for total symptoms and positive symptoms. In pairwise comparisons, symptom reductions for the PANSS total score and for positive and negative scales were larger for olanzapine than for quetiapine, risperidone, and ziprasidone.

Table 3.5b and Figure 3.5b display PANSS symptom change scores using LOCF methods to account for missing data among patients who discontinued treatment early. In LOCF analyses, in which patients who remained on treatment for a longer duration contributed more data and have more time on treatment to benefit, overall differences in symptom

Table 3.5a. PANSS change scores at 3 months, 6 months, and end of Phase 1/1A – observed cases

Variable	All	Olanzapine	Perphenazine	Quetiapine	Risperidone	Ziprasidone	p
3-Month visit							
	(N = 923)	(N = 233)	(N = 174)	(N = 206)	(N = 204)	(N = 106)	
PANSS Total Score	−6.22 (14.29)	−7.68 (13.60)	−6.20 (14.87)	−6.68 (14.42)	−4.87 (14.61)	−4.78 (13.78)	0.2387
PANSS Positive Score	−1.97 (5.04)	−2.67 (4.73)	−1.73 (5.38)	−1.85 (4.90)	−1.79 (5.22)	−1.41 (4.96)	0.1649
PANSS Negative Score	−1.41 (5.00)	−1.51 (4.87)	−1.52 (4.83)	−1.52 (5.12)	−0.91 (5.12)	−1.77 (5.08)	0.5737
6-Month visit							
	(N = 662)	(N = 189)	(N = 118)	(N = 132)	(N = 152)	(N = 71)	
PANSS Total Score	−8.21 (16.01)	−11.1 (14.56)	−7.49 (15.21)	−7.55 (16.39)	*−6.02 (18.00)	−7.75 (15.08)	0.0510
PANSS Positive Score	−2.70 (5.24)	−3.56 (5.00)	−2.43 (5.50)	−1.94 (4.86)	*−2.63 (5.79)	−2.46 (4.68)	0.0801
PANSS Negative Score	−1.84 (5.70)	−2.44 (5.50)	−1.76 (5.06)	−2.34 (6.14)	*−0.58 (6.00)	−2.14 (5.39)	0.0291
*End of Phase 1/1A**							
	(N = 1,067)	(N = 240)	(N = 200)	(N = 246)	(N = 253)	(N = 128)	
PANSS Total Score	−2.29 (17.89)	−6.65 (16.52)	−2.38 (17.80)	*−0.29 (17.24)	*−1.73 (19.37)	*1.03 (17.45)	0.0002
PANSS Positive Score	−0.73 (5.92)	−2.43 (4.95)	−0.78 (6.19)	*0.17 (5.90)	*−0.45 (5.96)	*0.19 (6.50)	0.0000
PANSS Negative Score	−0.60 (6.08)	−1.44 (6.40)	−0.82 (5.61)	*−0.36 (5.97)	*−0.26 (6.42)	*0.22 (5.53)	0.0790

Note: The End of Phase PANSS was conducted as part of a comprehensive set of measures whenever a phase was ended. Not all participants attended an End of Phase visit, for example those who dropped out.
p values from 1-way ANOVA test.
* Significantly different from Olanzapine (p < 0.05)

Table 3.5b. PANSS change scores at 3 months, 6 months, and end of Phase 1/1A – last observation carried forward

Variable	All (N = 1,447)	Olanzapine (N = 331)	Perphenazine (N = 260)	Quetiapine (N = 333)	Risperidone (N = 339)	Ziprasidone (N = 184)	p
3-Month visit							
PANSS Total Score	−4.27 (13.50)	−6.38 (13.00)	−4.85 (14.05)	−3.76 (13.51)	*−3.10 (13.51)	−2.74 (13.21)	0.0074
PANSS Positive Score	−1.39 (4.72)	−2.15 (4.37)	−1.41 (5.01)	−1.16 (4.75)	*−1.16 (4.75)	−0.88 (4.72)	0.0151
PANSS Negative Score	−0.97 (4.67)	−1.26 (4.66)	−1.32 (4.65)	−0.76 (4.69)	*−0.50 (4.68)	−1.20 (4.58)	0.1217
6-Month visit							
PANSS Total Score	−4.33 (14.57)	−7.83 (13.95)	−4.31 (14.26)	*−3.77 (14.20)	*−2.40 (15.46)	*−2.64 (14.06)	0.0000
PANSS Positive Score	−1.47 (4.93)	−2.54 (4.66)	−1.35 (5.17)	*−1.14 (4.79)	*−1.07 (5.18)	*−1.02 (4.65)	0.0003
PANSS Negative Score	−0.97 (5.02)	−1.59 (5.11)	−1.09 (4.75)	*−0.98 (5.10)	*−0.22 (5.07)	*−1.02 (4.85)	0.0124
End of Phase 1/1A							
PANSS Total Score	−4.69 (15.86)	−7.99 (15.55)	−4.47 (15.31)	*−3.63 (15.56)	*−3.88 (17.05)	*−2.43 (14.67)	0.0004
PANSS Positive Score	−1.42 (5.22)	−2.53 (4.87)	−1.34 (5.49)	*−0.91 (5.05)	*−1.26 (5.27)	*−0.73 (5.36)	0.0002
PANSS Negative Score	−1.12 (5.43)	−1.85 (5.89)	−1.07 (4.86)	*−1.04 (5.56)	*−0.66 (5.61)	*−0.88 (4.66)	0.0645

Note: *Significantly different from olanzapine ($p < 0.05$).
p values from 1-way ANOVA test.

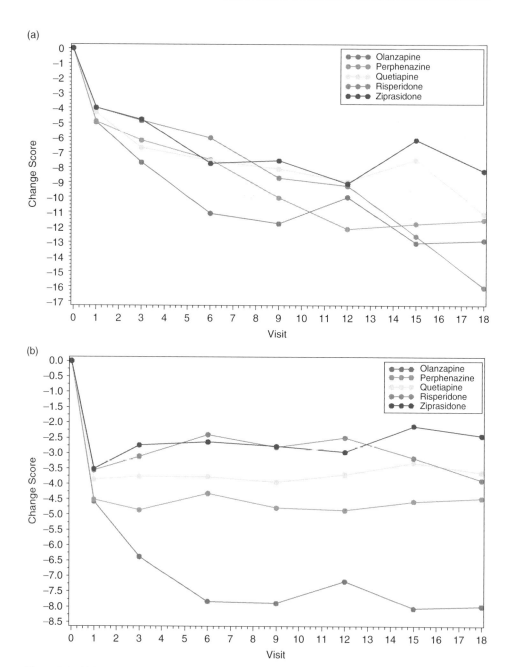

Figure 3.5. (a) Mean PANSS total change from baseline by treatment (OC). (b) Mean PANSS total change from baseline by treatment (LOCF). **See plate section for color version.**
Note: Scale of the two figures is different.

change scores were present in most instances. By 6 months, there were advantages for olanzapine over quetiapine, risperidone, and ziprasidone–but not perphenazine–for PANSS total score changes as well as for changes in positive and negative symptom scale scores.

Discussion and conclusions

In this chapter, we summarized effectiveness findings from all randomized phases of CATIE and the results of symptom reduction in Phase 1/1A. Olanzapine had an advantage in time to treatment discontinuation that was similar in magnitude compared to all other drugs in Phase 1/1A, but there was lower statistical power to detect differences in the comparisons to perphenazine and ziprasidone because fewer people were assigned perphenazine and ziprasidone than were assigned olanzapine, quetiapine, and risperidone. Also in Phase 1/1A, olanzapine showed no significant advantages over perphenazine in symptom reduction in any analyses, but had small advantages over each of the other newer medications in at least some analyses.

In Phase 2E, which enrolled mostly people who got inadequate symptom relief on the previous medication, clozapine had longer time to treatment discontinuation than risperidone and quetiapine. Although the difference between clozapine and olanzapine was not significant, and our data are limited because of small sample sizes and a lack of blinding for those taking clozapine, these results support previous work that has consistently found clozapine more effective when other drugs do not work well [8].

In Phase 2T, which enrolled a mix of people who had stopped the previous medication due to either inefficacy or intolerability, olanzapine and risperidone were more effective than quetiapine and ziprasidone. Secondary analyses suggested that olanzapine had an advantage for people with prior efficacy problems and risperidone had an advantage for people with prior tolerability problems.

In Phase 1B, which enrolled people who had discontinued perphenazine, olanzapine and quetiapine were more effective than risperidone. Quetiapine appeared to be particularly well tolerated in this situation, perhaps because it is substantially different from perphenazine and risperidone with regard to affinity for dopamine receptors and thus offered a tolerability advantage over these two drugs for some patients.

In our analyses of changes in symptoms, observed case symptom differences were smaller than LOCF differences, likely because of the large difference in time on treatment. Specifically, because patients stayed on olanzapine longer than other treatments in Phase 1, and because olanzapine showed an early advantage in symptom reduction, there was a larger olanzapine advantage in the LOCF analyses than in the observed case analyses. In observed case analyses, only patients continuing a medication (and likely benefiting from it) at a point in time contribute symptom measures.

In conclusion, the CATIE findings on effectiveness and symptom reduction are consistent with many careful meta-analyses [9–13]. Overall, clozapine is most effective. Olanzapine demonstrated strong efficacy but was not clearly better than perphenazine in any analysis. The older drug perphenazine was similar in effectiveness to the newer drugs. Unlike in the meta-analyses, risperidone did not stand out in CATIE. However, in Phase 2T, in which all participants began a new treatment, risperidone was similar to olanzapine in overall effectiveness and superior to both quetiapine and ziprasidone. Following discontinuation of perphenazine, quetiapine was superior to risperidone and similar to olanzapine. Ziprasidone was not a leader in the primary outcome or in symptom reduction in either randomized phase in which it was used. It is possible that the doses of quetiapine, risperidone, and ziprasidone were suboptimal; however, our *post hoc* analyses do not support the notion that dosing biases affected the study results [14].

In this chapter, we summarized the CATIE study findings on measures of effectiveness and efficacy. Other chapters report results of other outcome domains, including adverse effects, which add important information to aid interpretation of these primary findings.

References

1. Eisenberg L. The social imperatives of medical research. *Science* 1977;**198**:1105–10.

2. Heres S, Davis J, Maino K, *et al.* Why olanzapine beats risperidone, risperidone beats quetiapine, and quetiapine beats olanzapine: An exploratory analysis of head-to-head comparison studies of second-generation antipsychotics. *American Journal of Psychiatry* 2006;**163**:185–94.

3. Lieberman JA, Stroup TS, McEvoy JP, *et al.* Effectiveness of antipsychotic drugs in patients with chronic schizophrenia. *New England Journal of Medicine* 2005;**353**:1209–23.

4. Essock SM, Covell NH, Davis SM, *et al.* Effectiveness of switching antipsychotic medications. *American Journal of Psychiatry* 2006;**163**:2090–5.

5. Stroup TS, Lieberman JA, McEvoy JP, *et al.* Effectiveness of olanzapine, quetiapine, and risperidone in patients with chronic schizophrenia after discontinuing perphenazine: A CATIE study. *American Journal of Psychiatry* 2007;**164**:415–27.

6. McEvoy JP, Lieberman JA, Stroup TS, *et al.* Effectiveness of clozapine versus olanzapine, quetiapine, and risperidone in patients with chronic schizophrenia who did not respond to prior atypical antipsychotic treatment. *American Journal of Psychiatry* 2006;**163**:600–10.

7. Stroup TS, Lieberman JA, McEvoy JP, *et al.* Effectiveness of olanzapine, quetiapine, risperidone, and ziprasidone in patients with chronic schizophrenia following discontinuation of a previous atypical antipsychotic. *American Journal of Psychiatry* 2006;**163**:611–22.

8. Chakos M, Lieberman J, Hoffman E, *et al.* Effectiveness of second-generation antipsychotics in patients with treatment-resistant schizophrenia: A review and meta-analysis of randomized trials. *American Journal of Psychiatry* 2001;**158**:518–26.

9. Davis JM, Chen N and Glick ID. A meta-analysis of the efficacy of second-generation antipsychotics. *Archives of General Psychiatry* 2003;**60**:553–64.

10. Geddes J, Freemantle N, Harrison P, *et al.* Atypical antipsychotics in the treatment of schizophrenia: Systematic overview and meta-regression analysis. *British Medical Journal* 2000;**321**:1371–6.

11. Leucht S, Komossa K, Rummel-Kluge C, *et al.* A meta-analysis of head-to-head comparisons of second-generation antipsychotics in the treatment of schizophrenia. *American Journal of Psychiatry* 2009;**166**:152–63.

12. Leucht S, Pitschel-Walz G, Abraham D, *et al.* Efficacy and extrapyramidal side-effects of the new antipsychotics olanzapine, quetiapine, risperidone, and sertindole compared to conventional antipsychotics and placebo. A meta-analysis of randomized controlled trials. *Schizophrenia Research* 1999; **35**:51–68.

13. Leucht S, Wahlbeck K, Hamann J, *et al.* New generation antipsychotics versus low-potency conventional antipsychotics: A systematic review and meta-analysis. *Lancet* 2003;**361**:1581–9.

14. Rosenheck RA, Davis VG, Davis SM, *et al.* Can a nonequivalent choice of dosing regimen bias the results of flexible dose double blind trials? The CATIE schizophrenia trial. *Schizophrenia Research* 2009;**113**:12–8.

Chapter

4

Cost-effectiveness and cost-benefit analysis

Robert A. Rosenheck and Douglas L. Leslie

In the United States, second-generation antipsychotics have become the most widely used drugs in the treatment of schizophrenia, with total annual costs in 2007 of over $12 billion. Earlier studies of patients with chronic schizophrenia reported that these medications were not only more effective than older drugs with fewer side effects, but that they also lowered the risk of hospitalization, generating sufficient savings to offset their greater drug costs entirely [1–4]. However, many of these studies were based on non-experimental designs, and a small number of randomized trials showed either much smaller net savings [5,6] or even increased total costs [7,8]. Two more recent 12-month trials failed to find advantages for the newer drugs in either clinical effectiveness, reduced Parkinsonian side effects, or lowered costs [7,8], and an economic analysis showed increased costs to the California Medicaid program in association with the introduction of these medications [9]. A recent literature review of cost-effectiveness studies involving second-generation antipsychotics also failed to find evidence of greater cost-effectiveness for these agents [10].

To further evaluate the cost-effectiveness of these medications, the Clinical Antipsychotic Trial of Intervention Effectiveness (CATIE) schizophrenia trial included extensive data collection on health service use to allow estimation of health care costs incurred by study participants, along with several measures of effectiveness, including a disease-specific estimate of quality-adjusted life years (QALYs), that together would support a comparative analysis of the cost-effectiveness of one first-generation antipsychotic (perphenazine) and all four second-generation antipsychotics (olanzapine, risperidone, quetiapine, and ziprasidone), with the exception of clozapine, that were available in the US in 2001–2004 when CATIE was implemented [11]. (Ziprasidone was introduced soon after the study began; aripiprazole was introduced later and could not be included in the randomized phases of CATIE.) In the cost-effectiveness component of CATIE, we present pairwise comparisons of the five treatments on measures of health care costs, symptoms, and on several measures of effectiveness that address health-related quality of life. The primary objective of the cost-effectiveness component of CATIE was to compare alternative treatment initiation strategies, i.e., to determine whether choice of the first drug in the CATIE algorithm resulted in differences in cost-effectiveness, the amount of health benefit per dollar expended, over the entire study, including observations after medications had been changed. A comparison of the cost-effectiveness of treatments exclusively while patients were receiving the initially assigned treatment was also conducted.

While cost-effectiveness analysis evaluates the health benefits per additional dollar expended using measures of quality of life, cost-benefit analysis attempts to put a monetary

Antipsychotic Trials in Schizophrenia, ed. T. Scott Stroup and Jeffrey A. Lieberman. Published by Cambridge University Press. © Cambridge University Press 2010.

value on the health benefits of treatment and thus monetizes all outcomes. Accordingly, a cost-benefit analysis is also presented in this Chapter, in which both costs and benefits are expressed in dollars with a range of estimates for the dollar value of a QALY considered using the Net Health Benefit Approach [12].

Methods

The study design, procedures, and samples of CATIE have been described in previous chapters and will not be reiterated here.

Measures

The cost-effectiveness analysis of CATIE followed, as closely as possible, the methods recommended by the Public Health Services Task Force on Cost-Effectiveness in Health and Medicine [13]. The primary outcomes were total health care costs and Quality Adjusted Life Years (QALYs).

Service use

Service use was documented every month through a structured self-report questionnaire that recorded four kinds of hospital days (medical, surgical, psychiatric, and substance abuse) across six different facility types (state mental hospitals, private psychiatric hospitals, VA hospitals, non-federal general hospitals, community mental health centers, and detoxification facilities). Nights spent in nursing homes, halfway houses, board and care homes, and supervised apartments were also recorded. Use of 16 types of outpatient mental health care, including psychiatric and psycho-social rehabilitation services, were documented along with eight different types of medical or surgical outpatient visit, and use of both psychiatric and medical emergency room services.

Medication use was also documented each month and included study medications, concomitant psychotropic medications, and all ancillary medications for other medical conditions.

Costs

Antipsychotic medication costs were based on published wholesale prices for the specific capsule strengths used in CATIE [14], adjusted downward for discounts and rebates affecting patients whose medications would have been paid for by Medicaid (with costs about 25% less than wholesale prices) [15] or by the Department of Veterans Affairs (VA) (about 40% less than wholesale prices) [16]. Costs of over 200 different ancillary medications were estimated on the basis of average daily medication costs for specific agents in the 2002 MarketScan® data set, representing typical medication costs for privately insured patients [17].

The economic perspective for the cost evaluation is the total health care cost, including costs of all mental health and medical health service use, ancillary drugs, and study medications at the prescribed doses. Health service costs were estimated by multiplying the number of units of each type of service received by the estimated local unit cost of that service, and then summing the products across difference services. Unit costs estimated for each type of service were specific to each of the 24 states in which CATIE sites were geographically located. Where only national unit cost estimates were available, they were adjusted for state wage rates [18]. Cost estimates were derived from published sources documenting: inpatient costs in the various sectors in each state [19];

nursing home costs [20]; substance abuse treatment costs [21]; and residential treatment costs [22]. Unit costs of some services were estimated using claims data from the 2002 MarketScan® data set [17], a compilation of all mental health and medical insurance claims from over 500,000 private sector mental health service users, classified by diagnosis and CPT code. Some unit cost estimates were derived from VA administrative data files [23–26].

Unit costs estimated from published reports and public databases, as described above, were not specific to the agencies delivering services at each site. Estimates of service use were based on self-report data and could not be independently validated. Faulty recall of service use, however, was minimized by monthly assessments and by probing on many different types of service.

Since costs were estimated from the perspective of the total health system rather than of society as a whole, they do include the administrative cost of transfer (e.g. disability) payments [27], criminal justice costs [28], or productivity (employment earnings), although data were collected on these costs. Analysis of disability payments and incarceration showed scattered statistically significant differences between groups, but the dollar magnitude of the differences were small and thus not large enough to have substantially affected our results. Productivity was included as a benefit in the instrumental activity subscale of the Quality of Life Scale.

Effectiveness

Cost-effectiveness analysis requires a single measure of health related quality of life that reflects both health gains and health losses due to side effects. Although not accepted by all experts, the Public Health Service Task Force on Cost-effectiveness in Health and Medicine [13] specifically recommended that health states be expressed as QALYs, a year of life rated on a cardinal scale from 0 (worst possible health) to 1 (perfect health), as evaluated by members of the general public. The resulting measure of cost-effectiveness is the incremental cost-effectiveness ratio, the difference in total health costs between pairs of treatments divided by the difference in benefits, i.e., the net cost of each unit of benefit or the cost per QALY. Cost-benefit analysis, in which both costs and health benefits (QALYs) are expressed in dollars, allows one to compare treatments using a single monetized metric.

A series of studies [29–31] demonstrated a disease-specific method for evaluating QALYs in schizophrenia. First, a factor analysis of data on the Positive and Negative Syndrome Scale (PANSS) gathered from a sample of almost 400 patients [29] was used to identify positive, negative, and cognitive factors on the PANSS [32]. Then cluster analysis was used to identify eight disease-specific health states on the basis of these three factors. With input from expert clinicians, PANSS sub-scale scores for these eight health states were used to develop script and video materials to convey to lay individuals, representing the general public, the health impairments experienced in each schizophrenia state. Video materials were also created for five commonly co-occurring antipsychotic medication side effects (orthostatic hypotension, weight gain, tardive dyskinesia (TD), pseudo-parkinsonism and akathisia) [29]. Using these video presentations, the states were rated by 620 members of the general public using the standard gamble, the recommended method for QALY determination [13]. QALYs for the eight overall schizophrenia health states ranged from 0.44 to 0.88, while weights for the side effects ranged from a low of 0.857 for severe TD through 0.959 for weight gain and 1.0 when a side effect was not present. The final QALY estimate is the product of the QALY rating for the schizophrenia state and the QALY ratings for each side effect. Following the recommendations of the Public Health Task Force [13], this measure represents the health state of each subject on symptoms and side effects weighted for *societal* preferences.

To complement this primary measure of effectiveness, based as it is, on health state preferences of the general public, we also constructed a secondary measure based on the individual preferences of each CATIE participant at the time of each assessment, using methods that have been described in detail previously [33]. To construct this Patient Preference Weighted Index (PPWI), patients first ranked the importance of improvement to them in six domains: social life, work, energy, symptoms, confusion and side effects from 1 (most important) to 6 (least important). They then indicated how many times more important each domain was, to them personally, than the least important domain, with a possible range from 1–99. The weight for each domain was then standardized by dividing each score by the largest of the six scores for that person (possible range 0.01 to 1.0).

These personal patient domain preferences were then used to weight actual outcome data addressing each of the six domains. Measures of patient status in each domain were converted to standardized scores (z-scores), and averaged if there were more than one component measure. These scores were re-standardized, and then multiplied by the patient preference weights. Resulting measures for each of the six domains were themselves converted to standardized scores and averaged.

Specific domain measures were calculated as follows. Individual patient importance weights for: a) social life, were multiplied by the standardized score of the social activities subscale of the Quality of Life Scale (QOLS) [34]; weights for b) work, by the instrumental activities subscale of the QOLS; and weights for c) energy, by the average of three standardized measures: the intra-psychic activity subscale of the QOLS, the negative symptom factor from the PANSS [32], and the Calgary Depression scale [35]. Weights for d) symptoms, were applied to a standardized version of Lenert's positive symptom factor from the PANSS [29]; weights for e) confusion, to Lenert's standardized cognitive symptom factor [29]; and weights for f) side effects, to the average of three standardized measures of extrapyramidal symptoms [36–38] and of the Body Mass Index, a measure of obesity. Measures of symptoms and side effects were multiplied by –1 so that larger PPWI scores uniformly reflect better health. As noted above, the six patient-preference weighted domain scores were standardized (i.e., converted to z-scores) and averaged to yield a final PPWI that reflected the clinical status in six domains weighted by their importance to each patient at the time of each particular assessment.

Quality of life was also evaluated with two self-rated global measures: the Visual Analog Scale, on which patients rate their health on a scale from 0 (worst state of health) to 100 (perfect health) [29]; and the Lehman global quality of life item, on which patients rate their overall quality of life on a scale from 1 (terrible) to 7 (delighted) [39].

Statistical methods

For consistency and comparability, the statistical methods used in the analysis of continuous measures in the cost-effectiveness analysis were the same as those used in the original publication from CATIE. Two hundred and thirty-one patients with TD were excluded from assignment to perphenazine, and ziprasidone was added to the trial after 40% of the patients had been enrolled. Randomization took place under four separate regimens: including and excluding patients with TD, and including and excluding ziprasidone. Analyses were thus conducted on four different data sets with overlapping membership.

Each data set only included patients with an equal chance of being randomly assigned to the treatments under comparison. Perphenazine patients, in particular, were only compared to equivalent patients who did not have TD at baseline.

The primary comparison between the four treatments available at the beginning of the trial was an overall 3 degree of freedom test. This test was performed on Analytic Data Set I, excluding patients with TD and those randomized to ziprasidone. If the overall test was significant at $p < 0.05$, the three second-generation drugs were compared with perphenazine with a Hochberg adjustment for multiple comparisons [40] in which the smallest p-value was compared to $0.05/3 = 0.017$ and the largest to $p = 0.05$. Next, using Data Set II, which excludes perphenazine and includes TD patients, the three second-generation drugs were compared to each other via step-down testing. If the overall 2 degree of freedom test was significant at $p < 0.05$, an α of $p < 0.05$ was applied for all comparisons.

Data Sets III and IV were used to compare ziprasidone to the other four drugs among patients randomized after ziprasidone became available, but with TD patients excluded from the perphenazine comparison. Hochberg adjustment for four pair-wise comparisons was used to compare ziprasidone and perphenazine in Data Set III, and ziprasidone to the other three drugs using Data Set IV. The smallest p-value was considered significant if $p = 0.05/4 = 0.013$.

The central cost analysis was a paired comparison between treatment groups of average monthly costs from all 18 months using a mixed model including terms representing treatment group, the baseline value of the dependent cost variable, time (treated as a classification variable for months 1–18), site, a history of recent clinical exacerbation, and baseline-by-time interactions. The baseline-by-time term adjusts for baseline differences in characteristics of patients who dropped out early and thus are less well represented at later time points. Group-by-time interactions to evaluate differences in time trends between groups were also tested. A random subject effect and a first-order autoregressive covariance structure were used to adjust standard errors for the correlation of observations from the same individual.

Use of any hospital days in each month was examined using a dichotomous (0–1) measure analyzed with generalized estimation equations using GENMOD procedure of SAS©.

Because of the skewed distribution of service use (i.e., non-drug) cost data, log-transformed data were used in the analysis of both: a) non-drug health service costs and b) total costs, including medications, and both mean and median values are presented [41]. Adjusted average log-transformed costs were then re-transformed into average costs using the "smearing estimation" method of Duan [42], after testing the data for heteroscedasticity [43]. Untransformed monthly data were also averaged for each individual and compared with the Kruskal-Wallis non-parametric test.

The same mixed model analysis was used for effectiveness outcomes based on scores from months 1 and then quarterly from month 3 through 18, again using a random subject effect and a first-order autoregressive covariance structure. Measures contributing to the PPWI were available at months 1, 6, 12, and 18.

In addition to the analysis of effectiveness and costs, cost-benefit analysis was also conducted. In the cost-benefit analysis, treatments were compared using the method of net health benefits [12]. In this approach, a range of conventional estimates for the dollar value of a QALY are multiplied by the QALY estimate for each patient at each time point to estimate the monetized value of their health status at each observation. Following conventions used in policy making [44], we use estimates of $25,000/QALY/year ($2,083/month);

$50,000/QALY/year ($4,167/QALY/month) and $100,000/QALY/year ($8,333/QALY/month) in a sensitivity analysis. This yielded a monetized estimate of health status for each patient at each time point.

Monthly health care costs were then subtracted from these estimated health benefits to generate an estimate of "net health benefit" for each patient for each month at each of the three estimated monetary values of a QALY.

We then use mixed model regression analyses of the type described above to compare mean differences between the groups using monthly estimates of net health benefits from all time points and adjusting for time, site, and other factors, and with Hochberg adjustment for multiple comparisons as noted above [40].

Over the past decade, it has been increasingly recognized that policy makers typically have to make decisions even when findings do not meet the usual 5% standard of uncertainty used in scientific research and that it is important to know the probability that one treatment will be more cost-effective than another, even when the uncertainty is greater than 5% [45]. Using the method of Hoch *et al.* [46], we calculate the probability that the treatment with the greater net health benefits in each comparison is superior to each of the others at each of the three estimated monetary values of a QALY. This calculation was based on a one-tailed test based on the p-value representing the significance of differences between the least square means of each pair and was computed as 1-p/2 [46].

Results
Service use and cost

Analysis of all outcome data based on the intention to treat assignment, which attributes all costs to the initially assigned drug, showed that total medication costs for patients initially assigned to perphenazine were $200–$300/month (about 40%–50%) lower than drug costs for patients assigned to each of the four second-generation antipsychotics (Table 4.1, Figure 4.1) ($p < 0.0001$). Significant group-by-time statistical interactions ($p < 0.0001$) reflect the narrowing of differences in drug costs during the first 8 months, after which perphenazine remains consistently less costly ($p < 0.0001$ at each time point).

Data on drug treatment following the first *change* in treatment after randomization showed that virtually all treatments administered were second-generation drugs (range 96.1% to 99.6% across groups for all prescriptions following the first drug change) with a balanced distribution of agents across initial treatment groups (see Table 1 in Rosenheck *et al.*, 2006 [47]).

There were no significant differences in the proportion of patients who received inpatient care each month (see online supplemental Figure 1 in [46]), the single greatest source of cost among people with schizophrenia. The average total inpatient and residential treatment costs per month was also not significantly different between groups (Table 4.1, see on line supplemental Figure 2 in [46]), nor were there any significant differences in the sum of inpatient, residential, and outpatient health service costs (i.e., all non-drug costs – Table 4.1, online supplemental Figure 3 in [46]). Group by time interactions for these costs were not statistically significant, indicating continuous equivalence of these non-drug health service costs across groups over time.

When health service and drug costs were summed to generate total health care costs (the primary cost outcome), average total monthly health care costs were $300–$500 (20%–30%) lower for perphenazine than for second-generation antipsychotics (Table 4.1, Figure 4.2)

Table 4.1. Average monthly costs (including drug discounts and rebates) by treatment group over 18 months[1,2]. From [47] Reproduced with permission from the American Journal of Psychiatry.

	Olanzapine (O)	Perphenazine (P)	Quetiapine (Q)	Risperidone (R)	Ziprasidone (Z)	$F^{3,4}$ Chi-square[5]	Overall $p<$	Paired comparisons[6]
Total (N=)	328	256	326	332	182			
Data Set I (df=3): P vs. O, Q, and R (N=)	263	256	261	269				
Excluding patients with TD and patients on ziprasidone								
Monthly drug costs (3)	$595	$288	$523	$526	–	117.2	<0.0001	P < O,Q,R (all p < 0.0001*)
Experimental medications (3)	493	196	415	440	–	190.9	<0.0001	P < O,Q,R (all p < 0.0001*)
Concomitant medications (3)	103	93	108	86	–	1.1	0.34	ns
Monthly health service costs (4)	837	851	1,134	1,007	–	1.6	0.18	ns
Median (5)	121	89	132	129	–	5.1	0.16	ns
Inpatient and residential treatment costs (4)	556	531	753	692	–	2.1	0.09	ns
Outpatient, mental health/medical surgical svs. (4)	281	321	381	316	–	1.3	0.28	ns
Monthly total health costs (drugs and services) (4)	1,428	1,139	1,657	1,529	–	47.6	<0.0001	P < O,Q,R (all p < 0.0001*)
Median (5)	783	439	752	743	–	55.0	<0.0001	P < O,Q,R (all p < 0.0001*)

Table 4.1. (cont.)

	Olanzapine (O)	Perphenazine (P)	Quetiapine (Q)	Risperidone (R)	Ziprasidone (Z)	$F^{3,4}$ Chi-square[5]	Overall $p<$	Paired comparisons[6]
Data Set II (df=2): O vs. Q vs. R (N=)	328		326	332				
Including patients with TD but excluding those on zipr. or perph.								
Monthly drug costs (3)	616	–	518	540	–	23.2	<0.0001	O > Q,R (both p < 0.0001*)
Experimental medications (3)	506	–	410	437	–	36.0	<0.0001	O > Q,R (both p < 0.0001*); R > Q (p = 0.014*)
Concomitant medications (3)	111	–	109	104	–	0.4	0.64	Ns
Monthly health service costs (4)	902	–	1,230	1,095	–	1.7	0.19	ns
Median (5)	140	–	160	147	–	2.5	0.290	ns
Inpatient and residential treatment costs (4)	580	–	809	709	–	3.7	0.024	ns
Outpatient, mental health/medical surgical svs. (4)	322	–	421	386	–	0.1	0.87	ns
Monthly total health costs (drugs and services) (4)	1515	–	1,749	1,631	–	0.8	0.45	ns
Median (5)	825	–	775	800	–	0.5	0.80	ns

Data Set III: Z vs. P (N=)

Excluding patients with TD but including those on ziprasidone

	146		150		P vs. P
Monthly drug costs (3)	311	–	516	Not applicable	$P < Z$ ($p < 0.0001*$)
Experimental medications (3)	214	–	389	Not applicable	$P < Z$ ($p < 0.0001*$); $Z < R$ ($p < 0.0002*$)
Concomitant medications (3)	98	–	127	Not applicable	ns
Monthly health service costs (4)	947	–	1,220	Not applicable	$P < Z$ ($p < 0.04$)
Median (5)	89	–	129	Not applicable	$P < Z$ ($p < 0.03$)
Inpatient and residential treatment costs (4)	546	–	777	Not applicable	ns
Outpatient, mental health/medical surgical svs. (4)	402	–	443	Not applicable	ns
Monthly total health costs (drugs and services) (4)	1,258	–	1,737	Not applicable	$P < Z$ ($p < 0.0001*$)
Median (5)	475	–	715	Not applicable	$P < Z$ ($p < 0.0001*$)

Table 4.1. (cont.)

	Olanzapine (O)	Perphenazine (P)	Quetiapine (Q)	Risperidone (R)	Ziprasidone (Z)	$F^{3,4}$ Chi-square[5]	Overall $p<$	Paired comparisons[6]
Data Set IV: Z vs. O, Q, and R (N=)	177		181	174	178			
Including patients with TD and those on ziprasidone								
Monthly drug costs (3)	641	–	530	554	521	Not applicable		$Z < O$ ($p < 0.0001$*)
Experimental medications (3)	505	–	415	453	393	Not applicable		$Z < O$ ($p < 0.0001$*)
Concomitant medications (3)	137	–	115	102	128	Not applicable		ns
Monthly health service costs (4)	907	–	1,233	1,008	1,330	Not applicable		$Z > O$ ($p = 0.049$); $Z > R$ ($p = 0.038$)
Median (5)	132	–	165	121	147	Not applicable		$Z > O$ ($p = 0.024$); $Z > R$ ($p = 0.015$)
Inpatient and residential treatment costs (4)	584	–	798	603	839	Not applicable		ns
Outpatient, mental health/medical surgical svs. (4)	322	–	435	405	491	Not applicable		ns

| Monthly total health costs (drugs and services) (4) | 1,546 | – | 1,763 | 1,562 | **1,851** | Not applicable | ns |
| Median (5) | 931 | – | 819 | 770 | 771 | Not applicable | ns |

Notes: [1] Bolded values highlight treatment conditions of primary interest in each data set.

[2] All pairwise *p* values < 0.05 are presented. * = statistically significant using criteria for multiple comparisons.

[3] Statistical analysis of drug costs based on un-transformed data from months 1–18 where each patient has the data from each month they participated in data collection (N = 12,163 patient-month observations for Data Set I; 11,308 for Data Set II; 3,241 for Data Set III; and 7,732 for Data Set IV). Appropriate discounts and rebates applied to VA patients and patients whose care is funded by Medicaid.

[4] Statistical analysis of health service and total costs based on log transformed data from months 1–18 where each patient has the data from each month they participated in data collection (N = 12,163 patient-month observations for Data Set I; 11,308 for Data Set II; 3,241 for Data Set III; and 7,732 for Data Set IV).

[5] Kruskal-Wallis test.

[6] ns = paired comparisons examined with this data set were not significantly different.

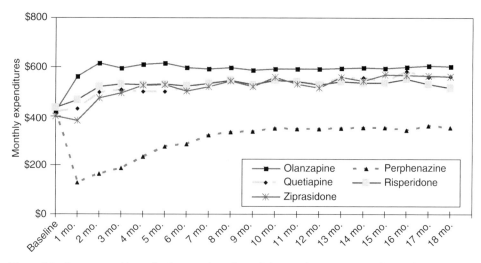

Figure 4.1. Average monthly medication costs (experimental drugs and concomitant medications). See plate section for color version. From [47] Reproduced with permission from the American Journal of Psychiatry. (Copyright 2006). American Psychiatric Association.

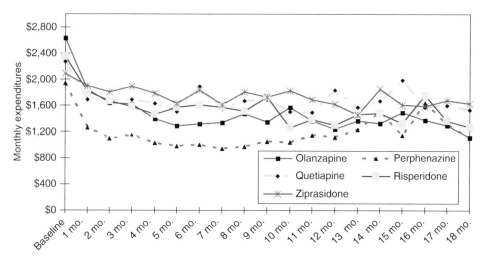

Figure 4.2. Average monthly costs: all healthcare costs including medications. See plate section for color version. From [47] Reproduced with permission from the American Journal of Psychiatry. (Copyright 2006). American Psychiatric Association.

($p < 0.0001$). The modest rise in total costs for the perphenazine group during the early months of the trial reflects increased drug costs as some perphenazine patients switched to second-generation antipsychotics, but there was no increase in non-drug costs among perphenazine patients over the study period. Significant group-by-time interactions reflected convergence in log-cost between groups, but perphenazine log-costs remained significantly lower than those of other groups ($p < 0.001$ at all time points). Although raw average cost data presented in Figure 4.2 overlap in the latter months of the trial, comparisons of log-transformed data for each specific month (online supplemental Tables 6, 7 in Rosenheck *et al.* [47]), which reduces the effect of outlier values, showed significantly lower costs for the perphenazine group at all time points. In a sensitivity analysis in which Medicaid or VA drug prices were applied to *all* patients (using 25% and 40% lower experimental drug costs, respectively), the advantage for perphenazine on cost comparisons remained statistically significant.

Drug costs for the olanzapine group were significantly higher than for the quetiapine, risperidone, and ziprasidone groups. Due to lower inpatient and outpatient costs for the olanzapine group (statistically significant only for inpatient costs in comparison to quetiapine), there were no significant differences in total health care costs between second-generation drugs.

Examination of median values revealed similar cost patterns, with significantly lower costs for the perphenazine group (Table 4.1).

Effectiveness

In the intention-to-treat analysis, significant improvement was observed from baseline to 18 months in the overall sample, with lower PANSS scores and higher QALYs and PPWI scores, as well as higher scores on the VAS and Lehman Quality of Life measures, over time.

Olanzapine showed the lowest PANSS scores but these were not significantly different than those for perphenazine after adjustment for multiple comparisons.

Perphenazine showed higher (i.e., better) QALY scores than other agents, but there was only one significant difference (perphenazine was significantly greater on QALYs than risperidone) (Table 4.2, Figure 4.3).

Phase 1-only analysis (initial drug assignment only)

When the analyses were limited to observations of patients while they received the first assigned medication (Phase 1), the patterns of statistically significant cost results did not change, although, as expected, without the additional costs of switching to second-generation antipsychotics, the savings for perphenazine in comparison to second-generation drugs in both medication costs and total health cost increased to $400–$600, i.e., by an additional $100–$200/month (Online supplemental table 4 in Rosenheck *et al.* [47]). Group-by-time interactions in total costs were not statistically significant, since there was less convergence of cost in Phase 1 during the latter months of the trial (i.e., excluding observations after the switch from perphenazine to second-generation drugs).

The pattern of statistically significant results on QALYs and other effectiveness measures were also unchanged in the analysis that only included observations on the initially randomized drug (Online supplemental table 5 in Rosenheck *et al.* [47]).

Adjusted outcomes and re-transformed log cost data

Least square means, adjusted for baseline values of the dependent cost measures (Online supplemental table 6 in Rosenheck *et al.* [47]), and re-transformed log-cost data (Online supplemental table 7 in Rosenheck *et al.* [47]) showed similar patterns of results to the raw mean cost data on both intention-to-treat analysis and the Phase 1 only analysis, with substantially and significantly lower costs for the perphenazine group.

Perphenazine, with significantly lower costs, and the slightly better, although not statistically significant, outcomes on the measure of QALYs, was the most cost-effective

Table 4.2. Comparison of effectiveness: mixed model analyses of monthly values by group[1,2]. From [47]. Reproduced with permission of the American Journal of Psychiatry. (Copyright 2006). American Psychiatric Association.

	Olanzapine (O)	Perphenazine (P)	Quetiapine (Q)	Risperidone (R)	Ziprasidone (Z)	F	p	Paired comparisons (6)
Total (N=)	328	256	326	332	182			
Data Set I (df=3): P vs. O, Q and R								
Excluding patients with TD and patients on ziprasidone (N=)								
PANSS Total Score[3]	64.8	66.8	67.3	68.8	–	6.46	<0.0002	O<P (0.03), P<R (0.03)
Quality-adjusted life years[4]	0.717	0.720	0.718	0.704	–	3.1	0.03	P>R (0.005*)
Patient Preference Weighted Index (PPWI)[5]	0.124	0.075	0.050	0.062	–	1.11	0.34	ns
Data Set II (df=2): O vs. Q vs. R	328		326	332				
Including patients with TD but excluding those on zipr. or perph. (N=)								
PANSS Total Score[3]	65.8	–	68.0	69.1	–	8.99	<0.0001	O < R (p<0.0001*), O < Q (p<0.005*)
Quality-adjusted life years[4]	0.705	–	0.705	0.698	–	1.1	0.33	ns
Patient Preference Weighted Index (PPWI)[5]	0.071	–	−0.005	0.022	–	2.05	0.13	ns
Data Set III: Z vs. P	146				150			
Excluding patients with TD but including those on ziprasidone (N=)								

PANSS Total Score[3]	67.2	–	–	68.0	Not applicable	ns
Quality-adjusted life years[4]	0.722	–	–	0.716	Not applicable	ns
Patient Preference Weighted Index (PPWI)[5]	0.120	–	–	0.124	Not applicable	ns
Data Set IV: Z vs. O, Q and R	177	181	174	178		
Including Patients with TD and those on ziprasidone (N=)						
PANSS Total Score[3]	63.2	67.1	68.4	**67.2**	Not applicable	ns
Quality-adjusted life years[4]	0.721	0.709	0.702	**0.710**	Not applicable	ns
Patient Preference Weighted Index (PPWI)[5]	0.100	0.060	0.062	**0.113**	Not applicable	ns

Notes: [1]Bolded values highlight treatment conditions of primary interest in each data set.
[2]All pairwise p values < 0.05 are presented. * = statistically significant using criteria for multiple comparisons.
[3]Least square means of PANSS scores from months 1, 3, 6, 9, 12, 15, 18 (N = 4,816 patient-month observations for Data Set I; 4,480 for Data Set II; 1,285 for Data Set III; and 3,802 for Data Set IV).
[4]Least squared means of QALYs (range 0–1): statistical analysis based on inverse transformation from month 1, 3, 6, 9, 12, 15, 18 (N = 4,777 patient-month observations for Data Set I; 4,454 for Data Set II; 1,270 for Data Set III; and 3,063 for Data Set IV).
[5]Least square means of PPWI (average z-scores weighted for patient preferences: interquartile range = −0.64 to +0.64) from months 6, 12, and 18 (N = 2,475 patient-month observations for Data Set I; 2,250 for Data Set II; 1,695 for Data Set III; and 1,613 for Data Set IV).
[6]ns = paired comparisons examined with this data set were not significantly different.

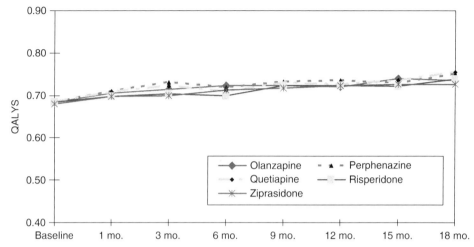

Figure 4.3. Quality-adjusted life years (QALYs). See plate section for color version. From [47] Reproduced with permission from the American Journal of Psychiatry. (Copyright 2006). American Psychiatric Association.

treatment. Computing the incremental cost-effectiveness ratio was not necessary since perphenazine was both more effective and less costly.

Cost-benefit analysis

Cost-benefit analysis using a range of estimates for the dollar value of one QALY from $25,000 to $100,000 found greater net health benefits for perphenazine than for any of the second-generation antipsychotics, with statistically significant differences from quetiapine and ziprasidone after adjustment for multiple comparisons in the intention-to-treat analysis and significant differences from all four second-generation drugs in the Phase 1 only analysis when the value of a QALY is estimated at $50,000 or greater (Table 4.3). These findings primarily reflect the substantially lower costs of perphenazine, which are augmented by the slightly higher, if not statistically significant, QALY scores. Thus, as the estimate of the dollar value of a QALY increases (Table 4.3), perphenazine performs increasingly, if only slightly, better than the other drugs in the cost-benefit analysis.

Using the Hoch method [46], perphenazine was determined to be superior to olanzapine on the measure of net health benefits with 86% probability, and was likely to be more cost-effective than the other second-generation drugs with greater than 95%–99% probability.

None of the second-generation antipsychotics were significantly superior to any of the others in the cost-benefit analysis on either the intent-to-treat analysis or the Phase 1-only analysis (Table 4.3).

Discussion

This study found that during the 18 months of the CATIE trial, initial assignment to a first-generation antipsychotic, perphenazine, was less costly and no less effective than assignment to each of four second-generation antipsychotics as measured by QALYs that combined measures of symptoms and side effects as well as on four other measures of symptoms or effectiveness. Several different analytic strategies all yielded the same pattern

Table 4.3. Cost benefit comparison of drug treatments using net health benefits analysis at three estimated dollar values per QALY[1]

Intention to treat (includes all data)

A. Estimate at $25,000/QALY (net health benefits of row medication less column medication)

	Olanzapine		Risperidone		Quetiapine		Ziprasidone	
Perphenazine	$159	ns	$272	ns	$469	b*	$529	b*
Olanzapine	–		$29	ns	$178	ns	$184	ns
Risperidone	–		–		$149	ns	$364	ns
Quetiapine	–		–		–		$123	ns

B. Estimate at $50,000/QALY (net health benefits of row medication less column medication)

	Olanzapine		Risperidone		Quetiapine		Ziprasidone	
Perphenazine	$164	ns	$292	a	$612	b*	$544	b*
Olanzapine	–		$47	ns	$178	ns	$192	ns
Risperidone	–		–		$131	ns	$343	ns
Quetiapine	–		–		–		$129	ns

C. Estimate at $100,000/QALY (net health benefits of row medication less column medication)

	Olanzapine		Risperidone		Quetiapine		Ziprasidone	
Perphenazine	$171	ns	$371	a	$472	b*	$573	b*
Olanzapine	–		$82	ns	$179	ns	$208	ns
Risperidone	–		–		$98	ns	$303	ns
Quetiapine	–		–		–		$137	ns

Phase 1 only (only observed on originally assigned drug)

A. Estimate at $25,000/QALY (net health benefits of row medication less column medication)

	Olanzapine		Risperidone		Quetiapine		Ziprasidone	
Perphenazine	$288	a*	$376	a*	$399	b*	$565	ns
Olanzapine	–		$13	ns	$3	ns	$114	ns
Risperidone	–		–		$10	ns	$340	ns
Quetiapine	–		–		–		$292	ns

B. Estimate at $50,000/QALY (net health benefits of row medication less column medication)

	Olanzapine		Risperidone		Quetiapine		Ziprasidone	
Perphenazine	$303	a*	$417	b*	$404	b*	$597	b*
Olanzapine	–		$3	ns	$13	ns	$123	ns
Risperidone	–		–		$10	ns	$331	ns
Quetiapine	–		–		–		$307	ns

Table 4.3. (cont.)

Phase 1 only								
C. Estimate at $100,000/QALY (net health benefits of row medication less column medication)								
	Olanzapine		Risperidone		Quetiapine		Ziprasidone	
Perphenazine	$328	a*	$496	b*	$412	a*	$654	b*
Olanzapine	–		$18	ns	($30)	ns	$142	ns
Risperidone	–		–		($48)	ns	$316	ns
Quetiapine	–		–		–		$334	ns

Notes: [1]Paired t-tests of least squared means, adjusted for time, baseline value of Net health benefits, site, exacerbation status at baseline, and the interaction of time and baseline status.
[2]Keys: a = $p < 0.05$; b = $p < 0.01$; ns = not significant; *Significant after Hochberg adjustment for multiple comparisons.

of significant results, including: a) analyses of all available outcome data, b) analyses limited to the period of treatment with the initially assigned drug (Phase 1), c) comparison of both means and medians using parametric and non-parametric statistics, respectively, d) examination of least square means of cost data as well as re-transformed log-cost data, and e) sensitivity analyses in which less expensive Medicaid and VA discounted drug prices were applied to all patients. Since in this study perphenazine was consistently and significantly less costly, and not less effective as measured by QALYs, than the next most effective treatment, calculation of the cost-effectiveness ratio was not performed [13]. Cost-benefit analysis using the Net Health Benefit Approach, also found perphenazine to be superior to the other medications tested in CATIE.

The original report from the CATIE trial identified an overall group-by-time interaction for the PANSS total score, suggesting improvement was greatest with olanzapine over some other treatments but diminished over time. However, specific pairwise treatment comparisons were not presented. In this chapter we have presented further details of paired comparisons between individual agents. Consistent with the original report, the paired comparisons on the PANSS reported here showed significant superiority of olanzapine over two other SGAs, risperidone and quetiapine. However, no significant difference was observed between olanzapine and perphenazine, the drugs with the lowest PANSS scores at each time point in the original report. On average, olanzapine scored an estimated 2.0 PANSS points lower than perphenazine, with a 95% confidence interval (CI) of the difference in least square means in mixed model analysis of –3.7 to –0.02 ($p = 0.03$, not significant after adjustment for multiple comparisons). Excluding all observations after the first medication change (i.e., the Phase 1 only analysis), the estimated mean difference was 1.5 points lower for olanzapine than perphenazine (95% CI = –3.3 to 0.03; $p = 0.11$). Thus, we can be 97.5% confident (one-tailed test) that the difference in mean PANSS scores between olanzapine and perphenazine in this study was less than 3.7 points (5% of the baseline value). Previous research suggests that a clinically significant improvement is typically associated with a 20% difference in the PANSS [48].

After the inclusion of data on side effects, weight gain, and symptoms in the measure of QALYs, perphenazine scored 0.003 higher than the next best drug (olanzapine), although the differences were not statistically significant (95% CI = 0.014 to –0.009). There were also no significant differences between any drugs on a complementary measure based on patient health state preferences (as contrasted with societal preferences) or on two patient-rated global measures of quality of life.

The data presented in the initial CATIE report suggesting lower rates of hospitalization for schizophrenia associated with olanzapine differ from those presented here, which show no differences in hospitalization between groups. While the earlier report was based exclusively on "serious adverse event" reporting of hospitalization, specifically for schizophrenia, data reported here were based on monthly, systematic questioning of patients about all types of hospitalization from each of several providers, and were specifically intended for cost purposes. The data presented in the earlier paper were thus neither as detailed nor as inclusive as the hospital utilization and related cost data presented here, which show no differences in inpatient utilization or cost.

There were no statistically significant differences among any pair of the four second-generation antipsychotics on either total costs, QALYs, or the other measures of effectiveness, with the exception of symptoms, on which olanzapine was superior to both risperidone and quetiapine. Olanzapine was superior to other second-generation antipsychotics, with the exception of risperidone, in cost-benefit analysis.

Strengths of this cost-effectiveness study are its large sample size, relatively long duration of follow-up, and recruitment of patients from diverse representative sites with minimal exclusion criteria – all of which increase the generalizability of the results. The study was also enhanced by the use of a rigorously developed algorithm for evaluating health states specific to schizophrenia in QALYs that takes both symptoms of schizophrenia and side effects into account.

At the time the study was initiated, it was widely believed that perphenazine increased the risk of TD, and differential randomization was used to minimize that risk. While a recent review suggested that second-generation antipsychotics are associated with less risk of TD than first-generation drugs [49], it noted that only 3 of 11 year-long studies were based on randomized trials and all used moderate-to-high doses of haloperidol for comparison. Results from CATIE are consistent with the results of other recent studies [6,7,50–53] that have questioned the extent to which the risk of either TD or pseudo-parkinsonism is greater with older drugs, especially when lower potency drugs are used in moderate doses. The maximum dose of perphenazine allowed in CATIE was 32 mg, about half the maximum clinically recommended dose (64 mg for inpatients). However, since patients in CATIE were outpatients during over 95% of assessments, the recommended outpatient maximum dose of 24 mg is more applicable. It is notable, however, that only 40% of perphenazine patients reached the maximally allowed 32 mg dose, the same percentage as reached maximal doses in the olanzapine and risperidone arms.

A recent cost-effectiveness analysis that combined cost-data from CATIE with TD incidence data from the review mentioned previously [54] estimated that it would cost over $50,000 for each case of TD avoided by use of second-generation antipsychotics instead of haloperidol. Additional data on the typical range of severity of TD and QALY-losses associated with TD suggested an incremental cost-effectiveness ratio of at least $600,000/QALY for the TD benefits of second-generation antipsychotics, a ratio that is far above the $50,000/QALY typically acceptable to policy makers [44].

Data loss from attrition was considerable. However, differences in loss-to-follow-up rates across treatments were generally small and not significantly different between olanzapine and perphenazine, the two most effective and least costly treatments, at 16 of 18 time points. In the comparisons between perphenazine and olanzapine, data were obtained at 65% of scheduled assessments for perphenazine and at 70% for olanzapine. To the extent that this difference introduces selection bias, it would tend to favor olanzapine since patients tend to do better at later assessments, a greater fraction of which were completed by patients in the olanzapine group. We also conducted a series of analyses to determine whether there were any differences between treatments in baseline characteristics (e.g., symptoms or substance abuse) that predicted duration of participation in the trial. If patients with severe symptoms at baseline were especially likely to drop out with one of the treatments, long-term findings could be systematically biased in favor of that treatment. However, there were no significant interactions between treatment assignment and any of the baseline characteristics in association with duration of participation in the trial. Differences between treatments in baseline predictors of drop out do not seem to have biased our results.

Furthermore, the failure to find significant differences between perphenazine and olanzapine on any effectiveness measure, other than the duration of treatment with the initially assigned antipsychotic, is not likely to be attributable to the lack of statistical power since differences of small magnitude (4 points on the PANSS and 0.016 QALYS) were found to be statistically significant in some comparisons involving both olanzapine and perphenazine and other treatments and 95% confidence interval analysis showed small differences between olanzapine and perphenazine on effectiveness measures.

It should also be reiterated that the comparisons with perphenazine only pertain to treatment of patients without TD at the time of treatment initiation. This, however, strengthened the ability to detect difference in TD outcomes since inclusion of patients with risk of the outcome at baseline adds noise to the analysis of that outcome. The results cannot, however, be generalized to other clinical populations such as first episode patients, refractory patients, the elderly, those with unstable medical problems, long-term institutionalized patients, patients who refuse to take medication, or patients with diagnoses other than schizophrenia. The relevance of these findings to first-generation antipsychotics other than perphenazine at modest doses, or to other second-generation drugs, and especially to clozapine, is also unknown. Furthermore, patients who believed that their current medication (whether first or second-generation) was uniquely effective for them were unlikely to have participated, and these results may not be applicable to patients who are satisfied with their current medication. A careful review of these and other limitations of CATIE [55] found them to be no different from those of other studies of second-generation antipsychotics, and thus they should not have precluded findings of distinct benefits to those drugs and are unlikely to have biased the results of the cost-effectiveness and cost-benefit analyses.

Conclusion

While the main CATIE analysis showed that patients stayed on olanzapine longer than two other second-generation antipsychotics, none of four second-generation antipsychotics showed any statistically significant advantage over the first-generation antipsychotic perphenazine on measures of symptoms, or on four other measures of quality of life presented here, and all four second-generation drugs incurred significantly greater costs than the older drug because of the higher cost of the medications themselves. The cost-benefit analysis presented here, which combines cost and benefit data in a single analysis, found perphenazine to be superior to each of the four second-generation antipsychotics with which it was compared.

References

1. Davis JM, Chen N and Glick ID. A meta-analysis of the efficacy of second-generation antipsychotics. *Archives of General Psychiatry* 2003;**60**:553–64.

2. Revicki DA, Luce BR, Weschler JM, Brown RE and Adler MA. Cost-effectiveness of clozapine for treatment-resistant schizophrenic patients. *Hospital & Community Psychiatry* 1990;**41**:850–4.

3. Reid WH and Mason M. Psychiatric hospital utilization in patients treated with clozapine for up to 4.5 years in a state mental health care system. *Journal of Clinical Psychiatry* 1998;**59**:189–94.

4. Hamilton SH, Revicki DA, Edgell ET, Genduso LA and Tollefson G. Clinical and economic outcomes of olanzapine compared with haloperidol for schizophrenia – results from a randomized clinical trial. *Pharmacoeconomics* 1999;**15**:469–80.

5. Essock SM, Frisman LK, Covell NH and Hargreaves W. Cost-effectiveness of clozapine compared with conventional antipsychotic medications for patients in State Hospitals *Archives of General Psychiatry* 2000;**5**:987–94.

6. Rosenheck R, Cramer J, Xu W, *et al.* A comparison of clozapine and haloperidol in the treatment of hospitalized patients with refractory schizophrenia. Department of Veterans Affairs Cooperative Study Group on Clozapine in Refractory Schizophrenia. *New England Journal of Medicine* 1997;**337**:809–15.

7. Rosenheck RA, Perlick D, Bingham S, *et al.* for the Department of Veterans Affairs Cooperative Study Group on the Cost-Effectiveness of Olanzapine. Effectiveness and cost of olanzapine and haloperidol in the treatment of schizophrenia: A randomized controlled trial. *Journal of the American Medical Association* 2003; **290**:2693–702.

8. Jones PB, Barnes TR, Davies L, *et al.* Randomized controlled trial of effect on quality of life of second-generation versus first-generation antipsychotic drugs in schizophrenia: Cost utility of the latest antipsychotic drugs in schizophrenia study (CUtLASS 1). *Archives of General Psychiatry* 2006;**63**:1079–87.

9. Duggan M. Do new prescription drugs pay for themselves? The case of second-generation antipsychotics. *Journal of Health Economics* 2005;**24**:1–31.

10. Polsky D, Doshi JA, Bauer MS, *et al.* Clinical trial-based cost-effectiveness analyses of antipsychotic use. *American Journal of Psychiatry* 2006;**163**:2047–56.

11. Stroup TS, McEvoy JP, Swartz MS, *et al.* The National Institute of Mental Health Clinical Antipsychotic Trials of Intervention Effectiveness (CATIE) project: Schizophrenia trial design and protocol development. *Schizophrenia Bulletin* 2003;**29**:15–31.

12. Stinnett AA and Mullahy J. Net health benefits: A new frame work for the analysis of uncertainty in cost-effectiveness analysis. *Medical Decision Making* 1998;**18**:(Suppl): S65–S80.

13. Gold MR, Siegel JE, Russell LB and Weinstein MC. *Cost Effectiveness in Health and Medicine.* New York, NY: Oxford University Press; 1996.

14. Medical Economics Company. *Drug Topics Red Book.* Montvale, NJ: Medical Economics Company; 1999.

15. Department of Health and Human Services, Office of Inspector General (2005) *Medicaid Drug Price Comparisons: Average Manufacturer Price to Published Prices* (http://oig.hhs.gov/oei/reports/oei-03–05–00200.pdf, accessed on 23 November, 2005).

16. Rosenheck RA, Leslie DL and Sernyak ME. From clinical trials to real-world practice: Use of atypical antipsychotic medication nationally in the Department of Veterans Affairs. *Medical Care* 2001;**39**:302–8.

17. Thompson Medstat Group. *Marketscan Communical Claims and Encounters Database.* Ann Arbor, MI: The Thompson Medstat Group; 2002.

18. Bureau of Labor Statistics, US Department of Labor. 2004–05 Edition, *Occupational*

Outlook Handbook, Bulletin 2540. Washington, DC: US Department of Labor; 2005.

19. National Association of State Mental Health Program Directors. *Table 19: SMNHA Mental Health—Controlled Expenditures Per Inpatient Day, All Civil (Voluntary and Involuntary) Patients in State Psychiatric Hospitals Receiving Mental Health Services by Age and State, FY 2002.* Alexandria, VA: National Association of State Mental Health Program Directors; 2002.

20. Grabowski DC, Feng Z, Intrator O and Mohr V. Recent trends in state nursing home payment policies. *Health Affairs (Millwood)* Web Exclusives 2004;**4**:W4–363–73.

21. US Department of Health and Human Services. June 18. *The ADSS Cost Study: Costs of Substance Abuse Treatment in the Specialty Sector.* Washington, DC: US Department of Health and Human Services; 2004.

22. Kasprow WJ, Rosenheck R, DiLella D, Cavallaro L, Harelik N. *Health Care for Homeless Veterans Programs: The Seventeenth Annual Report.* West Haven, CT: US Department of Veterans Affairs, North East Program Evaluation Center, VA Connecticut Health Care System; 2004.

23. Barnett PG. Review of methods to determine VA health care costs. *Medical Care* 1999;**37**(Suppl):AS9–AS17.

24. Greenberg G and Rosenheck RA. *National Mental Health Program Performance Monitoring System: Fiscal Year 2002 Report.* West Haven, CT: Northeast Program Evaluation Center; 2003.

25. Neale M, Rosenheck R, Martin A, Morrissey J and Castrodonatti J. *Mental Health Intensive Case Management (MHICM): The Sixth National Performance Monitoring Report: FY 2003.* West Haven, CT: Northeast Program Evaluation Center; 2004.

26. Resnick S, Rosenheck RA, Corwel L and Medak S. *Seventh Progress Report on the Compensated Work Therapy/Veterans Industries Program. Fiscal Year 2003.* West Haven,

CT: Northeast Program Evaluation Center; 2004.

27. Frisman LK and Rosenheck RA. How transfer payments are treated in cost-effectiveness and cost-benefit analysis. *Administration and Policy in Mental Health* 1996;**23**:533–46.

28. US Department of Justice. In: K. Maguire and T. Flanagan, eds. *Office of Justice Programs, Bureau of Justice Statistics Sourcebook of Criminal Justice Statistics–1990 (NCJ-130580).* Washington, DC: USGPO; 1991.

29. Lenert L, Sturley AP, Rapaport MH, *et al.* Public preferences for health states with schizophrenia and a mapping function to estimate utilities from positive and negative syndrome scale scores. *Schizophrenia Research* 2004;**71**:155–65.

30. Lenert L, Sturly AP and Rupnow M. Toward improved methods for measurement of utility: Automated repair of errors in utility elicitations. *Medical Decision Making* 2003;**23**:1–9.

31. Mohr PE, Cheng CM, Claxton K, *et al.* The heterogeneity of schizophrenia in disease states. *Schizophrenia Research* 2004;**71**:83–95.

32. Kay SR, Fiszbein A and Opler L. The positive and negative syndrome scale (PANSS) for schizophrenia. *Schizophrenia Bulletin* 1987;**13**:261–76.

33. Rosenheck RA, Stroup S, Keefe R, *et al.* Measuring outcome priorities and incorporating preferences in mental health status assessment of people with schizophrenia. *British Journal of Psychiatry* 2005;**187**:529–36.

34. Heinrichs DW, Hanlon ET and Carpenter WT. The quality of life scale: An instrument for rating the schizophrenic deficit syndrome. *Schizophrenia Bulletin* 1984;**10**:388–98.

35. Addington D, Addington J and Maticka-Tyndale E. A depression rating scale for schizophrenics. *Schizophrenia Research* 1996;**3**:247–51.

36. Barnes T. A rating scale for drug-induced akathisia. *British Journal of Psychiatry* 1989;**131**:672–6.

37. Guy W. Abnormal involuntary movements. In: W. Guy ed., *ECDEU Assessment Manual for Psychopharmacology. (DHEW No. ADM 76–338)* Rockville, MD: National Institute of Mental Health; 1976.

38. Simpson GM and Angus JW. A rating scale for extrapyramidal side effects. *Acta Psychiatrica Scandinavica. Supplementum* 1970;**212**:11–9.

39. Lehman A. A quality of life interview for the chronically mentally ill. *Evaluation and Program Planning* 1988;**11**:51–62.

40. Hochberg Y. A sharper Bonferroni procedure for multiple tests of significance. *Biometrika* 1988;**75**:800–2.

41. Tabachnick B and Fidell L. *Using Multivariate Statistics (4th Edition)*. Boston, MA: Allen and Bacon; 2000.

42. Duan N. Smearing estimate: A nonparametric retransformation method. *Journal of the American Statistical Association* 1983;**78**:605–10.

43. Manning WG and Mullahy J. Estimating log models: To transform or not to transform? *Journal of Health Economics* 2001;**20**:461–94.

44. Neumann PJ. *Using Cost-effectiveness Analysis to Improve Health Care.* New York: Oxford University Press; 2005.

45. Briggs A and Fenn P. Confidence intervals or surfaces? Uncertainty on the cost-effectiveness plane. *Health Economics* 1998;**7**:723–40.

46. Hoch J, Briggs A and Willan A. Something old, something new, something borrowed, something blue: A framework for the marriage of health economics and cost effectiveness analysis. *Health Economics* 2002;**11**:415–30.

47. Rosenheck RA, Leslie D, Sindelar J, *et al.* Cost-effectiveness of second generation antipsychotics and perphenazine in a randomized trial of treatment for chronic schizophrenia. *American Journal of Psychiatry* 2006;**163**:2080–9.

48. Cramer JA, Rosenheck R, Xu W, Henderson W, Thomas J and Charney D. Detecting improvement in quality of life and symptomatology in schizophrenia. *Schizophrenia Bulletin* 2001;**27**:227–35.

49. Correll CU, Leucht S and Kane JM. Lower risk for tardive dyskinesia associated with second-generation antipsychotics: A systematic review of 1-year studies. *American Journal of Psychiatry* 2004;**161**:414–25.

50. Halliday J, Farrington S, Macdonald S, MacEwan T, Sharkey V and McCreadie R. Nithsdale Schizophrenia Surveys: Movement disorders. *British Journal of Psychiatry* 2002;**181**:422–7.

51. Lee PE, Sykora K, Gill SS, *et al.* Antipsychotic medication and drug-induced movement disorder: A population-based cohort study in older adults. *Journal of the American Geriatric Society* 2005;**53**:1374–9.

52. Rochon PA, Stukel TA, Sykora K, *et al.* Atypical antipsychotics and parkinsonism. *Archives of Internal Medicine* 2005;**165**:1882–8.

53. Woods S, Saksa JR, Walsh B, Sullivan MC, Morganstern H and Glazer W (under review). *Tardive Dyskinesia in a Community Mental Health Center: 2000–2005.*

54. Rosenheck RA. Considerations for evaluating the cost-effectiveness of reducing tardive dyskinesia with second generation antipsychotics. *British Journal of Psychiatry* 2007;**191**:238–45.

55. Rosenheck RA, Swartz M, McEvoy J, *et al.* Changing perspectives on second generation antipsychotics: Reviewing the cost-effectiveness component of the CATIE trial. *Expert Review of Pharmacoeconomics and Outcomes Research* 2007;**7**:103–11.

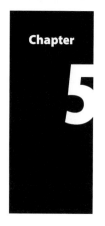

Chapter

5

Psychosocial functioning in patients with chronic schizophrenia: findings from the NIMH CATIE study

Marvin S. Swartz

Introduction

Reduction of psychotic symptoms is a key goal of schizophrenia treatment, but may not translate into meaningful improvement in the day-to-day functioning of affected patients. Psychosocial functioning is strongly correlated with cognitive functioning and negative symptoms, but these domains are also among the most illusive targets of schizophrenia treatment [1,2]. As a result, despite the clear importance of psychosocial functioning in achieving recovery, improvement in this domain is a severe challenge in schizophrenia treatment [3]. Demonstrable improvement in social relationships, performance of key social roles, and community living skills may substantially lag behind symptomatic improvement [4–6].

The introduction of second-generation antipsychotics (SGAs) was accompanied by hopes and expectations that they would be superior to first-generation antipsychotics (FGAs) in improving psychosocial functioning [6]. The reasoning was that the putative superior efficacy and reduced side effect burden of SGAs relative to FGAs, would improve social functioning. For example, extrapyramidal symptoms and sedation may make instrumental daily activities difficult; negative symptoms may reduce interest and initiative, and positive symptoms may cause further disorganization and social rejection.

The many diverse approaches to evaluating psychosocial functioning and quality of life for individuals with schizophrenia make comparisons across schizophrenia studies difficult. However, the Quality of Life Scale (QLS) [7] is the most widely used clinician-rated scale of psychosocial functioning and assesses social functioning, interpersonal relationships, vocational functioning, and psychological well-being. The scale was originally developed to measure a schizophrenic deficit syndrome, but is now used widely as a proxy measure of community functioning. The alternative to such a proxy measure, direct observational measures of day-to-day functioning in the community, is not feasible to assess in most clinical studies.

Clinical trials of psychosocial functioning comparing FGAs and SGAs on the QLS have had inconsistent findings [4–6,8–14]. Most early studies evaluating psychosocial functioning with the QLS compared clozapine, risperidone, and olanzapine, but many of these studies had multiple design limitations, including small sample sizes, lack of appropriate controls, relatively short follow-up, and possible bias due to industry sponsorship. Few trials prior to the CATIE and Cost Utility of the Latest Antipsychotic Drugs in Schizophrenia Study (CUtLASS) studies [13,14] evaluated the long-term effectiveness of SGAs and FGAs in

Antipsychotic Trials in Schizophrenia, ed. T. Scott Stroup and Jeffrey A. Lieberman. Published by Cambridge University Press. © Cambridge University Press 2010.

head-to-head comparisons. Prior to CUtLASS and CATIE, there was scant evidence of superiority in psychosocial functioning of one SGA over another or of SGAs over FGAs, although one recent review concluded that SGAs were superior to older agents in functional gains [6].

The CUtLASS study was a randomized trial of SGAs and FGAs in the United Kingdom [13]. In CUtLASS I, 227 individuals with schizophrenia and related disorders aged 18 to 65 years were assessed for an antipsychotic medication change due to inadequate treatment response or adverse effects. These individuals, who were judged not to be treatment resistant, were randomly prescribed to a medication within the FGA or SGA drug class (other than clozapine), with the choice of the specific drug within the class made by the treating psychiatrist. The primary outcome of CUtLASS was the QLS, with other key outcomes including schizophrenia symptoms, adverse side effects, patient satisfaction, and costs of care. The study found no significant differences in QLS scores during the first year of the study, but did find a trend toward greater improvements in QLS and symptom scores with FGAs. There were no differences in patient satisfaction, and treatment costs were comparable. Thus, contrary to expectations, SGAs were not superior and arguably inferior to FGAs in psychosocial functioning outcomes.

The current chapter reviews findings from the CATIE study as it compared the effects of olanzapine, perphenazine, quetiapine, risperidone, and ziprasidone on psychosocial functioning as measured on the QLS [14–26]. In assessing psychosocial functioning, we hypothesized that improvement would be significantly different among treatments. However, we also recognized that many CATIE patients had discontinued their first study medication earlier than might be expected to result in functional gains. In order to maximize the opportunity for treatment to result in meaningful improvements in psychosocial functioning, we reasoned that 12 months of uninterrupted antipsychotic treatment would allow enough time for adjunctive psychosocial and rehabilitative treatments to take effect, for new skills and competencies to develop, for key interpersonal relationships and role functioning to improve and thus provide the best test of pharmacologic benefit. We also planned to evaluate changes at other QLS assessment intervals at months 6 and 18. We also planned comparisons of the four QLS subscale scores at all time points.

Method
Study design and measures
The CATIE study was initiated by the National Institute of Mental Health (NIMH) to determine the comparative effectiveness of antipsychotic drugs. Its rationale, design, and methods are described in Chapters 1 and 2 of this volume.

For the Psychosocial Functioning Study presented in this chapter, we hypothesized that there would be significant differences among olanzapine, perphenazine, quetiapine, risperidone, and ziprasidone in improvement in psychosocial functioning as measured by the QLS total scale [7].

The QLS [7] is a widely used clinician-rated scale of social functioning, interpersonal relationships, and psychological well-being, originally developed to measure a schizophrenic deficit syndrome. The scale was administered at 6, 12, and 18 months and contains 21 items with four subscales: interpersonal relations (household, friends, acquaintances, social activity, social network, social initiative, withdrawal, sociosexual relations), instrumental roles (occupational or educational role, work functioning, work level, and satisfaction), intrapsychic foundations (sense of purpose, motivation, curiosity, anhedonia, aimless inactivity, empathy, emotional interaction), and common objects and activities (commonplace objects, commonplace activities). All items are rated on a seven-point scale and a total score is calculated by taking the mean of 21 items, with higher scores indicating higher functioning. Subscales are similarly calculated by taking the mean of the subscale items.

Analyses for this evaluation also included extrapyramidal symptoms [27], scores on the Positive and Negative Syndrome Scale (PANSS) [28], clinical status based on the clinician-rated Clinical Global Impression Scale (CGI-S) [29], substance use [30], depressive symptoms [31], attitudes toward medication [32], self-rated health status based on the 12-item questionnaire from the Medical Outcomes Study (SF-12) [33], and neurocognitive functioning [18,24].

Statistical analysis

In order to ensure consistency and comparability with other CATIE analyses, the statistical methods in this study were comparable to those used in the original publication and described in Chapter 2 [19]. Analytic approaches to evaluating QLS treatment gains were dictated, in part, by availability of the 6-month time points at which the QLS was measured. The primary analysis was the comparison of changes across treatment groups from baseline to month 12 in the QLS. Secondary analyses comparably focused on changes in the four QLS subscale scores as well as QLS total and subscale changes at months 6 and 18. Analysis of covariance (ANCOVA) was utilized to compare changes across treatment groups with adjustments for baseline score, whether the patient had required crisis stabilization in the three months prior to study entry and tardive dyskinesia status where applicable. All comparisons involving perphenazine were limited to the cohort of patients without tardive dyskinesia. Because ziprasidone was added after approximately 40% of the patients had been enrolled, ziprasidone comparisons are secondary and were limited to the cohort of patients who underwent randomization after ziprasidone was added. There were four datasets for comparison: Analytic Sets I and II (for pre-ziprasidone patients without and with tardive dyskinesia respectively), Analytic Sets III and IV (for post-ziprasidone patients without and with tardive dyskinesia respectively). For example, because patients with tardive dyskinesia might differ from non-tardive dyskinesia patients and could not receive perphenazine, comparisons for those patients only include patients with TD who were randomly assigned to SGAs only and separately evaluated cohorts before and after ziprasidone was included in the trial. Adjustments for multiple treatment comparisons were adjusted with a Hochberg modification of the Bonferroni adjustment [34].

Predictors of change in QLS scores were identified with Pearson and Spearman correlations, t-tests, and analysis of variance and stepwise regression techniques and mixed models that included patient demographics, baseline antipsychotic use, substance abuse, site characteristics (type and measure of urbanicity), and baseline and change from baseline scores measuring symptoms, neurocognitive functioning, extrapyramidal symptoms, and depression, as well as outpatient service use during the 12 months, and compliance with study drug.

Results
Characteristics and dispositions of patients

The characteristics and follow-up of study patients were described previously [19–21] and in Chapters 1 and 3. This analysis was limited to the roughly one third of patients (N = 455)

Table 5.1. Demographic and baseline characteristics of patients with quality of life data

Variable	Baseline data and month 12 data available (N = 455)	Baseline data available but month 12 data not available (N = 985)	p Value for comparing patients with month 12 data vs. without	
	Mean (SD) or N (%)	Mean (SD) or N (%)	T or Chi-square statistic	p Value
Age (years)	41.9 (11.1)	40.0 (11.0)	−2.98	0.003
Patient's education (years)	12.1 (2.2)	12.1 (2.3)	0.41	0.68
Duration since first prescribed antipsychotic medication (years)	14.9 (11.5)	14.2 (10.3)	−1.05	0.29
PANSS (total score)	72.8 (18.0)	76.9 (17.2)	4.15	<0.001
DAI (total score)	5.7 (3.4)	4.7 (4.1)	−4.60	<0.001
Calgary	3.9 (4.0)	4.8 (4.5)	3.81	<0.001
Sex				
Male	345 (75.8)	723 (73.4)	0.96	0.33
Female	110 (24.2)	262 (26.6)		
Race				
White	282 (62.0)	586 (59.6)	0.73	0.39
Other	173 (38.0)	397 (40.4)		
Ethnic origin				
Hispanic	50 (11.0)	117 (11.9)	0.24	0.62
Marital status				
Married	44 (9.7)	123 (12.5)	3.52	0.17
Previously married[1]	143 (31.4)	275 (27.9)		
Never married	268 (58.9)	587 (59.6)		
Employment status				
Unemployed	376 (82.8)	836 (85.8)	2.15	0.14
Alcohol abuse				
No use	231 (50.8)	516 (52.4)	6.06	0.05
Use	92 (20.2)	149 (15.1)		
Abuse	132 (29.0)	320 (32.5)		
Drug abuse				
No use	272 (59.8)	520 (52.8)	14.88	<0.001

Table 5.1. (cont.)

Variable	Baseline data and month 12 data available (N = 455)	Baseline data available but month 12 data not available (N = 985)	p Value for comparing patients with month 12 data vs. without	
	Mean (SD) or N (%)	Mean (SD) or N (%)	T or Chi-square statistic	p Value
Use	90 (19.8)	170 (17.3)		
Abuse	93 (20.4)	295 (29.9)		
Drug use				
Use or abuse	183 (40.2)	465 (47.2)	26.17	0.01
Baseline antipsychotic medications				
Olanzapine alone	114 (25.1)	206 (20.9)	3.04	0.08
Quetiapine alone	26 (5.7)	68 (6.9)	0.74	0.39
Risperidone alone	109 (24.0)	163 (16.6)	10.81	<0.001
Any combination including olanzapine, quetiapine, or risperidone	33 (7.3)	92 (9.3)	1.76	0.18
All others	62 (13.6)	165 (16.8)	2.34	0.13
None	111 (24.4)	291 (29.5)	4.06	0.04
Baseline QLS and domain scores QLS	2.86 (1.1)	2.68 (1.0)	−3.02	0.003
Interpersonal Relations	2.66 (1.4)	2.47 (1.3)	−2.62	0.009
Instrumental Roles	1.97 (1.7)	1.65 (1.6)	−3.48	<0.001
Intrapsychic foundations	3.19 (1.2)	3.06 (1.2)	−1.86	0.06
Common objects and activities	3.39 (1.2)	3.33 (1.2)	−0.92	0.36

Notes: [1]Previously married includes widowed, divorced or separated.
Reprinted with permission from the American Journal of Psychiatry (2007), American Psychiatric Press [14].

in Phase 1 who completed the QLS at baseline and also completed the 12 month QLS assessment while still on the initial study medication. Table 5.1 compares the baseline demographic and clinical characteristics of this retained cohort at 12 months and those who completed the QLS at baseline, but were unavailable at 12 months (N = 985).

The group still on the initial drug and evaluated for psychosocial functioning at 12 months had several characteristics likely associated with clinical stability and treatment retention. They were older, had less severe psychopathology as reflected in lower PANSS total scores, had more favorable attitudes toward antipsychotic medication as reflected in

Table 5.2. Post-baseline characteristics of patients with quality of life data

Variable	Baseline data and month 12 data available (N = 455)	Baseline data available but month 12 data not available (N = 985)	p Value for comparing patients with month 12 data vs. without	
	Mean (SD) or N (%)	Mean (SD) or N (%)	T or Chi-square statistic	p Value
Time to discontinuation (months)	17.6 (2.0)	3.8 (3.3)	−98.33	<0.001
Compliance at month 12	91.5 (11.4)		N/A	N/A
Overall study compliance	91.2 (11.2)	73.8 (32.7)	−14.63	<0.001
Mean modal dose (capsules)	2.8 (1.0)	2.6 (0.9)	−4.67	<0.001
% Reaching max. dose	222 (40.0)	233 (30.1)	13.99	<0.001

Reprinted with permission from the American Journal of Psychiatry (2007), American Psychiatric Press [14].

higher Drug Attitudes Inventory scores [32], had fewer depressive symptoms as rated on the Calgary Depression Scale [31], were less likely to use or abuse alcohol and/or illicit drugs, were more likely to have been on risperidone prior to randomization, and less likely to have been on no antipsychotics. The QLS total score and the subscales of interpersonal relations and instrumental roles were also higher, indicating psychosocial functioning at baseline.

As seen in Table 5.2, this sample at 12 months, as expected, also had far longer time to discontinuation in Phase 1 compared to those discontinued or who were unavailable at 12 months (17.6 versus 3.8 months) and had higher mean rates of compliance during this phase of treatment (91.2 versus 73.8%). Mean modal dose in capsules was higher for those available at 12 months (2.8 versus 2.6 capsules), and a larger proportion of those available at 12 months achieved a maximum dose of four capsules (40.0 versus 30.1%).

Table 5.3 demonstrates aggregate QLS scores and their changes across combined treatment groups at baseline, 6, 12, and 18 months. This table also demonstrates the level of patient attrition from Phase 1 at these time points: 45% remained at 6 months, approximately one third at 12 months, and approximately one quarter at 18 months. At baseline, the highest QLS subscale scores are seen in the common objects and activities scale which are indicative of participation in mainstream vocational, recreational, or instrumental task-related activities. In comparison, the next highest scores are seen in the intrapsychic functioning scale thought to measure a sense of purpose, motivation, and curiosity. Lower scores are seen in the instrumental relations scale, reflecting social interactions and initiative-taking. Lowest scores are found in the instrumental roles scale reflecting occupational and educational functioning. These scores generally reflect that the initial CATIE sample was a moderately impaired and vocationally disabled

Table 5.3. Quality of life outcomes for all treatment groups combined

	N	Mean	SD
Baseline			
Quality of Life Scale	1,440	2.74	1.1
Interpersonal Relations		2.53	1.3
Instrumental Roles		1.75	1.6
Intrapsychic Foundations		3.10	1.2
Common Objects and Activities		3.35	1.2
Month 6			
Quality of Life Scale	652	2.98	1.1
Interpersonal Relations		2.78	1.3
Instrumental Roles		2.09	1.8
Intrapsychic Foundations		3.31	1.2
Common Objects and Activities		3.54	1.1
Month 12			
Quality of Life Scale	458	3.05	1.2
Interpersonal Relations		2.86	1.4
Instrumental Roles		2.25	1.8
Intrapsychic Foundations		3.33	1.3
Common Objects and Activities		3.57	1.2
Month 18			
Quality of Life Scale	361	3.15	1.2
Interpersonal Relations		2.96	1.4
Instrumental Roles		2.25	1.9
Intrapsychic Foundations		3.45	1.3
Common Objects and Activities		3.75	1.2

Notes: Mean scores are for all items in scale or subscale, range 0–6, with 0 indicating extremely poor and 6 indicating fully adequate functioning.
SD = Standard Deviation.

population with chronic schizophrenia. Of note, the greatest gains in psychosocial functioning occurred between baseline and 6 months, less so at 12 and 18 months. By 18 months, retained patient total scores increased 0.41 from baseline, reflecting a small effect size. Greatest gains are seen in instrumental roles and common objects and activities subscales.

In order to examine relative rates of improvement in functioning from baseline, patients still on their initial medication at 12 months were stratified by their baseline QLS scores (data not shown). Patients with a low functioning baseline score of less than 2.0 made the largest gains (mean = 0.71, SD = 0.96, $p < 0.01$), but only represent 23% of the retained

12-month sample. Those with a QLS of 2.0 to less than 3.0 (34% of the sample) made more modest gains (mean $= 0.32$, SD $= 0.97$, $p < 0.01$) and represent roughly one-third (34%) of the retained 12 month sample. Those highest functioning at baseline scoring 3.0 or above, on average made no gains, declined somewhat, and represent 43% of the 12-month retained sample. As a result, the sample for this assessment of functioning at 12 months included only one quarter of the patients who were most likely to improve.

QLS changes after 12 months of treatment

Changes in QLS total score from baseline to 12 months, adjusted for baseline QLS score and whether the patient had required hospitalization or crisis stabilization in the 3 months prior to study entry are seen in Table 5.4. Changes in functioning were evaluated on the basis of the appropriate comparison data set and are shown in boldface to illustrate the source of comparison for each medication. The four cohort datasets created for comparison included: patients *without* tardive dyskinesia randomized *before* inclusion of ziprasidone (Analytic Set I: **P** vs. O, Q, R), patients *with* tardive dyskinesia randomized *before* inclusion of ziprasidone (Analytic Set II: **O** vs. Q vs. R), patients *without* tardive dyskinesia randomized *after* inclusion of ziprasidone (Analytic Set III: **Z** vs. P), patients *with* tardive dyskinesia randomized *after* inclusion of ziprasidone (Analytic Set IV: **Z** vs. O, Q, R).

There were no significant differences between the treatment groups in the amount of change in the QLS total score or subscales at 12 months. Within treatment groups, psychosocial functioning improved at the level of $p < 0.05$ or greater (Data Set II) for the olanzapine (0.19) and risperidone (0.26) treatment groups. Improvement was comparable for the perphenazine (0.19) (Data Set I) and the ziprasidone treatment groups (0.26) (Data Set IV) but was less for the quetiapine (0.09) (Data Set II) treatment group. The perphenazine and ziprasidone groups had smaller sample sizes that reduced the power to demonstrate differences at the level of $p < 0.05$. Several subscale improvements at the level of $p < 0.05$ or greater can be seen (see Table 5.4). Evaluated by the metric of effect sizes, all improvements within treatment groups were small to modest.

Psychosocial functioning (QLS) changes at 6 and 18 months were also examined (data not shown), and there were no significant differences between the treatment groups in the amount of change in the QLS total score or subscales at 6 months or 18 months. Within treatment groups at 6 months, psychosocial functioning improved at the level of $p < 0.05$ or greater for the olanzapine (0.26) and risperidone (0.21) and quetiapine (0.16) treatment groups (Data Set II). In addition, in the non-TD group, perphenazine statistically approached this level of improvement (0.17, $p = 0.055$) (Data Set I). Similar improvement was also seen with ziprasidone (0.27) (Data Set IV).

At 18 months, there were no significant differences between treatment groups in the amount of change in the QLS total score or subscales. Within treatment groups at 18 months, psychosocial functioning improved at the level of $p < 0.05$ or greater for the olanzapine (0.35), quetiapine (0.52), and risperidone (0.42) treatment groups (Data Set II), but not for perphenazine (0.14) (Data Set I) or ziprasidone (0.11) (Data Set IV). Finally, mixed model analyses encompassing the month 6, 12, and 18 time points also confirmed the findings of a lack of differences between treatment groups in improvement in functioning.

Because the QLS is a proxy measure of psychosocial functioning, we sought to examine whether other potential indicators of improvement in psychosocial functioning not captured in the QLS showed evidence of change. Change from baseline to 12 months was examined for

Table 5.4. Change from baseline to month 12 in Quality of Life Scale and domain scores by treatment

	OLZ (O) Mean (SD)	PERP (P) Mean (SD)	QUET (Q) Mean (SD)	RISP (R) Mean (SD)	ZIPR (Z) Mean (SD)	F	p value	Value paired comparison
Data Set I: P vs. O, Q, R Excluding patients with TD and patients on Z	N = 113	N = 74	N = 71	N = 86				
Quality of Life Scale	0.20 (0.9)*	0.19 (1.1)	0.01 (1.0)	0.26 (0.9)*	–	0.59	0.62	n.s.
Interpersonal Relations	0.21 (1.1)*	0.14 (1.4)	–0.08 (1.4)	0.36 (1.1)**	–	1.28	0.28	n.s.
Instrumental Roles	0.28 (1.8)	0.45 (1.6)*	0.37 (1.7)	0.10 (1.7)	–	0.53	0.66	n.s.
Intrapsychic Foundations	0.14 (1.1)	0.16 (1.2)	–0.09 (1.2)	0.22 (1.1)	–	0.44	0.72	n.s.
Common Objects and Activities	0.18 (1.1)	0.11 (1.2)	0.20 (1.1)	0.22 (1.1)	–	0.02	0.99	n.s.
Data Set II: O vs. Q vs. R Including patients with TD, excluding patients on Z or P	N = 145		N = 82	N = 107				
Quality of Life Scale	0.19 (0.9)*	–	0.09 (1.0)	0.26 (1.0)**	–	0.64	0.53	n.s.
Interpersonal Relations	0.20 (1.1)*	–	–0.01 (1.4)	0.32 (1.2)**	–	1.71	0.18	n.s.
Instrumental Roles	0.24 (1.8)	–	0.39 (1.7)*	0.15 (1.7)	–	0.13	0.88	n.s.
Intrapsychic Foundations	0.15 (1.1)	–	0.03 (1.3)	0.21 (1.2)	–	0.30	0.74	n.s.
Common Objects and Activities	0.09 (1.1)	–	0.20 (1.1)	0.30 (1.1)**	–	0.92	0.40	n.s.

Data Set III: Z vs. P
Excluding patients with TD, including patients on Z

	N = 65		N = 34		N = 38	
Quality of Life Scale	0.13 (0.9)	–	0.39 (1.2)	–	0.36 (0.9)*	Not applicable
Interpersonal Relations	0.16 (1.1)	–	0.28 (1.5)	–	0.58 (1.5)*	Not applicable
Instrumental Roles	0.40 (1.8)	–	0.86 (2.0)*	–	0.35 (1.5)	Not applicable
Intrapsychic Foundations	–0.01 (1.1)	–	0.40 (1.2)	–	0.17 (1.0)	Not applicable
Common Objects and Activities	0.05 (1.3)	–	0.21 (1.1)	–	0.11 (1.1)	Not applicable

Data Set IV: Z vs. O, Q, R
Including patients with TD and patients on Z

	N = 46	N = 53	N = 47	
Quality of Life Scale	0.03 (1.0)	0.15 (1.0)	**0.26 (1.0)**	Not applicable
Interpersonal Relations	–0.17 (1.4)	0.16 (1.1)	**0.40 (1.5)**	Not applicable
Instrumental Roles	0.36 (1.6)	0.14 (1.6)	**0.23 (1.6)**	Not applicable
Intrapsychic Foundations	0.07 (1.1)	0.12 (1.2)	**0.08 (1.1)**	Not applicable
Common Objects and Activities	0.14 (1.3)	0.10 (1.2)	**0.24 (1.1)**	Not applicable

Notes: [1]Bolded values highlight treatment conditions of primary interest in each data set.
[2]Results (for descriptive purposes) for testing the within sample mean different from zero are denoted as follows: * $\leq$ 0.05 and ** $\leq$ 0.01.

residential status, competitive employment, instrumental activities of daily living, and leisure activities (data not shown). Overall, these indicators were consistent with findings from the QLS in that there were no differences between treatment groups in change from baseline for any of these alternate indicators of psychosocial functioning at 12 months. At baseline, 79% of the entire cohort were living independently; of patients retained in Phase 1 at 12 months, 88.7% had no change in residential status from baseline to 12 months, while 6.9% had some improvement and 4.4% had some decline. In addition, few changes were seen in employment, instrumental and social or leisure activities. Resnick and colleagues examine these employment findings in greater depth in Chapter 7 and elsewhere [35].

Correlates of change in psychosocial functioning

We also sought to examine predictors of QLS changes over time independent of medication regimen. Correlations between selected baseline demographic and clinical factors and change in QLS total scores from baseline to 12 months are shown in Table 5.5. Among these baseline measures, higher QLS baseline scores were correlated with less improvement— higher functioning patients improved less. In addition, use or abuse of illicit substances was correlated with less and non-urban residence was correlated with greater QLS improvement. Improvement was unrelated to use of adjunctive medications such as antidepressants or anxiolytics. We also examined correlations with clinical measures assessed over time that might also predict QLS changes. Improvements on PANSS positive symptoms, Calgary Depression symptoms, extrapyramidal symptoms, and Clinical Global Impression – Severity scales were all correlated with more QLS improvement. However, due to content overlap between certain QLS domains and the PANSS negative and general psychopathology scales, the total PANSS, negative, and general psychopathology scores, these relationships could not be meaningfully evaluated.

In order to further evaluate unique predictors of QLS change, multivariable regression modeling was used to identify predictors of change in psychosocial functioning among the predictors examined in Table 5.5. The multivariable model included controls for clinical exacerbation at baseline, trial site, treatment group, whether the patient had tardive dyskinesia and whether the patient entered the trial after the introduction of ziprasidone. However, none of these adjustments were significant at the level of $p < 0.05$ (see Table 5.6). The strongest positive predictor of improvement was lower baseline QLS score, explaining 13% of the total variation in the QLS change scores. Those who were lowest functioning at baseline made the greatest gains. Other significant positive predictors of improvement included female gender, avoidance of illicit substances, non-urban residence, higher baseline neurocognitive functioning, improvement in extrapyramidal symptoms, and improvement in illness severity as measured on the CGI-S. In comparison to the baseline QLS score, all of these parameters together explain only an additional 11% of the total variation in the QLS change scores.

As a clinician-rated measure, the QLS may not be sensitive enough to detect self-perceived changes in functioning. In an effort to confirm these QLS findings using self, and not clinician, report of functioning, changes from baseline to 12 months in self-rated physical and mental well-being as measured on the SF-12 were also examined (analyses not shown). As expected the QLS and SF-12 physical well-being measures were modestly correlated and the QLS more strongly correlated with mental well-being ($r = 0.10$, $p < 0.05$ and $r = 0.47$, $p < 0.01$ respectively). Consistent with the

Table 5.5. Correlations with Quality of Life Scale change from baseline to month 12

	N	Correlation	p Value
Baseline parameters			
Baseline Total QLS Score	455	−0.36	<0.01
Illicit substance abuse	455	−0.13	<0.01
Non-urban residence	455	0.10	0.04
Female Gender	455	0.06	0.21
Baseline PANSS (Positive)	453	0.04	0.45
Baseline Neurocognitive Score	429	0.05	0.26
Post-Baseline Parameters (12 month change)			
PANSS (Positive) Change	453	−0.19	<0.01
Calgary Depression Score Change	454	−0.14	<0.01
Extrapyramidal Symptom Score Change	454	−0.10	<0.01
CGI-S Score Change	454	−0.23	<0.01

Notes: All baseline parameters in this table have a p value < 0.10 for predicting QOL change from baseline to month 12 based on an ANCOVA model adjusting for crisis stabilization in the 3 months prior to study entry, Site group, TD status, and baseline QLS total score. PANSS = Positive and Negative Syndrome Scale, CGI-S = Clinical Global Impressions-Severity Scale.

Table 5.6. Prediction model of Quality of Life Scale change from baseline to month 12

Parameter, listed in order of entry into a forward selection model	Partial R^2	df	p Value
Baseline Total QLS Score	0.136	1	<0.01
CGI-S Score Change	0.034	1	<0.01
Illicit substance abuse	0.017	1	<0.01
Non-urban residence	0.018	1	<0.01
Baseline Neurocognitive score	0.015	1	<0.01
Gender	0.015	1	<0.01
Extrapyramidal Symptom Change	0.007	1	0.05
Overall $R^2 = 0.28$			

Notes: The following design variables were also included in the above final model: crisis stabilization in the 3 months prior to study entry ($p = 0.80$), Site group ($p = 0.24$), TD status ($p = 0.07$), ziprasidone cohort indicator ($p = 0.86$), and Phase 1/1A randomized treatment ($p = 0.49$). R^2 for all design variables together $= 0.04$

prior QLS results, there were no differences between treatment groups on the SF-12 at 12 months or the secondary time points of 6 and 18 months. Thus, even from the perspective of the patient, there were no differences in psychosocial functioning across medication regimens.

QLS changes in the efficacy pathway (Phase 2E)

Given the evidence, albeit mixed, that clozapine is particularly efficacious for refractory patients [36,37], the clozapine arm of the CATIE study was of particular interest in examining improvements in psychosocial functioning among patients who discontinued Phase 1 due to inefficacy. Because only 99 patients chose to enter the efficacy pathway, the analysis was restricted to the relatively small number of patients with a QLS assessment at baseline and after approximately 12 months of treatment (N = 24) and 6 months in this phase (N = 50) (analyses not shown). Comparisons were made between clozapine treated patients versus all others treatment groups combined, including olanzapine, quetiapine, and risperidone. In a previous report, these groups were found to be demographically and clinically comparable [21]. The clozapine group had some-what lower baseline QLS scores, so that comparisons with the other combined treatment groups were adjusted for baseline QLS differences. Once these adjustments were made, there were no significant differences between clozapine and other groups in QLS change scores at 6 and 12 months. The QLS changes for clozapine were comparable to those for olanzapine and risperidone in Phase 1.

QLS changes in the tolerability pathway (Phase 2T)

Similar analyses were conducted in the tolerability pathway, which included patients who discontinued Phase 1 due to intolerability or were unwilling to enter the efficacy pathway with its possibility of clozapine treatment. The primary analysis was restricted to the relatively small number of patients randomized after ziprasidone had been added to the study and who had a QLS assessment available at baseline and at approximately 12 months of treatment (N = 67) and secondarily at 6 months (N = 151) (analyses not shown). There were no significant differences between treatment groups in QLS change scores at 6 and 12 months, and QLS changes were comparable to those in Phase 1.

Correlations between QLS and quality adjusted life years

The QLS measure and Quality Adjusted Life Years (QALYs) utilized for the evaluation of cost-effectiveness (see Chapter 4) were different measures. The QLS was based on clinician ratings of psychosocial functioning; the QALY measure was a composite score based on PANSS psychopathology scores and side effect ratings [26]. There were no differences in QALYs across treatment groups in Phase 1 of the trial. We examined correlations between these measures and, as expected, the 12 month QALY and the QLS total score were moderately correlated ($r = 0.38$, $p < 0.001$) as were change from baseline in QLS and QALYs at 12 months ($r = 0.32$, $p < 0.001$).

Discussion

Our goal was to examine the potential improvements in community functioning achievable if chronically ill schizophrenia patients were treated with assigned medication regimens for 12 months. From previous CATIE analyses, we recognized that most patients would not continue the initial medication for a year. However, we reasoned that the best test of potential gains from a particular medication would come from a consistent period of drug treatment, even if these findings were not generalizable to all patients initiated on a particular regimen. We also recognized that the high rate of treatment discontinuation in

Phase 1—roughly 75%—would limit the statistical power to detect gains at 12 months. With these caveats, we examined QLS change at 12 months as our primary outcome of interest, but also examined QLS changes at 6 and 18 months. Although previous head-to-head comparisons of antipsychotics in improving psychosocial outcomes were limited [4–6,8–12], we hypothesized that there would be differences in community functioning across treatment groups.

We found no significant differences *between* medication groups and no distinct superiority of any antipsychotic in improving psychosocial functioning, findings consistent with those from the CUtLASS study [38]. There were improvements within treatment groups compared to baseline, but improvements were largely comparable across medication groups. At 12 months, there were relatively modest improvements for the olanzapine (0.19), risperidone (0.26), perphenazine (0.19), and ziprasidone (0.26) treatment groups, and somewhat less improvement for quetiapine (0.09), although the quetiapine treatment group did roughly as well as other groups at 6 and 18 months.

Multivariate models of improved functioning identified several modestly strong predictors of improvement. Women were more likely to improve than men, possibly because they have better social supports or are less likely to have gains impeded by drug use [39–41]. As expected, illicit drug users did far worse, probably due to their poor treatment compliance, involvement with drug-using peer networks, and related behaviors that undermined opportunities for rehabilitation [22,23]. Patients from non-urban communities also made greater gains possibly because they lived in less adverse social environments and encountered fewer barriers to improvement. Improvements in extrapyramidal symptoms were also associated with better functioning, likely because reducing the stigma of these symptoms promoted better community re-integration and reduced a barrier to more normal community functioning. Patients who had better neurocognitive functioning at baseline also made greater QLS gains, most likely because better neurocognitive functioning facilitates gains in community functioning [25]. A clear implication of these findings is that, if neurocognitive functioning does not improve, other functional gains are unlikely [42,43].

While patients did make greater symptomatic gains on clozapine in the Phase 2E efficacy pathway, their gains in psychosocial functioning were disappointing. The sample size in the efficacy pathway was small, and once adjustments were made for baseline functioning, clozapine-related improvements were roughly comparable to those seen in Phase 1.

The earliest post-baseline QLS assessment point occurred 6 months into Phase 1 and many patients with poor psychosocial functioning discontinued their initial treatment before reaching this milepost. Unfortunately, patients with the lowest quartiles of functioning on the QLS at baseline had the greatest potential for gains, but were far more likely to discontinue treatment early. This low functioning group, with the greatest potential for improvement, comprised less than a quarter of the 12-month sample. Conversely, higher baseline functioning patients comprised approximately 40% of the 12-month sample, and made little to no gains, due to an apparent ceiling effect [42]. Longer retention of these lower functioning patients in their initial treatment group might have resulted in stronger gains.

The apparent ceiling among higher functioning patients could be a result of the limited gains achievable without improvements in neurocognitive functioning or the lack of sufficiently effective or aggressive rehabilitative interventions during the trial. Although the study design included a limited psychoeducational intervention intended to improve treatment adherence, and other rehabilitative and treatment services were provided by the patients' usual treatment providers, overall the psychosocial interventions were not intensive and varied according to local service availability. More substantial gains in functioning probably require more intensive rehabilitative services, for example cognitive rehabilitation and more effective treatment retention [43–45]. For chronically ill patients, in the absence of vigorous rehabilitative services [35,44], effective medication may be necessary but insufficient to improve real-world community functioning.

References

1. Norman RM, Malla AK, McLean T, et al. The relationship of symptoms and level of functioning in schizophrenia to general wellbeing and the Quality of Life Scale. *Acta Psychiatrica Scandinavica* 2000;**102**:303–9.

2. Priebe S. Social outcomes in schizophrenia. *British Journal of Psychiatry* 2007; **191**:s15–s20.

3. Rosenheck RA, Stroup S, Keefe R, et al. Measuring outcome priorities and incorporating preferences in mental health status assessment of people with schizophrenia. *British Journal of Psychiatry* 2005;**187**:529–36.

4. Lambert M and Naber D. Current issues in schizophrenia: Overview of patient acceptability, functioning and quality of life. *CNS Drugs* 2004;**18** (Suppl):5–17.

5. Karow A and Naber D. Subjective well-being and quality of life under antipsychotic treatment. *Psychopharmacology* 2002;**162**:3–10.

6. Awad AG and Voruganti LNP. Impact of atypical antipsychotics on quality of life in patients with schizophrenia. *CNS Drugs* 2004;**18**:877–93.

7. Heinrichs DW, Hanlon TE, Carpenter WT Jr. The Quality of Life Scale: An instrument for rating the schizophrenic deficit syndrome. *Schizophrenia Bulletin* 1984;**10**:388–98.

8. Meltzer HY, Burnett S, Bastani B and Ramirez LF. Effects of six months of clozapine treatment on quality of life of chronic schizophrenic patients. *Hospital & Community Psychiatry* 1990;**41**:892–7.

9. Essock SM, Hargreaves WA, Covell NH, et al. Clozapine's effectiveness for patients in state hospitals: Results from a randomized trial. *Psychopharmacology Bulletin* 1996;**32**:683–97.

10. Rosenheck R, Cramer J, Xu W, et al. A comparison of clozapine and haloperidol in hospitalized patients with refractory schizophrenia: Department of Veterans Affairs cooperative study group on clozapine in refractory schizophrenia. *New England Journal of Medicine* 1997;**337**:809–15.

11. Tran PV, Hamilton SH, Kuntz AJ, et al. Double-blind comparison of olanzapine vs. risperidone in the treatment of schizophrenia and other psychotic disorders. *Journal of Clinical Psychopharmacology* 1997;**17**:407–18.

12. Hamilton SH, Revicki DA, Genduso LA, et al. Olanzapine vs. placebo and haloperidol: Quality of life and efficacy results of the North American double-blind trial. *Neuropsychopharmacology* 1998;**18**:41–9.

13. Jones PB, Barnes TRE, Davies L, et al. Randomized controlled trial of the effect on quality of life of second- vs first-generation antipsychotic drugs in schizophrenia: Cost utility of the latest antipsychotic drugs in schizophrenia study (CUtLASS 1) *Archives of General Psychiatry* 2006;**63**:1079–87.

14. Swartz MS, Perkins DO, Stroup TS, et al. Effects of antipsychotic medications on psychosocial functioning in patients with chronic schizophrenia: Findings from the NIMH CATIE Study. *American Journal of Psychiatry* 2007;**164**:428–36.

15. Stroup TS, McEvoy JP, Swartz MS, et al. The National Institute of Mental Health Clinical Antipsychotic Trials of Intervention Effectiveness (CATIE) project: Schizophrenia trial design and protocol development. *Schizophrenia Bulletin* 2003;**29**:15–31.

16. Swartz MS, Perkins DO, Stroup TS, *et al.* Assessing clinical and functional outcomes in the Clinical Antipsychotic Trials of Intervention Effectiveness (CATIE) Schizophrenia Trial. *Schizophrenia Bulletin* 2003;**29**:33–43.

17. Davis SM, Koch GG, Davis CE, *et al.* Statistical approaches to effectiveness measurement and outcome-driven re-randomizations in the Clinical Antipsychotic Trials of Intervention Effectiveness (CATIE) studies. *Schizophrenia Bulletin* 2003;**29**:73–80.

18. Keefe RS, Mohs RC, Bilder RM, *et al.* Neurocognitive assessment in the Clinical Antipsychotic Trials of Intervention Effectiveness (CATIE) project schizophrenia trial: Development, methodology, and rationale. *Schizophrenia Bulletin* 2003;**29**:45–55.

19. Lieberman JA, Stroup TS, McEvoy JP, *et al.* Effectiveness of antipsychotic drugs in patients with chronic schizophrenia. *New England Journal of Medicine* 2005;**353**:1209–23.

20. Stroup TS, Lieberman JA, McEvoy JP, *et al.* Effectiveness of olanzapine, quetiapine, risperidone, and ziprasidone in patients with chronic schizophrenia after discontinuation of a previous atypical antipsychotic. *American Journal of Psychiatry* 2006;**163**:611–22.

21. McEvoy JP, Lieberman JA, Stroup TS, *et al.* Effectiveness of clozapine, quetiapine and risperidone in patients with chronic schizophrenia who failed prior atypical antipsychotic treatment. *American Journal of Psychiatry* 2006;**153**:600–10.

22. Swartz MS, Wagner HR, Swanson JW, *et al.* Substance use in persons with schizophrenia: Baseline prevalence and correlates from the NIMH CATIE study. *Journal of Nervous and Mental Disease* 2006;**194**:164–72.

23. Swartz MS, Wagner HR, Swanson JW, *et al.* Substance use and psychosocial functioning in schizophrenia among new enrollees in the NIMH CATIE Study. *Psychiatric Services* 2006;**57**:1110–6.

24. Keefe RS, Bilder RM, Harvey PD, *et al.* Baseline neurocognitive deficits in the CATIE Schizophrenia Trial. *Neuropsychopharmacology* 2006;**4**:1–14.

25. Keefe RS, Bilder RM, Harvey PD, *et al.* Neurocognitive effects of antipsychotic medications in patients with chronic schizophrenia. *Archives of General Psychiatry* 2007;**64**:633–47.

26. Rosenheck R, Leslie D, Sindelar J, *et al.* Cost-effectiveness of first and second generation antipsychotics in the treatment of chronic schizophrenia. *American Journal of Psychiatry* 2006;**163**:2080–9.

27. Tracy K, Adler LA, Rotrosen J, *et al.* Interrater reliability issues in multicenter trials. Part I: Theoretical concepts and operational procedures in VA Cooperative Study #394. *Psychopharmacology Bulletin* 1997;**33**:53–57.

28. Kay SR, Fiszbein A and Opler LA. The positive and negative syndrome scale (PANSS) for schizophrenia. *Schizophrenia Bulletin* 1987;**13**:261–76.

29. Guy W. *ECDEU Assessment Manual for Psychopharmacology – Revised (DHEW Publ No. ADM 76–338)*. Rockville, MD: U.S. Department of Health, Education, and Welfare. Public Health Service, Alcohol, Drug Abuse, and Mental Health Administration, NIMH Psychopharmacology Research Branch, Division of Extramural Research Programs; 1976. pp 218–22.

30. Drake RE, Osher FC, Noordsy DL, *et al.* Diagnosis of alcohol use disorders in schizophrenia. *Schizophrenia Bulletin* 1990;**16**:57–67.

31. Addington D, Addington J, Maticka-Tyndale E, *et al.* Reliability and validity of a depression rating scale for schizophrenics. *Schizophrenia Research* 1992;**6**:201–8.

32. Hogan T, Awad AG and Eastwood R. A self-report scale predictive of drug compliance in schizophrenics: Reliability and discriminative validity. *Psychological Medicine* 1983;**13**:177–83.

33. Ware J Jr, Kosinski M and Keller SD. A 12-item short-form health survey: Construction of scales and preliminary tests of reliability and validity. *Medical Care* 1996;**34**:220–33.

34. Hochberg Y. A sharper Bonferroni procedure for multiple tests of significance. *Biometrika* 1988;**75**:800–802.

35. Resnick SG, Rosenheck RA, Canive J, *et al.* Employment outcomes in a randomized trial of second-generation antipsychotics and perphenazine in the treatment of individuals with schizophrenia. *The Journal of Behavioral Health Services & Research* 2008;**35**:215–25.

36. Tuunainen A, Wahlbeck K and Gilbody SM. Newer atypical antipsychotic medication in comparison to clozapine: A systematic review of randomised trials. *Schizophrenia Research* 2002;**56**:1–10.

37. Wahlbeck K, Cheine M and Essali MA. Clozapine versus typical neuroleptic medication for schizophrenia. *Cochrane Database of Systematic Reviews* 2000;**2**: CD000059.

38. Jones PB, Barnes TR, Davies L, *et al.* Randomized controlled trial of the effect on quality of life of second- vs. first-generation antipsychotic drugs in schizophrenia: Cost utility of the latest antipsychotic drugs in schizophrenia study (CUtLASS 1). *Archives of General Psychiatry* 2006;**63**:1079–87.

39. Pinikahana J, Happell B, Hope J, *et al.* Quality of life in schizophrenia: A review of the literature from 1995 to 2000. *International Journal of Mental Health Nursing* 2002;**11**:103–11.

40. Siegel SJ, Irani F, Brensinger CM, *et al.* Prognostic variables at intake and long-term level of function in schizophrenia. *American Journal of Psychiatry* 2006;**163**:433–41.

41. Hafner H. Gender differences in schizophrenia. *Psychoneuroendocrinology* 2003;**28**(Suppl 2):17–54.

42. Carter CS. Understanding the glass ceiling for functional outcome in schizophrenia *Am J Psychiatry* 2006;**163**:356–358.

43. Carpenter WT Jr. Targeting schizophrenia research to patient outcomes. *American Journal of Psychiatry* 2006;**163**:353–5.

44. Lehman AF, Kreyenbuhl J, Buchanan RW, *et al.* The schizophrenia patient outcomes research team (PORT): Updated treatment recommendations 2003. *Schizophrenia Bulletin* 2004;**30**:193–217.

45. Lehman AF, Lieberman JA, Dixon LB, *et al.* American Psychiatric Association. Steering Committee on Practice Guidelines. Practice guideline for the treatment of patients with schizophrenia, second edition. *American Journal of Psychiatry* 2004;**161**(Suppl):1–56.

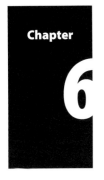

Chapter

6

Neurocognition

Richard S. E. Keefe

Introduction

Neurocognition is commonly impaired in patients with schizophrenia [1,2] in all stages of the illness and varying levels of severity [3,4]. While these impairments may appear prior to the onset of psychosis [5–7], their severity in chronic schizophrenia patients is about 1.5 [8–10] to 2.0 [11] standard deviations below the healthy population. Neurocognitive impairment is a central clinical feature of schizophrenia, as it is associated with pre-morbid history, concurrent brain functioning, and functional outcomes, and is under consideration as a possible component of the diagnosis for schizophrenia in DSM-V and ICD-11 [12,13].

Despite the centrality of cognition in schizophrenia, there are no proven pharmacologic treatments currently available. Spurred by the NIMH Measurement and Treatment Research to Improve Cognition in Schizophrenia (MATRICS) initiative, a pathway for FDA approval of compounds to improve cognition is being established including an approved battery of tests, the MATRICS Consensus Cognitive Battery (MCCB), and numerous clinical trials are underway to identify new treatments. While these studies utilize newly established methods primarily developed to assess cognition in stable patients with schizophrenia, the methods for assessing cognition in patients who require a change in antipsychotic may differ. Most published studies of cognition have used samples of convenience that have included groups of patients who can complete extensive research protocols due to their chronic institutionalization or who are available because they have entered a clinical trial or other specialized research study, and have thus been carefully screened with extensive exclusion criteria, such as the absence of substance abuse and medical co-morbidities. These studies thus present a relatively narrow view of a filtered group of patients who may not reflect the profile of neurocognitive deficits, symptoms, and substance abuse found in the overall population of patients with schizophrenia. Due to these limitations, important questions about cognition in the majority of patients with schizophrenia remain. These issues have implications for the methodology that will be used for assessing cognition in clinical practice in patients with schizophrenia, including not only the neurocognitive measures that will be employed, but also what kinds of patients may enter these trials.

This NIMH-sponsored study, Clinical Antipsychotic Trials of Intervention Effectiveness (CATIE), compared the neurocognitive effects of olanzapine, perphenazine, quetiapine, risperidone, and ziprasidone in patients with chronic schizophrenia. Because of the large sample size that was assessed and the inclusion of many patients who would have been

Antipsychotic Trials in Schizophrenia, ed. T. Scott Stroup and Jeffrey A. Lieberman. Published by Cambridge University Press. © Cambridge University Press 2010.

excluded in traditional trials, including those with co-morbidities such as medical disorders and substance abuse, the CATIE sample affords us an opportunity to evaluate cognitive impairment in schizophrenia in a unique manner.

This chapter will describe the cognitive findings from the CATIE project, including analyses of the baseline cognitive assessments in 1,331 patients, one of the largest schizophrenia cohorts to be studied with neuropsychological measures, and the effects of treatment on these measures in over 800 patients randomized to five different antipsychotic treatments.

Neurocognitive methods in multi-site studies of schizophrenia

As listed in Table 6.1, multi-site trials present a large number of challenges that need to be met for cognitive data to be reliably and efficiently collected [14]. Sites and testers must be trained and certified on the test battery and related procedures. Data review processes must be established, followed, and maintained throughout the course of the study. Plans must be in place for adding replacement testers or new sites during the study. Test selection must address the scientific hypotheses of the investigators yet be efficient to implement without excessive missing data. Finally, the data analytic plan should focus on a single or small number of outcome measures to reduce statistical errors or reduced statistical power.

Table 6.1. Concerns for schizophrenia cognitive enhancement clinical trials using standard neuropsychological tests*

Rater training and certification is essential

Are testers qualified?

Excluding unqualified testers

Educating testers prior to certification

All testers will require certification

Are the necessary procedures supported by sponsors?

Is the importance of these procedures acknowledged by site investigators?

Data review processes

When cognition is the primary outcome measure, all data reviewed centrally

Less intensive data review is risky, and must include random checks throughout trial

Intervention during a trial

Prior to study initiation, procedures must be in place for adding testers and sites

Task considerations for clinical trials

Increased task complexity can increase missing data rate

Simplify instructions for testers and patients

Additional concerns with computerized tests

Automatized procedures can hide problems indigenous to schizophrenia clinical trials

Note: *Modified from Keefe and Harvey, by permission of Oxford University Press [14].

The CATIE schizophrenia trial methodologies addressed all of these issues in the manner described below.

Neurocognitive advisory group

The choice of tests for a neurocognitive battery is often controversial. Since the CATIE project promised to yield a rich database, it was important that the batteries of tests chosen for the project receive consensus approval from the leaders in schizophrenia and dementia research. The CATIE project also included a trial of antipsychotics for psychosis and/or agitation in individuals with Alzheimer's disease [15]. It was determined that consensus approval of the batteries and the neurocognitive approach for the trials would be particularly important given that numerous independent investigators may desire access to the neurocognitive database for ancillary studies. Thus, the first step in determining the methodology for neurocognitive assessment in the CATIE Project was to appoint and convene a Neurocognitive Advisory Group (NAG), in concert with NIMH staff and the External Scientific Advisory Board. The NAG was composed of the following individuals: Richard Keefe, director; Richard Mohs, co-director; Robert Bilder, Michael Green, Terry Goldberg, Philip Harvey, Herbert Meltzer, James Gold, and Mary Sano.

Assessment training

Overview

The aim of the CATIE Neurocognitive Assessment Unit training program was for testers and investigators to achieve a thorough understanding of the rationale and methods of the neurocognitive assessment protocol. Considerable preparation preceded the production of manuals and training materials. The basic manuals and data forms not only documented the planned procedures for each study, but also served as source documents for training in-house and site staff. The proper training of site personnel responsible for collecting, editing, and transmitting data is essential for ensuring a high-quality study. Accordingly, prior to enrollment of subjects at any of the sites, the Neurocognitive Assessment Unit trained site investigators and staff on all aspects of study design and implementation of neurocognitive assessments. Our philosophy was that training in multi-site studies is most effective when it occurs in close temporal proximity to those critical points in the study timeline when site staff must acquire specific knowledge and skills in order to implement study tasks. Based on protocol design and site participation in multiple protocols, approximately 100 sites required neurocognitive tester certification: 65 in the schizophrenia trial, and 35 in the dementia trial.

Specifics of training plan

All potential neurocognitive testers completed a Tester Evaluation Form to ensure that they had sufficient experience to collect accurate cognitive data from the relevant patient populations. Potential testers were scheduled for group and individual training by the Neurocognitive Assessment Unit staff at the Investigator's Meeting. To help approved testers prepare for the meeting and training, each site was sent copies of the neurocognitive assessment manual and instructional videotape prior to the meeting. The manual included descriptions of how to administer and score each test, score sheets if required, and detailed instructions for preparing and sending the raw test materials for data entry. The videotape demonstrating the test procedures for each test in the battery served as a training and reference tool. It was also useful as a training aid for new testers who did not attend the initial training meetings. Testers were informed that prior to the collection of neuro-cognitive data at their site, they would need to be certified for their ability to complete each of the tests of the test battery.

Training meeting

The details of the final batteries were presented during the Neurocognitive Assessment Training at the Investigator's Meeting. Testers from each investigative site were present at this meeting to learn, practice, and become expert in the administration and scoring procedures for the diagnosis-specific neurocognitive batteries. The meeting included a presentation of all testing and scoring procedures to the group. Following this presentation, testers had opportunities to practice the tests in small groups supervised by psychologists fully familiar with the entire battery. Although many of the testers had extensive experience with the tests in the battery, or with psychological assessment in general, they were required to pass certification procedures for the CATIE neurocognitive battery, as even highly qualified psychologists can develop idiosyncratic data collection methods that may threaten inter-rater reliability.

Certification of testers

Testers were told that they would be expected to master the testing procedures prior to the initiation of the trial at their site. To verify mastery of all testing procedures, all testers met individually with a Neurocognitive Assessment Unit evaluator to determine whether they were satisfactorily proficient with the neurocognitive testing batteries. Each potential tester administered the complete neurocognitive battery to the neurocognitive evaluator, who demonstrated some of the challenges that could be expected of testing patients with schizophrenia. A list of particularly important challenges was made prior to the meeting as a reference for evaluators, so that each potential tester would be given the opportunity to be tested similarly. For example, testers were challenged by "patients" who deviated from the rules in various ways, or who had sudden decrements in performance. Testers who failed the initial certification procedures were given an opportunity to practice test adminis-tration and scoring procedures during the meeting, and then later attempt to be re-certified. Certified testers were sent a document indicating that they were permitted to conduct neurocognitive testing for the CATIE Project.

Following initial certification, each tester was required to send the computer test files, source documents, and summary score sheets from the first five completed assessments. Data collection and scoring procedures were audited by following each measure from the raw testing material or response sheet, through the relevant scoring procedures, to the recording of the data on summary score sheets, to the online data from the computer database. These results were reviewed by the Neurocognitive Assessment Unit personnel, and any errors were corrected with a full explanation of the necessary changes. Testers were required to complete five consecutive testing sessions without error.

Post-meeting certification

A small number of testers were not able to attend the initial Investigator's Meeting. Arrangements were made for these testers to follow the same procedures as those who attended the meeting, with the exception that Neurocognitive Assessment Unit personnel visited these sites to conduct the same certification procedures as had been completed at the meeting. These procedures and the necessary documents are made available to new sites via the CATIE Project website.

Several sites requested the certification of an additional tester, and this was encouraged to handle vacations, sickness, and other potential absences of the primary tester. For additional testers, or if the tester at a site changed, the new personnel underwent the same evaluation procedures as described above.

Initial and ongoing site interaction and assessment

The performance of neurocognitive testers was monitored during the study, and any adminis- tration and scoring problems were addressed and resolved as they occurred. Neurocognitive Assessment Unit personnel were available on a daily basis to answer questions or issues that may occur at the sites. Raw data from each site were entered directly into the database using a web-based data entry system. As an additional check on the quality of neurocognitive data, the Neurocognitive Assessment Unit made random requests for testers to send the source documents and summary scores for patients tested in the study. These scores were compared to those recorded in the electronic data base for the study.

Spanish-speaking subjects. A manual for Spanish-speaking subjects in the United States was developed with assistance from a cross-cultural neuropsychologist, Dr. Lidia Artiola. For those tests not available in Spanish, test instructions, materials, and procedures were translated into Spanish. Sites with testers who planned to test patients in Spanish were required to demonstrate testing competency in Spanish and English.

Assessment of primary language. In patients for whom English is not primary, English testing was allowed to proceed if a sixth-grade reading level using the Wide Range Achievement Test, third edition (WRAT-III) Reading test [16] was demonstrated.

Pervasive developmental disorder. Patients who received a diagnosis of pervasive devel- opmental disorder (mental retardation) were excluded.

Adjunctive medications. Regarding adjunctive medications during the trial, medications used continually, such as anticholinergics, were acceptable. Medications that are used on an as needed basis, such as one-time use of benzodiazapines for anxiety, may interfere with test performance, and could not be given on the day of testing.

Neurocognitive assessment battery

The neurocognitive assessment battery for this trial was developed as a result of the meetings of the Neurocognitive Advisory Group and the Neurocognitive Assessment Unit. A number of guidelines were used to facilitate the selection of tests. These guidelines are based on the suggestions of Mohs [17], Davidson and Keefe [18], and Keefe *et al.* [19] regarding the use of neurocognitive measures to assess treatment response. Similar to the MATRICS Project guidelines [20], the CATIE guidelines included the following: 1) adequate psychometric properties of the procedure, including minimal ceiling and floor effects in the diagnostic group being studied; 2) reliability in the specific diagnostic group being studied; 3) known deficits compared to normal controls in the diagnostic group being studied; 4) minimal test–retest practice effects and/or availability of alternate forms; 5) ease of administration to reduce examiner error across sites; 6) brevity; 7) relevance to the clinical population being studied; 8) relevance to specific hypotheses about the effect of second-generation antipsychotic treatment on cognition in the group being studied; 9) relation to important outcome variables, such as community functioning; 10) previous suggestions that second-generation or first-generation antipsychotic treatments have a possible positive or negative impact on the functions measured by the test; and 11) if possible, available normative data. Adherence to these guidelines resulted in the battery of tests listed and described in Table 6.2.

The CATIE neurocognitive battery of tests was administered at baseline, and then again after 2, 6, and 18 months of treatment. The following assessments were completed at the baseline visit only: education level; previous experience with the tests in the neurocognitive battery; and the WRAT-III Reading subtest. If for some reason these assessments could not be completed at the baseline visit, they were completed at a subsequent visit.

Computerized assessments

One discussion point among the Advisory Group members was the risks and benefits of computerized versus pencil-and-paper testing. Several group members expressed concerns about computerized testing given their previous experiences with computerized tests often resulting in more missing data points than non-computerized tests. We ultimately chose a combination of the two methods. To minimize some of the difficulties caused by tests administered from variable computers and software platforms, we purchased 65 desktop computers, developed and installed the software for the computerized tests at the Neuro-cognitive Assessment Unit, and shipped the test-ready computers to each site. This method allowed us to maintain a consistency of computerized test conditions across sites, and ensured that novel software–hardware interaction difficulties would be minimized through the course of the study. The baseline data suggested that the computerized tests had more missing data points than the non-computerized tests (Table 6.3).

Findings from study of the baseline neurocognitive data

The CATIE schizophrenia trial presented an excellent opportunity to assess the severity of neurocognitive performance and the relation of neurocognitive deficits to symptoms and demographic factors in patients who may better represent typical patients with schizophrenia, including those who often do not participate in research protocols or clinical trials. Since the number of subjects available for analysis (N = 1,331) was larger than any previous study of cognitive performance in schizophrenia, it provided a unique opportunity to conduct analyses not possible with smaller samples: comparison of competing models of the structure of neurocognitive deficits in schizophrenia; determination of the magnitude of the correlations of neurocognitive deficits with symptom severity; and determination of the specific contributions of each test added to a battery for generating an estimate of overall neurocognitive functioning.

Statistical characteristics of measures

For each collected and calculated measure, the mean, standard deviation, median, mode, skewness, and kurtosis were determined. All variables except the Facial Emotion Discrimination Task were judged to have reasonable normality such that subsequent analyses could proceed. While three of the individual measures that were used to derive cognitive outcome measures (e.g., the no-delay visuospatial working memory test performance) were skewed,

Table 6.2. Neurocognitive tests used in the CATIE schizophrenia trial*

1. Cognitive domain	2. Type of test	3. Description of test and measures used for domain summary scores
Processing Speed	1. Controlled Oral Word Association Test (Benton *et al*, 1978)	Generate as many words as possible beginning with F, A, and S in three separate trials of 60 seconds. *Measure*: mean number of words
	2. Category Instances (Benton *et al*, 1978)	Name as many words as possible in 60 seconds within each of three categories (animals, fruits, vegetables). *Measure*: mean number of words
	3. Grooved Pegboard (Lafayette, 1989)	Insert pegs in a certain order into 25 randomly positioned slots using dominant hand. Insert as many pegs as possible in two 45-second trials. *Measure*: mean number of pegs
	4. Wechsler Adult Intelligence Scale-Revised, Digit Symbol Test (Wechlser *et al*, 1974)	Each numeral (1 through 9) is associated with a different simple symbol. Copy as many symbols associated with the numerals as possible in 90 seconds. *Measure*: number of symbols correctly copied
Reasoning	1. Wisconsin Card Sorting Test, 64-card computerized version (Kongs *et al*, 2000)	A complex task of categorization, set shifting, and response to feedback from the tester. Only 64 cards were presented at each testing session. *Measure*: Mean of perseverative errors (sign reversed) and categories z-scores
	2. WISC-III Mazes (Wechsler, 1991)	Use a pencil to attempt to draw through a series of 9 timed mazes without entering into blind alleys. *Measure*: raw score
Verbal Memory	Hopkins Verbal Learning Test (Brandt and Benedict, 1991)	Recall as many words as possible from a list of 12 words read aloud by the tester. The procedure was repeated three times. *Measure*: total number of words recalled
Working Memory	1. Computerized Test of Visuospatial Working Memory (Lyons-Warren *et al*, 2004)	Focus on cross in center of computer screen while dot appears at random locations on the screen. Then watch shapes appear on screen and press space bar when diamond shape appears. When the cross reappears, point to where dot appeared in beginning. Distance between response and dot is measured. There are three conditions (no delay, 5-sec delay and 15-sec delay) and 8 trials of each condition. *Measure*: Mean error distance of

Table 6.2. (cont.)

1. Cognitive domain	2. Type of test	3. Description of test and measures used for domain summary scores
		delay conditions minus no-delay error distance (sign reversed)
	2. Letter-Number Sequencing Test (Gold et al, 1997)	Clusters of letters combined with numbers (e.g., N6G2) are read aloud by the tester, and the patient reorganizes the cluster so that the numbers are listed first, from lowest to highest, followed by the letters in alphabetical order. Measure: number of correct sequences
Vigilance	Continuous Performance Test (CPT) (Cornblatt & Keilp, 1994)	Respond to a series of numbers on a computer screen at a rate of one per second by lifting a finger from a mouse key whenever the current number is identical to the previous number. Three 150-trial conditions of increasing difficulty are administered (2, 3, and 4-digit numbers respectively). Measure: mean response sensitivity (d-prime)
Social Cognition	Facial Emotion Discrimination Test (Kerr & Neale, 1993)	Two pictures of different human faces displaying emotions are presented concurrently. Patients declare whether the faces are displaying the same or different emotions in thirty trials. Measure: number of correct responses

Notes: *From Keefe RSE, Bilder RM, Harvey PD, et al. [21].
Used with permission of Nature Publishing Group.

Benton AL, Hamscher K (1978). Multilingual Aphasia Examination Manual (revised). University of Iowa: Iowa City, IA.

Brant J, Benedict R (1991). Hopkins Verbal Learning Test. Psychological Assessment Resources: Lutz, FL.

Cornblatt BA, Keilp JG (1994). Impaired attention, genetics, and the pathophysiology of schizophrenia. Schizophr Bull 20: 31–46.

Gold JM, Carpenter C, Randolph C, Goldberg TE, Weinberger DR (1997). Auditory working memory and Wisconsin Card Sorting Test performance in schizophrenia. Arch Gen Psychiatry 54: 159–165.

Kerr SL, Neale JM (1993). Emotion perception in schizophrenia: specific deficit of further evidence of generalized poor performance? J Abnorm Psychol 102: 312–318.

Kongs SK, Thompson LL, Iverson GL, Heaton RK (2000). Wisconsin Card Sorting Test-64 Card Version Professional Manual. Psychological Assessment Resources, Inc.: Lutz, FL.

Lafayette Instrument Company (1989). Grooved Pegboard Instruction Manual, Model 32025. Lafayette Instrument Company: Lafayette, Indiana.

Lyons-Warren A, Lillie R, Hershey T (2004). Short and long-term spatial delayed response performance across the lifespan. Dev Neuropsych 26: 661–678.

Wechsler D (1974). Wechsler Adult Intelligence Scale, Revised edn. Psychological Corporation: San Antonio, TX.

Wechsler D (1991). Wechsler Intelligence Scale for Children, 3rd edn. Harcourt Publishers, NY.

Table 6.3. Number of patients (of 1,331 total) in the CATIE schizophrenia trial for whom data were missing at baseline based upon the reasons and whether the test was computerized**

Reason for missing data	Number of patients missing data	
	Non-computerized tests (N = 7)	Computerized tests (N = 3)
Patient refused test	38	119
Patient did not understand instructions	4	215*
Computer malfunction	0	135
Tester error	14	11
Unknown	18	37

Notes: Computerized tests included bundled versions of the 64-card Wisconsin Card Sorting Test, Visuospatial Working Memory Test, and Identical Pairs Continuous Performance Test.
*Only two patients did not understand computerized WCST test instructions.
**From Keefe and Harvey, by permission of Oxford University Press [14].

all of the measures that comprised the domain scores (described below), the domain scores themselves, and the composite scores (described below) had skewness indices of between 0.45 and −0.25, suggesting considerable normality. Scores that were judged to reflect a patient's inability to complete the task were set to "missing" in the data set; some scores generated queries to the tester to ensure validity (see Appendix II of Keefe *et al.*) [21] for a description of scores that were queried or set to "missing"). The data collected from the Facial Emotion Discrimination Test had a ceiling effect and positive skew that was so severe that it would be likely to reduce the sensitivity of the battery to treatment effects, so it was eliminated from further analyses.

Domain summary scores

All test measures were first converted to standardized z-scores by setting the mean of each measure to 0 and the standard deviation to 1 based upon the entire patient sample. The Controlled Oral Word Association Test and Category Instances summary measures were averaged together to form one summary test score referred to as verbal fluency. For domains that had more than one measure, summary scores were determined by calculating the mean of the z-scores for the measures that comprised the domain (as described in Table 6.2), then converting the mean to a z-score with mean of 0 and standard deviation of 1. This process resulted in nine test summary scores and five domain scores (after excluding facial emotion discrimination) that correspond to five of the seven domains in the MATRICS consensus battery [22].

Baseline results

Table 6.4 presents raw score performance data for each collected and calculated neurocognitive measure. The table also includes comparison data from normative samples for measures with normative data judged to be of sufficient size and quality.

The principal components analysis (PCA) suggested that a single component best described the data, as the Eigenvalue of the first principal component was 4.07, accounting

Table 6.4. Neurocognitive performance in patients with schizophrenia and comparison to available normative data

Variable	Schizophrenia patients			Normative data		Group difference in mean*
	N	Mean	SD	Mean	SD	
WRAT-3 Reading	1,294	43.10	8.49	49.0	7.00	−0.84
COWAT – F words	1,331	9.88	4.06			
COWAT – A words	1,331	7.95	3.66			
COWAT – S words	1,331	10.08	4.28			
COWAT Sum	1,331	27.91	10.63	38.93	12.17	−0.91
Category Instances (Animals)	1,332	13.91	4.88			
Category Instances (Fruits)	1,331	10.14	3.38			
Category Instances (Vegetables)	1,332	8.64	3.44			
Category Instances Sum	1,331	32.69	9.95			
WISC-III Mazes	1,319	17.54	5.98			
Letter-Number Sequencing	1,323	10.21	4.47			
Hopkins Verbal Learning Test Trial 1	1,331	4.75	1.74	7.63	1.77**	−1.63
Hopkins Verbal Learning Test Trial 2	1,331	6.48	2.14	9.79	1.67**	−1.98
Hopkins Verbal Learning Test Trial 3	1,331	7.50	2.45	10.74	1.31**	−2.47
Facial Emotion Discrimination Test	1,331	24.59	3.37			
WAIS-R Digit Symbol	1,327	37.43	13.41	53.50	14.00	−1.15
Grooved Pegboard Trial 1	1,323	11.75	3.93	15.36	4.24	−0.85
Grooved Pegboard Trial 2	1,323	13.30	4.02			
CPT d′, two digit	1,095	2.37	1.05			
CPT d′, three digit	1,099	1.79	0.93			
CPT d′, four digit	1,081	1.01	0.76			
Visuospatial Working Memory Test no delay condition	1,211	2.31	2.93			
Visuospatial Working Memory Test 5-sec condition	1,211	28.28	19.08			
Visuospatial Working Memory Test 15-sec condition	1,211	30.46	19.11			
Visuospatial Working Memory Test (mean 5 & 15 sec) minus no delay	1,211	27.06	17.59			
Wisconsin Card Sorting Test-64, perseverative errors	1,263	13.66	10.18	8.50	6.30	0.82

Table 6.4. *(cont.)*

Variable	Schizophrenia patients			Normative data		Group difference in mean*
	N	Mean	SD	Mean	SD	
Wisconsin Card Sorting Test-64, categories completed	1,260	2.13	1.60	3.56	1.47	−0.97
Wisconsin Card Sorting Test-64, categories completed + additional cards in final category	1,261	2.33	1.69			

Abbreviations: COWAT = Controlled Oral Word Association Test, WISC-III – Wechsler Intelligence Test for Children, third edition, WAIS-R = Wechsler Adult Intelligence Test, Revised edition, CPT = Continuous Performance Test, Identical Pairs.
Notes: *Based upon normative data z-score; all between-group comparisons were statistically significant at least $p < 0.0001$, except VVMT no delay, which was not significant.
**SDs were estimated from Table 6.2 in the HVLT manual (Brandt and Benedict, 1991). Four age groups were pooled resulting in an age range of 20–60 years. The normative standard deviation was estimated by squaring individual SDs from each age group, dividing them by N-1 for that group, summing them, dividing by total N and taking the square root. From: Keefe *et al*, 2006 [21]. Reprinted with permission of Nature Publishing Group.

for 45.2% of the overall variance in test scores, with no other principal component greater than 1.0. Since this one component accounted for a relatively low percentage of the overall variance, two-, three-, and four-component solutions were examined. These extractions followed by Varimax rotations, which emphasize differences among components, did not adequately explain the data structure.

Structural equation modeling analyses compared a null model (no structure), a unifactorial model including the nine individual tests as one factor, a unifactorial model including the five pre-defined domain scores as a single factor, and a five-factor model that included the tests from each of the five cognitive domains as separate factors (see Figure 6.1). The unifactorial model based upon a mean of the five domain scores was the best fit, and significantly better than any of the other models. Thus, it is recommended that all future analyses using a composite score from these data will be calculated by averaging the five domain scores.

Several analyses were completed to address the issues of whether a meaningful overall composite score can be calculated from a briefer set of tests. In one analysis, we sequentially eliminated the tests that were most likely to produce missing values. This analysis suggested that a significant increase in sample size (from 1,035 to 1,297) was possible if the three computerized tests are eliminated, yet the Pearson correlation between the composite score and an unweighted mean generated from all of the non-computerized tests was 0.951 (df = 1,295, $p < 0.0001$). Another analysis investigated the shortest amount of testing time that could provide a composite score that was as meaningful as the full battery of tests. The results of a stepwise multiple regression predicting an unweighted mean of all standardized test scores with variable entry based upon the estimated amount of time that a test takes to administer are presented in Table 6.5. The most striking aspect of this analysis is that the overwhelming majority of the variance in the composite score was accounted for by a few tests that take only about 25 minutes to complete.

Pearson correlations of the neurocognitive domain scores and the composite score with demographic and clinical characteristics, including symptoms, suggested very little difference

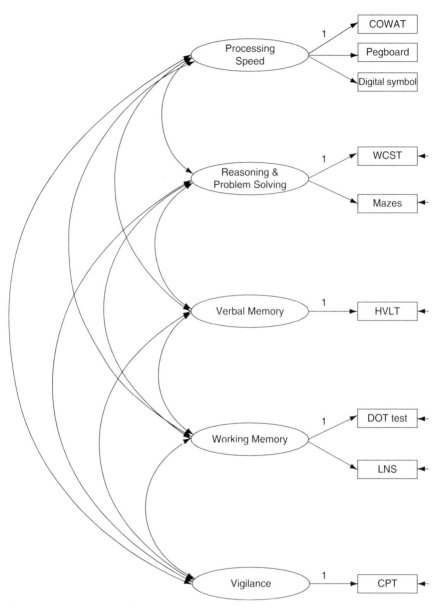

Figure 6.1. Comparison of different models of the structure of cognitive performance at baseline of the CATIE trial. A null model failed to fit the data. A unifactorial model based on the nine tests was an improvement in fit; chi-square(27) = 192.18, $p < 0.001$; CFI = 0.94, GFI = 0.97; RMSEA = 0.077. A unifactorial model including the five pre-defined domain scores was a considerable improvement in fit over the unifactorial model from the nine tests chi-square(22) = 152.27, $p < 0.001$; CFI = 0.98, GFI = 0.97; RMSEA = 0.080. A five-factor model that included the tests from each of the five cognitive domains as separate factors was a significantly poorer fit compared to the unifactorial model from the five pre-defined domain scores chi-square(14) = 78.04, $p < 0.001$.

Table 6.5. Stepwise multiple regression predicting unweighted mean of variables from each test. Order of entry from least to most estimated test administration time*

Variable entered	Estimated test		
	Total R^2	R^2 Change	Admin time (min)
WAIS-R Digit Symbol	0.610	0.610	3.4
HVLT Total Recall	0.722	0.112	4.1
Grooved Pegboard	0.790	0.068	5.0
Letter-Number Sequencing	0.867	0.078	5.9
Verbal Fluency	0.888	0.021	8.0
WISC-R Mazes	0.934	0.046	11.2
Continuous Performance Test	0.956	0.022	13.4
Visuospatial Working Memory Test	0.978	0.022	13.4
WCST	1.000	0.022	20.0

Abbreviations: WAIS-R = Wechsler Adult Intelligence Test, Revised edition, HVLT = Hopkins Verbal Learning Test, WISC-III = Wechsler Intelligence Test for Children, third edition, WCST = Wisconsin Card Sorting Test.
*From Keefe RSE, Bilder RM, Harvey PD, et al. [21]. Reprinted with permission of Nature Publishing Group.
Notes: F-statistic for all steps was greater than 193.0; all p values < 0.0001; N = 1,035.

between neurocognitive domains. The magnitude of the correlations with age, education, and duration of illness were in the medium range, defined by Cohen [23] as r = 0.30, while the other correlations were smaller. The correlations with negative symptoms were in the range defined by Cohen as small (r = 0.10) to medium (r = 0.30). Of particular note, all of the correlations between the neurocognitive measures and Positive and Negative Syndromes Scale (PANSS) positive symptoms were non-significant and less than r = 0.08.

Discussion and conclusion of baseline findings

Neurocognition can be assessed adequately in the vast majority of patients with schizophrenia, even when including patients with substance abuse and other co-morbid conditions. An acceptable composite score could be derived for over 90% of the patients in the CATIE trial. However, some tests, particularly computerized tests, were more likely to yield missing data in this study. It was determined that, while most patients can complete all tests in a 90-minute battery, it is likely that most of the variance in neurocognitive composites scores for this type of assessment can be completed with a small number of tests, requiring less time and resources. While the data from this study suggested that neurocognition is best described as a single factor, this conclusion needs to be tempered by the limitations of the test battery, which included only 11 tests. More comprehensive neurocognitive assessments may yield a more complex factor structure [24]. Finally, the domains of cognition and overall composite score showed medium correlations with symptoms and near-zero correlations with positive symptoms. Given that this patient cohort included "all-comers" and that over 90% of patients completed testing, these data provide impressive support for the notion that positive symptoms and neurocognitive impairment are largely independent in patients with schizophrenia.

The effects of antipsychotic medications on cognition: CATIE and beyond

The effects of antipsychotic medications on cognition remain controversial. While many studies [10,23–60] and meta-analyses [19,61,62] have suggested that second-generation antipsychotic treatment provides greater neurocognitive benefit to schizophrenia patients than first-generation, "typical" antipsychotics, many of these studies have had substantial limitations or flaws, such as small sample sizes, short duration of treatment, no comparator or a comparator of relatively high doses of first-generation antipsychotic treatment, and inattention to important clinical factors such as the relationship of cognitive improvement with symptom change, anticholinergic treatment, and change in extrapyramidal symptoms [19,61–63]. The CATIE study enabled us to address these issues in a large sample of patients. Our primary cognitive hypothesis for the CATIE schizophrenia treatment study was that neurocognitive response would be significantly different among these treatments. To maximize the statistical power for testing this hypothesis, our primary statistical tests focused on change in a single composite score after 2 months of treatment, during which improvement in neurocognition was expected to occur based upon previous studies. An additional hypothesis was that neurocognitive improvement in the early stages of treatment would predict treatment effectiveness as measured by time to all-cause discontinuation.

Results for the effects of treatment on neurocognition in the CATIE schizophrenia trial

The enrollment, allocation, and follow-up of study patients were described previously [64,65] and are found in other chapters in this volume. A total of 1,493 patients were enrolled in the study and randomized to treatment. Data from 33 subjects at one site were excluded prior to analysis due to questions about data integrity. The 1,331 patients who were tested at baseline were found in previously published analyses to be very similar on demographic measures to the total number of 1,460 patients who were entered into the study [21], and this also applies to the cohort of 817 patients who completed neurocognitive testing at baseline and at the primary endpoint 2 months post-baseline and comprise the primary cohort for the cognitive treatment analyses. At baseline, 25% of patients reported being antipsychotic-free, 60% of patients were on second-generation antipsychotics, 10% were on first-generation antipsychotics, and 5% were on a combination of first- and second-generation antipsychotics. The percentages of patients who were randomized to the same drug they reported being on at baseline are as follows: olanzapine, 30%; perphenazine, 0%; quetiapine, 10%; risperidone, 24%; ziprasidone, 4%. The primary cohort was representative of the population of chronic schizophrenia patients except there were fewer females (25%). Patients who completed testing at baseline and 18 months were very similar to the primary cohort.

Mean modal doses (mg/d) during the entire course of Phase I for the patients who had neurocognitive test data at baseline and 2 months were olanzapine (21.0), perphenazine (21.5), quetiapine (566.3), risperidone (4.1), and ziprasidone (121.9). Because time to treatment discontinuation differed between treatments [67], the percentage of patients who provided neurocognitive data at the 2-month assessment also differed between treatments, as follows: olanzapine, 68%; perphenazine, 65%; quetiapine, 59%; risperidone, 58%; and ziprasidone, 55%.

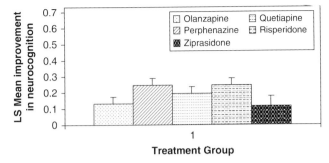

Figure 6.2. Least-squares (LS) mean improvement in neurocognitive composite score after two months of antipsychotic treatment, adjusted for baseline score and whether the patient had required crisis stabilization in the 3 months prior to study entry. Patients with tardive dyskinesia were not included in the data presented in this figure. Only the ziprasidone data were from data collected when ziprasidone became available, after 40% of the patients had already been entered into the study [65]. Reprinted with permission of Archives of General Psychiatry (2007).

Neurocognitive changes after 2 months of treatment

Change in the neurocognitive composite score from baseline to 2 months, the primary outcome measure in this study, showed improvement in each of the treatment groups. In patients without tardive dyskinesia (TD), treatment resulted in the following composite score improvements: olanzapine, 0.13 $(p < .002)$, perphenazine, 0.25, $(p < .0001)$ quetiapine, 0.18 $(p < .0001)$, risperidone 0.26 $(p < .0001)$. (Least-square means are presented in Figure 6.2.) There was no overall difference among the treatment groups $(p = 0.20)$. When TD patients were included in the analysis, and TD was used as an additional covariate in the analysis, the results were very similar. Within the cohort of 463 patients who underwent randomization after ziprasidone was added to the trial, the results were similar and there were no statistically significant between groups. Patients randomized to ziprasidone had improvements of 0.12 $(p < .06)$ when TD patients were excluded and 0.18 $(p < .001)$ when they were included. There was also no significant disparity between the groups in improvement across the neurocognitive domains (all p's > 0.08). Treatment analyses were also completed with site, WRAT Reading score, years of education, and baseline alcohol and substance use included in the model. These covariates did not produce statistics that differed from the unadjusted analyses.

A model of prediction of improvement in neurocognitive composite score from baseline to 2 months ($R^2 = 0.19$) suggested that lower baseline composite score $(p < .0001)$, higher WRAT Reading score $(p < 0.0001)$, presence of substance abuse at baseline $(p = 0.002)$, better compliance $(p = 0.003)$, greater improvement in PANSS negative symptom scale scores at 1 month $(p = 0.007)$, absence of tardive dyskinesia $(p = 0.01)$, and site $(p = 0.01)$ were all significant predictors of greater cognitive improvement.

Neurocognitive changes after 6 months of treatment

There were 523 patients who completed neurocognitive testing at baseline and then 6 months later while still receiving the medication to which they had been randomized. In the original analytic plan, the comparisons at 6 months were considered exploratory and, thus, not eligible for statistical thresholds for significance. However, for completeness, here we present these exploratory results. The neurocognitive composite score improved $(p < 0.001)$ for each of the treatment groups from baseline to 6 months of treatment. There were no differences among the groups on the change in the neurocognitive composite score ($p = 0.35$) or any of the neurocognitive domains (all p's > 0.01).

Neurocognitive changes after 18 months of treatment

A total of 303 patients were tested at 18 months while still receiving the medication to which they had originally been randomized. Thus, 37% of the patients from the 2-month analyses were included. The 303 patients represent only 21% of the 1,460 patients entered into the trial. There were no significant differences on the composite score or any of the individual domains (all p's > 0.05), suggesting that the patients in these analyses are representative of the entire cohort in terms of baseline neurocognition. The percentage of patients who provided neurocognitive data at the 18-month assessment differed between treatments, as follows: olanzapine, 29%; perphenazine, 23%; quetiapine, 18%; risperidone, 21%; and ziprasidone, 18%.

In the original analytic plan, the comparisons at 18 months were considered exploratory and, thus, not eligible for statistical thresholds for significance. Again, for completeness, we present these exploratory results. In patients without TD, there were improvements in the neurocognitive composite score from baseline in all of the treatment groups. The improvement in the composite score from month 2 to month 18 was 0.11 (t = 3.20, df = 273, $p = < 0.01$), suggesting that most of the cognitive improvement occurred in the first 2 months of treatment.

There were overall differences among treatments in composite score change ($p < 0.05$). Pairwise comparisons suggested that improvement in the neurocognitive composite score was greater in the perphenazine group (0.49) than in the olanzapine (0.15; $p = 0.0017$) group or the risperidone group (0.28; $p = 0.036$). The ziprasidone and quetiapine groups did not differ from any of the other treatments.

Some of the overall differences between groups were explained by the differences in the reasoning domain, although this difference would not have met the criteria for formal statistical significance after controlling for multiple comparisons. The perphenazine group tended to improve more than the other treatment groups (see Table 6.4). In comparisons among the second-generation treatments that included patients with TD, there were no overall differences between the groups.

Associations between cognitive change from baseline and other clinical changes

The Pearson correlations between change in neurocognitive composite score from baseline and change in PANSS symptom factors from baseline were quite small. The correlations between change in neurocognitive composite score from baseline to 2 months and the 1-month and 3-month changes from baseline in extrapyramidal symptoms (Simpson-Angus mean score), tardive dyskinesia (AIMS global severity score), akathisia (Barnes global score) were r < 0.05 with all p values greater than 0.05. The correlation between neurocognitive change and compliance was 0.07 ($p = 0.04$). The 151 patients who were receiving anticholinergic medications at baseline had neurocognitive change of 0.169, which did not differ from the 666 patients who were not receiving anticholinergic medications at baseline, who had a mean change of 0.224. However, for the 38 patients who had anticholinergic medications added during the first 2 months of treatment, composite scores worsened (mean change = −0.049; SD = 0.46) at the 2-month assessment, compared to other patients whose composite scores improved (mean change = 0.190; SD = 0.56) ($p = < 0.01$).

Neurocognitive predictors of treatment discontinuation

Cox proportional hazards regression analyses suggested that change from baseline to 2 months in the neurocognitive composite score was not a significant predictor of time until all-cause discontinuation. However, there was a suggestion of a treatment interaction for this analysis ($p < 0.10$). Neurocognitive improvement predicted time to all-cause discontinuation in patients treated with quetiapine ($p = 0.021$; hazard ratio [HR] for 0.25 SD improvement in composite score $= 0.98$; 95% CI $= 0.954$ to 0.996) and ziprasidone ($p = 0.009$; HR $= 0.957$; 95% CI $= 0.925$ to 0.989), but not the other treatments. Inclusion of change in PANSS score, compliance, and other baseline covariates found previously to predict time to discontinuation did not reduce the statistical significance for the quetiapine group. The prediction of time to discontinuation due to inefficacy produced similar results.

Discussion and conclusions from the CATIE neurocognition treatment trial

All of the antipsychotic treatment groups had a small improvement in neurocognition as measured by the primary outcome measure for this study, that is, change in a composite score derived from 11 neurocognitive tests assessed at baseline and after 2 months of treatment. However, there was no significant difference among the groups. Quite surprisingly, exploratory analyses suggested that, after 18 months of treatment, there might be differences among the treatments, with the older antipsychotic perphenazine demonstrating the most neurocognitive improvement. This result contradicts many other studies in which second-generation antipsychotic medications appeared to provide greater cognitive benefit than first-generation antipsychotics [10,25–62]. This failure to document a neurocognitive advantage of second-generation antipsychotics suggests that the positive findings from prior reports may not generalize well to the type of everyday clinical practice examined in the CATIE trial.

The contrast between the current results and those reported previously may be explained in part by methodological differences between the studies. First, the current study included neurocognitive treatment data on 817 patients, more than twice as many as the largest previous trial. It is possible that smaller studies are susceptible to results that are less stable and generalizable. Second, in contrast to many previous studies that used high dosages of first-generation antipsychotics, usually haloperidol, a high-potency drug known to have increased risk of extrapyramidal symptoms and anticholinergic treatment which may impair cognition [19,61–66], this study used perphenazine as the representative of the older antipsychotic medications. That choice may have reduced the extrapyramidal symptoms and need for anticholinergic treatment associated with haloperidol and other high potency first-generation antipsychotics [64,66], especially since the dose range of 8–32 mg, equivalent to 2.5–10 mg haloperidol, was lower than in most early studies [67–69]. Perphenazine, a phenothiazine, has been available since the late 1950s. It was selected for CATIE because it is a moderate potency first-generation antipsychotic and causes only mild sedative effects and EPS in the dose range selected. Although it has never been considered to be an atypical antipsychotic, one of its metabolites, n-dealkylperphenazine (DAPZ) has relatively high affinity for serotonin 2A receptors, which by some definitions may confer atypical properties [70]. Therefore, prior studies may have documented, at least in part, negative effects associated with high dose haloperidol treatment rather than an intrinsic, specific cognitive enhancement effect associated with some of the second-generation drugs versus the older medications. It will be important for clinicians using perphenazine or other first-generation antipsychotics to carefully consider these dosage implications. Third, compared to most clinical trials [71], the present study had broad inclusion and minimal exclusion criteria, and allowed co-morbid conditions, concomitant medications, and current substance abuse. It was conducted at a variety of clinical settings where people with schizophrenia are treated. These "real-world" features of the study, which were intended to make the results more widely applicable [71], may also account for the differences in results between this and previous studies. While single-site trials that are limited to research centers and highly screened patients may be more sensitive to the cognitive changes associated with treatment, and may offer hope for the potential neurocognitive benefit of these medications, the current results may more accurately reflect clinical reality.

An additional difference between this study and previous studies that found advantages for the newer drugs for neurocognitive functioning is that at least 60% of patients in this study reported being on atypical antipsychotic treatment prior to randomization. This is substantially higher than in many of the earlier studies, which were completed when treatment with second-generation antipsychotics was less common. However, only 16% of patients were randomized to the same drug they reported being on at baseline. Although the inclusion in our statistical analyses of patients' report of their antipsychotic medication prior to randomization did not change the study results, it is possible that some of the potential neurocognitive benefit of the second-generation treatments examined in this study had already been realized prior to the initiation of the randomized treatment. If so, treatment effects may have been attenuated, but this would not explain the surprisingly beneficial effect of perphenazine. The best way to address this question would be to complete studies on first-episode patients who have never received antipsychotic medication. Two studies completed since the CATIE neurocognition treatment study shed light on this question. First, a comparison of olanzapine, quetiapine, and risperidone in first-episode patients using the identical neurocognitive test battery of the CATIE trial produced very similar results, with all treatments having a very modest effect on cognition [72]. Most recently, in the European Union First Episode Schizophrenia Trial (EUFEST), a comparison of open-label haloperidol (1–4 mg/d), amisulpride (200–800 mg/d), olanzapine (5–20 mg/d), quetiapine (200–750 mg/d), or ziprasidone (40–160 mg/d) produced similar results with no differences between treatments, even in antipsychotic-naïve patients [73]. These data support the findings from CATIE that the impact of antipsychotic medications on neurocognition varies little across treatments.

Since the neurocognitive benefit of treatment in this study was small, the possibility that neurocognitive improvement was due solely to practice effects or expectation biases cannot be ruled out. The amount of improvement reported in CATIE was demonstrated in a study by Goldberg et al. in a sample of first-episode schizophrenia patients treated with second-generation antipsychotics, as well as in a control sample of healthy individuals [74]. In the EUFEST trial, the changes between the baseline and 6-month testing ranged from 0.56 ES to 0.33 ES, depending on the individual test, slightly larger than the CATIE trial. Although in the study reported by Goldberg et al. patients were tested more often than in the EUFEST study, it is still possible that at least part of the observed improvement might be the result of practice. In studies of antipsychotic medications, practice and placebo effects in schizophrenia are impossible to disentangle from treatment effects. However, a double-blind study using the CATIE battery to determine the effects of donepezil and placebo in a highly refined sample of 226 schizophrenia patients stabilized on second-generation antipsychotics suggested that patients on placebo, who had negative symptom improvement, also had neurocognitive effect size improvements of 0.22 standard deviations after being tested twice over 6 weeks on the same test battery used in this study, suggesting a practice or placebo effect [75] consistent with the improvements reported in the CATIE trial. However, it is important to note that higher doses of haloperidol may blunt working memory performance [76] and procedural learning, which are likely mediators of practice-related performance improvements [77,78] and may have conferred an advantage for the newer drugs in some previous studies, while patients treated with lower doses of haloperidol have demonstrated learning improvements, especially in first-episode samples [10,79]. Thus, while practice effects or expectation biases may be present in patients with schizophrenia on some tests, they may be adversely affected by certain treatments. However, this suggestion is not supported by the EUFEST data since the cognitive improvement in patients receiving a low dose of haloperidol was not significantly different from that of the second-generation antipsychotics [73]. Nevertheless, it is still conceivable that higher doses of haloperidol might exert a deleterious effect on cognitive performance.

Recent findings from the CATIE trial, EUFEST, and other antipsychotic trials have suggested minimal neurocognitive improvement effects in patients treated with conventional or second-generation antipsychotics. New treatments that specifically target cognition are sorely needed. The NIMH MATRICS Project and related efforts have stimulated interest from government and industry, and several studies are under way to explore new treatments for cognitive impairment in schizophrenia [80,81]. In addition, cognitive remediation strategies have recently demonstrated cognitive benefits for patients with schizophrenia [82,83]. Although these strategies have yet to be introduced into standard clinical practice, they hold the promise that effective treatments for cognition in schizophrenia may be developed.

References

1. Saykin AJ, Gur RC, Gur RE, et al. Neuropsychological function in schizophrenia. Selective impairment in memory and learning. Archives of General Psychiatry 1991;48:618–24.

2. Braff DL, Heaton R, Kuck J, et al. The generalized pattern of neuropsychological deficits in outpatients with chronic schizophrenia with heterogeneous Wisconsin Card Sorting Test results. Archives of General Psychiatry 1991;48:891–8.

3. Brickman AM, Paul RH, Cohen RA, et al. Category and letter verbal fluency across the adult lifespan: Relationship to EEG theta power. Archives of Clinical Neuropsychology 2005;20:561–73.

4. Saykin AJ, Shtasel DL, Gur RE, et al. Neuropsychological deficits in neuroleptic naive patients with first-episode schizophrenia. Archives of General Psychiatry 1994;51:124–31.

5. Davidson M, Reichenberg A, Rabinowitz J, et al. Behavioral and intellectual markers for schizophrenia in apparently healthy male adolescents. American Journal of Psychiatry 1999;156:1328–35.

6. Reichenberg A, Weiser M, Rapp MA, et al. Elaboration on premorbid intellectual performance in schizophrenia: Premorbid intellectual decline and risk for schizophrenia. Archives of General Psychiatry 2005;62:1297–304.

7. Fuller R, Nopoulos P, Arndt S, et al. Longitudinal assessment of premorbid cognitive functioning in patients with schizophrenia through examination of standardized scholastic test performance. American Journal of Psychiatry 2002;159:1183–9.

8. Heinrichs RW and Zakzanis KK. Neurocognitive deficit in schizophrenia: A quantitative review of the evidence. Neuropsychology 1998;12:426–45.

9. Bilder RM, Goldman RS, Robinson D, et al. Neuropsychology of first-episode

schizophrenia: Initial characterization and clinical correlates. *American Journal of Psychiatry* 2000;**157**:549–59.

10. Keefe RSE, Seidman LJ, Christensen BK, *et al.* Comparative effect of atypical and conventional antipsychotic drugs on neurocognition in first-episode psychosis: A randomized, double-blind trial of olanzapine versus low doses of haloperidol. *American Journal of Psychiatry* 2004;**161**:985–95.

11. Gold JM, Queern C, Iannone VN, *et al.* Repeatable battery for the assessment of neuropsychological status as a screening test in schizophrenia I: Sensitivity, reliability, and validity. *American Journal of Psychiatry* 1999;**156**:1944–50.

12. Green MF. What are the functional consequences of neurocognitive deficits in schizophrenia? *American Journal of Psychiatry* 1996;**153**:321–30.

13. Harvey PD, Howanitz E, Parrella M, *et al.* Symptoms, cognitive functioning, and adaptive skills in geriatric patients with lifelong schizophrenia: A comparison across treatment sites. *American Journal of Psychiatry* 1998;**155**:1080–6.

14. Keefe RS and Harvey PD. Implementation considerations for multi-site clinical trials with cognitive neuroscience tasks. *Schizophrenia Bulletin* 2008;**34**:656–63.

15. Schneider LS, Tariot PN, Dagerman KS, *et al.* Effectiveness of atypical antipsychotic drugs in patients with Alzheimer's disease. *New England Journal of Medicine* 2006;**355**:1525–38.

16. Jastak S and Wilkinson GS. *Wide Range Achievement Test-Revised 3.* Wilmington, DE: Jastak Associates; 1993.

17. Mohs RC. Assessing cognitive function in schizophrenics and patients with Alzheimer's disease. *Schizophrenia Research* 1995;**17**:115–21.

18. Davidson M and Keefe RK. Cognitive impairment as a target for pharmacological treatment in schizophrenia. *Schizophrenia Research* 1995;**17**:123–9.

19. Keefe RS, Silva SG, Perkins DO, *et al.* The effects of atypical antipsychotic drugs on neurocognitive impairment in

schizophrenia: A review and meta-analysis. *Schizophrenia Bulletin* 1999;**25**:201–22.

20. Nuechterlein KH, Green MF, Kern RS, *et al.* The MATRICS consensus cognitive battery: Part 1. Test selection, reliability, and validity. *American Journal of Psychiatry* 2008;**165**:203–13.

21. Keefe RS, Bilder RM, Harvey PD, *et al.* Baseline neurocognitive deficits in the CATIE schizophrenia trial. *Neuropsychopharmacology* 2006; **31**:2033–46.

22. Green MF, Nuechterlein KH, Gold JM, *et al.* Approaching a consensus cognitive battery for clinical trials in schizophrenia: The NIMH-MATRICS conference to select cognitive domains and test criteria. *Biological Psychiatry* 2004;**56**:301–7.

23. Cohen J. *Statistical Power Analysis for the Behavioral Sciences.* New York: Academic Press; 1977.

24. Nuechterlein KH, Barch DM, Gold JM, *et al.* Identification of separable cognitive factors in schizophrenia. *Schizophrenia Research* 2004;**72**:29–39.

25. Keefe RSE, Seidman LJ, Christensen BK, *et al.* Two-year neurocognitive effects of olanzapine or low-dose haloperidol in first-episode psychosis. *Biological Psychiatry* 2006;**59**:97–105.

26. Kern RS, Green MF, Marshall BD Jr, *et al.* Risperidone vs. haloperidol on reaction time, manual dexterity, and motor learning in treatment-resistant schizophrenia patients. *Biological Psychiatry* 1998;**44**:726–32.

27. Kivircik Akdede BB, Alptekin K, Kitis A, Arkar H and Akvardar Y. Effects of quetiapine on cognitive functions in schizophrenia. *Progress in Neuro-psychopharmacology & Biological Psychiatry* 2005;**29**:233–8.

28. Wagner M, Quednow BB, Westheide J, *et al.* Cognitive improvement in schizophrenic patients does not require a serotonergic mechanism: Randomized controlled trial of olanzapine vs. amisulpride. *Neuropsychopharmacology* 2005;**30**:381–90.

29. McGurk SR, Carter C, Goldman R, *et al.* The effects of clozapine and risperidone on spatial working memory in schizophrenia. *American Journal of Psychiatry* 2005;**162**:1013–6.

30. Harvey PD, Meltzer H, Simpson GM, *et al.* Improvements in cognitive function following a switch to ziprasidone from conventional antipsychotics, olanzapine, or risperidone in outpatients with schizophrenia. *Schizophrenia Research* 2004;**66**:101–13.

31. McGurk SR, Lee MA, Jayathilake K and Meltzer HY. Cognitive effects of olanzapine treatment in schizophrenia. *Medscape General Medicine* 2004;**6**:27.

32. Harvey PD, Green MF, McGurk SR, *et al.* Changes in cognitive functioning with risperidone and olanzapine treatment: A large-scale, double-blind, randomized study. *Psychopharmacology* 2003;**169**:404–11.

33. Harvey PD, Napolitano JA, Mao L and Gharabawi G. Comparative effects of risperidone and olanzapine on cognition in elderly patients with schizophrenia or schizoaffective disorder. *International Journal of Geriatric Psychiatry* 2003;**18**:820–9.

34. Harvey PD, Siu CO and Romano S. Randomized, controlled, double-blind, multicenter comparison of the cognitive effects of ziprasidone versus olanzapine in acutely ill inpatients with schizophrenia or schizoaffective disorder. *Psychopharmacology* 2003;**172**:324–32.

35. Stip E, Remington GJ, Dursun SM, *et al.* Canadian multicenter trial assessing memory and executive functions in patients with schizophrenia spectrum disorders treated with olanzapine. *Journal of Clinical Psychopharmacology* 2003;**23**:400–4.

36. Sharma T, Hughes C, Soni W, *et al.* Cognitive effects of olanzapine and clozapine treatment in chronic schizophrenia. *Psychopharmacology* 2003;**169**:398–403.

37. Velligan DI, Prihoda TJ, Sui D, *et al.* The effectiveness of quetiapine versus conventional antipsychotics in improving cognitive and functional outcomes in standard treatment settings. *Journal of Clinical Psychiatry* 2003;**64**:524–31.

38. Bilder RM, Goldman RS, Volavka J, *et al.* Neurocognitive effects of clozapine, olanzapine, risperidone, and haloperidol in patients with chronic schizophrenia or schizoaffective disorder. *American Journal of Psychiatry* 2002;**159**:1018–28.

39. Good KP, Kiss I, Buiteman C, *et al.* Improvement in cognitive functioning in patients with first-episode psychosis during treatment with quetiapine: An interim analysis. *British Journal of Psychiatry* 2002;**181**:45–9.

40. Vaiva G, Thomas P, Llorca PM, *et al.* SPECT imaging, clinical features, and cognition before and after low doses of amisulpride in schizophrenic patients with the deficit syndrome. *Psychiatry Research* 2002;**115**:37–48.

41. Velligan DI, Newcomer J, Pultz J, *et al.* Does cognitive function improve with quetiapine in comparison to haloperidol? *Schizophrenia Research* 2002;**53**:239–48.

42. Chua L, Chong SA, Pang E, Ng VP and Chan YH. The effect of risperidone on cognitive functioning in a sample of Asian patients with schizophrenia in Singapore. *Singapore Medical Journal* 2001;**42**:243–6.

43. Fleming K, Thyrum P, Yeh C, *et al.* Cognitive improvement in psychotic subjects treated with "seroquel" (Quetiapine Fumarate): An exploratory study. *Journal of Clinical Psychopharmacology* 2001;**21**:527–9.

44. Potkin SG, Fleming K, Jin Yi, *et al.* Clozapine enhances neurocognition and clinical symptomatology more than standard neuroleptics. *Journal of Clinical Psychopharmacology* 2001;**21**:479–83.

45. Purdon SE, Labelle A and Boulay L. Neuropsychological change in schizophrenia after 6 weeks of clozapine. *Schizophrenia Research* 2001;**48**:57–67.

46. Purdon SE, Malla A, Labelle A and Lit W. Neuropsychological change in patients with schizophrenia after treatment with

quetiapine or haloperidol. *Journal of Psychiatry & Neuroscience* 2001;**26**:137–49.

47. Smith RC, Infante M, Singh A, *et al*. The effects of olanzapine on neurocognitive functioning in medication-refractory schizophrenia. *International Journal of Neuropsychopharmacology* 2001;**3**:239–50.

48. Purdon SE, Jones BD, Stip E, *et al*. Neuropsychological change in early phase schizophrenia during 12 months of treatment with olanzapine, risperidone and haloperidol. The Canadian Collaborative Group for research in schizophrenia. *Archives of General Psychiatry* 2000;**57**:249–58.

49. Lee MA, Jayathilake K and Meltzer HY. A comparison of the effect of clozapine with typical neuroleptics on cognitive function on neuroleptic responsive schizophrenia. *Schizophrenia Research* 1999;**37**:1–11.

50. Galletly CA, Clark CR, McFarlane AC and Weber DL. Effects of clozapine for non-treatment-resistant patients with schizophrenia. *Psychiatric Services* 1999;**50**:101–3.

51. Kern RS, Green MF, Barringer MD, *et al*. Risperidone versus haloperidol on secondary memory: Can newer medications aid learning? *Schizophrenia Bulletin* 1999;**25**:223–32.

52. Manschreck TC, Redmond DA, Candela SF and Maher BA. Effects of clozapine on psychiatric symptoms, cognition, and functional outcome in schizophrenia. *The Journal of Neuropsychiatry and Clinical Neurosciences* 1999;**11**:481–9.

53. Meltzer HY and McGurk SR. The effects of clozapine, risperidone, and olanzapine on cognitive function in schizophrenia. *Schizophrenia Bulletin* 1999;**25**:233–55.

54. Rossi A, Mancini F, Stratta P, *et al*. Risperidone, negative symptoms and cognitive deficit in schizophrenia: An open study. *Acta Psychiatrica Scandinavica* 1997;**95**:40–3.

55. Serper MR and Chou JCY. Novel neuroleptics improve attentional functioning in schizophrenia patients:

56. Fujii DE, Ahmed I, Jokumsen M, *et al*. The effects of clozapine on cognitive functioning in treatment-resistant schizophrenic patients. *The Journal of Neuropsychiatry and Clinical Neurosciences* 1997;**9**:240–5.

57. Hoff AL, Faustman WO, Wieneke M, *et al*. The effects of clozapine on symptom reduction, neurocognitive function, and clinical management in treatment-refractory state hospital schizophrenic inpatients. *Neuropsychopharmacology* 1996;**15**:361–9.

58. Lee MA, Thompson P and Meltzer H. Effects of clozapine on cognitive function in schizophrenia. *Journal of Clinical Psychiatry* 1994;**55**:82–7.

59. Buchanan RW, Holstein C and Breier A. The comparative efficacy and long-term effect of clozapine treatment on neuropsychological test performance. *Biological Psychiatry* 1994;**36**:717–25.

60. Hagger C, Buckley P, Kenny JT, *et al*. Improvement in cognitive functions and psychiatric symptoms in treatment-refractory schizophrenic patients receiving clozapine. *Biological Psychiatry* 1993;**34**:702 12.

61. Harvey PD and Keefe RS. Studies of cognitive change in patients with schizophrenia following novel antipsychotic treatment. *American Journal of Psychiatry* 2001;**158**:176–84.

62. Woodward ND, Purdon SE, Meltzer HY, *et al*. A meta-analysis of neuropsychological change to clozapine, olanzapine, quetiapine, and risperidone in schizophrenia. *International Journal of Neuropsychopharmacology* 2005;**8**:457–72.

63. Carpenter WT and Gold JM. Another view of therapy for cognition in schizophrenia. *Biological Psychiatry* 2002;**51**:969–71.

64. Lieberman JA, Stroup TS, McEvoy JP, *et al*. Effectiveness of antipsychotic drugs in patients with chronic schizophrenia. *New England Journal of Medicine* 2005;**353**:1209–23.

65. Keefe RS, Bilder RM, Davis SM, *et al*. Neurocognitive effects of antipsychotic

Ziprasidone and aripiprazole. *CNS Spectrums* 1997;**2**:56–9.

medications in patients with chronic schizophrenia in the CATIE trial. *Archives of General Psychiatry* 2007;**64**:633 47.

66. Rosenheck RA. Open forum: Effectiveness versus efficacy of second-generation antipsychotics: Haloperidol without anticholinergics as a comparator. *Psychiatric Services* 2005;**56**:85–92.

67. Hoyberg OJ, Fensbo C, Remvig J, *et al.* Risperidone versus perphenazine in the treatment of chronic schizophrenic patients with acute exacerbations. *Acta Psychiatrica Scandinavica* 1993;**88**:395–402.

68. Fruensgaard K, Wollenberg J, Hansen KM, Fensbo C and Sihm F. Loxapine versus perphenazine in psychotic patients. A double-blind, randomized, multicentre trial. *Current Medical Research and Opinion* 1978;**5**:601–7.

69. Van Putten T, Marder SR, Wirshing WC, *et al.* Neuroleptic plasma levels. *Schizophrenia Bulletin* 1991;**17**:197–216.

70. Sweet RA, Pollock BG, Mulsant, *et al.* Pharmacologic profile of perphenazine's metabolites. *Journal of Clinical Psychopharmacology* 2000;**20**:181–7.

71. Haro JM, Edgell ET, Jones PB, *et al.* The European Schizophrenia Outpatient Health Outcomes (SOHO) study: Rationale, methods and recruitment. *Acta Psychiatrica Scandinavica* 2003;**107**:222–32.

72. Keefe RS, Sweeney JA, Gu H, *et al.* Effects of olanzapine, quetiapine, and risperidone on neurocognitive function in early psychosis: A randomized, double-blind 52-week comparison. *American Journal of Psychiatry* 2007;**164**:1061–71.

73. Davidson M, Galderisi S, Weiser M, *et al.* Cognitive effects of antipsychotics drugs in first-episode schizophrenia and schizophreniform disorder: A randomized, open-label clinical trial (EUFEST). *American Journal of Psychiatry* (In press).

74. Goldbert GE, Goldman RS, Burdick KE, *et al.* Cognitive improvement after treatment with second-generation antipsychotic medications in first-episode

schizophrenia: Is it a practice effect? *Archives of General Psychiatry* 2007;**64**:1115–22.

75. Keefe RS, Malhotra AK, Meltzer H, *et al.* Efficacy and safety of donepezil in patients with schizophrenia or schizoaffective disorder: A 12-week, randomized, double-blind, placebo-controlled trial. *Neuropsychopharmacology* 2008;**33**:1217–28.

76. Castner SA, Williams GV, Goldman-Rakic PS. Reversal of antipsychotic-induced working memory deficits by short-term dopamine D1 receptor stimulation. *Science* 2000;**287**:2020–2.

77. Robbins TW. The 5-choice serial reaction time task: Behavioural pharmacology and functional neurochemistry. *Psychopharmacology* 2002;**163**:362–80.

78. Harvey PD, Moriarty PJ, Serper MR, *et al.* Practice-related improvement in information processing with novel antipsychotic treatment. *Schizophrenia Research* 2000;**46**:139–48.

79. Harvey PD, Rabinowitz J, Eerdekens M, *et al.* Treatment of cognitive impairment in early psychosis: A comparison of risperidone and haloperidol in a large long-term trial. *American Journal of Psychiatry* 2005;**162**:1888–95.

80. Buchanan RW, Davis M, Goff D, *et al.* A Summary of the FDA-NIMH-MATRICS workshop on clinical trial designs for neurocognitive drugs for schizophrenia. *Schizophrenia Bulletin* 2005;**31**:5–19.

81. Green MF, Nuechterlein KH, Kern RS, *et al.* Functional co-primary measures for clinical trials in schizophrenia: Results from the MATRICS psychometric and standardization study. *American Journal of Psychiatry* 2008;**165**:221–8.

82. McGurk SR, Twamley EW, Sitzer DI, *et al.* A meta-analysis of cognitive remediation in schizophrenia. *American Journal of Psychiatry* 2007;**164**:1791–802.

83. Medalia A, Revheim N and Casey M. The remediation of problem-solving skills in schizophrenia. *Schizophrenia Bulletin* 2001;**27**:259–67.

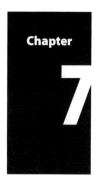

Chapter 7

Vocational outcomes

Sandra G. Resnick and Robert A. Rosenheck

For many, becoming a "worker" in the competitive economy is an important developmental milestone and an acquisition of a valued social role [1]. Employment provides more than fiscal benefits, as being a worker often provides both social integration and daily structure. For individuals with schizophrenia, becoming a worker can lead to improvements in well-being [2], self-esteem [3], and provide an identity beyond "patient" [4].

It has been hypothesized that appropriate symptom management through psychopharmacology is critical for work success. A corollary to this hypothesis is that the second-generation antipsychotic medications (SGAs) will lead to greater work success as compared to treatment with first-generation agents (FGAs). If newer antipsychotic agents lead to greater symptom improvement, reduced side effects, and improved neurocognition, then this may in turn result in improvements in employment [5,6].

Several studies have already examined the differential effects of FGAs and SGAs on employment. The conclusions to be drawn from these studies are equivocal, as most involved small samples and brief follow-up periods, and used observational or retrospective methods which may not control for confounding factors that affect the relationship between medication and outcomes [5]. When compared to FGAs, greater employment was observed in some studies of risperidone [7] and olanzapine [8], and an observational study showed an association between use of SGAs and higher income [6]. However, several other studies failed to demonstrate benefits of SGAs on employment [9–11].

The data from the Clinical Antipsychotic Trials of Intervention Effectiveness (CATIE) schizophrenia trial provided an opportunity to prospectively examine the differential effect of FGAs and SGAs on employment outcomes. A baseline analysis suggested that increased severity of schizophrenia-specific symptoms, greater neurocognitive deficits, and lower scores on a measure of intrapsychic functioning were significant barriers to employment [12]. If SGAs lead to greater improvement on these measures, they could lead to improved employment outcomes as well.

This chapter describes the results from Phase 1 of CATIE that examined the relationship between assignment to five different antipsychotic medications and two outcomes: employment and participation in psychiatric rehabilitation. We hypothesized that outcomes would be superior for those assigned to one of the four SGAs (olanzapine, quetiapine, risperidone, ziprasidone) as compared to those assigned to perphenazine. We also examined participation in psychiatric or psychosocial rehabilitation (PSR), which includes participation in vocational rehabilitation.

Antipsychotic Trials in Schizophrenia, ed. T. Scott Stroup and Jeffrey A. Lieberman. Published by Cambridge University Press. © Cambridge University Press 2010.

Methods

Details of the CATIE study were described previously [13] and in Chapters 1 and 2. This report focuses on Phase 1, in which 1,460 participants were randomly assigned to one of five medications: olanzapine, perphenazine, quetiapine, risperidone, or ziprasidone. Included in these analyses were 1,121 individuals with schizophrenia for whom employment data were available at both baseline and at least one follow-up point.

Measures

Baseline background and demographic variables included age, gender, ethnicity, education level, receipt of public support income, severity of schizophrenia and depressive symptoms, co-morbid psychiatric diagnoses, quality of life, presence/absence of movement medication side effects, and a composite neurocognitive functioning score. The quality of life and neurocognitive measures are described in detail in Chapters 5 and 6, respectively.

Three dependent variables were used in the analyses presented here. The first and primary dependent variable is a dichotomous measure of employment status. Participants were categorized as working if they reported at least 1 day worked for pay, or an average of at least 1 hour worked per week, over the prior 30 days. These measures were concordant in 99% of cases.

The second dependent variable is a dichotomous measure representing participation in PSR, defined as self-report of at least one visit in the previous month in any of the following service types: PSR, vocational rehabilitation, or supported employment. The third dependent variable is a continuous measure of earned income in the 30 days prior to each interview.

Data analysis
Bivariate comparisons

Chi-square analyses and t-tests were conducted on all study variables between those included in the final sample and those excluded because of missing data. Bivariate comparisons of baseline demographic and clinical variables were then conducted by medication assignment in order to assess baseline group equivalence among those with follow-up data. Where group differences were identified, the variables for which differences were observed were included as covariates in the subsequent analyses.

Primary analyses

Two sets of repeated measures models were used to examine the relationships between medication assignment and both paid employment and participation in PSR. General estimation equation modeling [14] was used to adjust estimates for the correlation of data from the same subjects. General estimation equation modeling uses all available data assigned to its actual date of collection and, thus, is preferable to other methods for analyzing longitudinal data.

A third set of analyses examined the relationship between medication assignment and earned income. Mixed-models analysis with an autocorrelation variance, that is, co-variance matrix, was used to examine earned income at each time point.

Because randomization took place under four separate regimens (including and excluding individuals with tardive dyskinesia (TD), including and excluding individuals randomized to ziprasidone), analyses are conducted on four different Analytic Sets with overlapping membership described in Chapter 2 and elsewhere [15]. Each Analytic Set includes participants with an equal chance of being randomly assigned to the treatments under comparison.

The primary comparison between the four treatments available at the beginning of the trial (e.g., prior to FDA approval of ziprasidone) was an overall 3-degree of freedom test. This test was performed on Analytic Set I, which excluded participants with TD and those randomized to ziprasidone. The three SGAs (olanzapine, quetiapine, risperidone) were compared with perphenazine with a Hochberg adjustment for multiple comparisons [16] in which the smallest p value was compared to $0.05/3 = 0.017$ and the largest to $p < 0.05$.

Next, using Analytic Set II (including participants with TD but excluding those randomized to perphenazine) the SGAs (olanzapine, quetiapine, risperidone) were compared to each other at $p < 0.05$.

Analytic Sets III and IV were used to compare ziprasidone to the other four drugs among participants randomized after ziprasidone became available, but with participants with TD excluded from comparisons with perphenazine. Hochberg adjustment for four pairwise comparisons was used to compare ziprasidone and perphenazine in dataset III, and ziprasidone to the other three drugs using dataset IV. The smallest p value was considered significant if $p < 0.05/4 = 0.013$.

Exploratory analyses

We conducted two sets of exploratory analyses to further examine the relationship between participation in PSR and employment. First, bivariate comparisons were made to examine baseline differences between the group of those who reported having worked at least once during the study period and those who had not. Variables that discriminated between the two groups (were significant in bivariate comparisons) were entered into three multivariate models to identify baseline predictors of employment status, earned income, and participation in PSR in the total combined sample.

For the final set of analyses, the two exploratory models from above were repeated with the addition of participation in PSR as a time-varying, lagged independent variable. Thus, participation in PSR was evaluated as a predictor of employment and earnings *at the next assessment point.*

Results

Sample characteristics and bivariate comparisons

Participants were assigned to perphenazine (N = 213), olanzapine (N = 273), quetiapine (N = 244), risperidone (N = 258), or ziprasidone (N = 133). The sample was an average of 41 years old (SD = 11.0), had slightly greater than a high school education (M = 12.1, SD = 2.3), were predominantly male (74%), White (61%), and never married (59%). There were no significant differences on study variables between those included in the final sample (N = 1,121) and those excluded due to missing data (n = 339).

Chi-square analyses and t-tests compared all selected background and demographic baseline variables between medication groups (Table 7.1). There was a significant overall difference between groups in this sample only on the percentage of individuals with a co-occurring depressive disorder as assessed by the SCID at baseline ($\chi^2(4) = 11.89$, $p = 0.02$). No other group differences were observed, including duration of participation. Overall, almost 60% of participants remained on initial study medication for 6 months or

Table 7.1. Baseline characteristics of participants

	Perphenazine N = 213 n (%)	Olanzapine N = 273 n (%)	Quetiapine N = 244 n (%)	Risperidone N = 258 n (%)	Ziprasidone N = 133 n (%)	Total N = 1,121 n (%)
Male	157 (73.7%)	195 (71.4%)	189 (77.5%)	190 (73.6%)	96 (72.2%)	827 (73.8%)
Race (N = 1,120)						
White	128 (60.1%)	160 (58.6%)	163 (66.8%)	154 (59.7%)	82 (62.1%)	687 (61.3%)
Black	72 (33.8%)	98 (35.9%)	73 (29.9%)	92 (35.7%)	42 (31.8%)	377 (33.7%)
Other	13 (6.1%)	15 (5.5%)	8 (3.3%)	12 (4.7%)	8 (6.1%)	56 (5.0%)
Hispanic	19 (8.9%)	33 (12.1%)	36 (14.8%)	25 (9.7%)	15 (11.3%)	128 (11.4%)
Public support income	89 (41.8%)	90 (33.0%)	86 (35.3%)	76 (29.5%)	51 (38.4%)	392 (35.0%)
None Any public support	124 (58.2%)	183 (67.0%)	158 (64.8%)	182 (70.5%)	82 (61.7%)	729 (65.0%)
Never married	123 (57.8%)	154 (56.4%)	149 (61.1%)	158 (61.2%)	77 (57.9%)	661 (59.0%)
	Perphenazine N = 213 n (%)	**Olanzapine N = 273 n (%)**	**Quetiapine N = 244 n (%)**	**Risperidone N = 258 n (%)**	**Ziprasidone N = 133 n (%)**	**Total N = 1,121 n (%)**
Current co-morbidities						
Alcohol use disorder	17 (8.0%)	14 (5.1%)	18 (7.4%)	17 (6.6%)	7 (5.3%)	73 (6.5%)
Drug use disorder	29 (13.6%)	27 (9.9%)	18 (7.4%)	25 (9.7%)	13 (9.8%)	112 (10.0%)
Major depression[1]	23 (10.8%)	29 (10.6%)	16 (6.6%)	31 (12.0%)	23 (17.3%)	122 (10.9%)
Any paid employment	176 (82.6%)	226 (82.8%)	193 (79.1%)	218 (84.5%)	107 (80.5%)	920 (82.1%)
None Part-time	22 (10.3%)	21 (7.7%)	28 (11.5%)	23 (8.9%)	20 (15.0%)	114 (10.2%)
Full-time	15 (7.0%)	26 (9.5%)	23 (9.4%)	17 (6.6%)	6 (4.5%)	87 (7.8%)
Any participation in PSR						
No	161 (75.6%)	211 (77.3%)	183 (75.3%)	184 (71.6%)	98 (73.7%)	837 (74.8%)
Yes	52 (24.4%)	62 (22.7%)	60 (24.7%)	73 (28.4%)	35 (26.3%)	282 (25.2%)

123

Table 7.1. (cont.)

	Perphenazine N = 213 n (%)	Olanzapine N = 273 n (%)	Quetiapine N = 244 n (%)	Risperidone N = 258 n (%)	Ziprasidone N = 133 n (%)	Total N = 1,121 n (%)
Movement side effects (n = 940)[2]						
Tardive dyskinesia	6 (2.9%)	13 (6.0%)	12 (3.7%)	8 (3.74%)	7 (6.7%)	46 (4.9%)
Akathisia	23 (11.0%)	39 (18.0%)	25 (12.9%)	30 (14.0%)	15 (14.3%)	132 (14.0%)
EPS	4 (1.9%)	9 (4.2%)	4 (3.3%)	7 (3.3%)	6 (5.7%)	30 (3.2%)
	M (SD)	M (SD)	M (SD)	M (SD)	M (SD)	M (SD)
Age	40.5 (10.8)	41.4 (10.6)	41.1 (11.4)	41.2 (11.2)	40.3 (11.1)	41.0 (11.0)
Years education (N = 1,116)	12.2 (2.1)	12.3 (2.1)	12.1 (2.5)	12.0 (2.1)	12.0 (2.7)	12.1 (2.3)
PANSS Total (N = 1,120)	73.6 (18.3)	75.0 (18.0)	75.7 (17.1)	76.6 (16.6)	76.3 (18.6)	75.4 (17.6)
Positive	17.6 (6.0)	18.3 (5.3)	18.7 (5.5)	18.5 (5.6)	18.3 (5.8)	18.3 (5.6)
Negative	20.1 (6.4)	20.1 (6.5)	19.9 (6.6)	20.5 (6.1)	20.3 (6.4)	20.2 (6.4)
General	35.9 (9.7)	36.6 (9.5)	37.1 (9.2)	37.6 (8.7)	37.6 (9.7)	36.9 (9.3)
Depression (Calgary)	1.6 (0.6)	1.6 (0.6)	1.5 (0.5)	1.6 (0.6)	1.6 (0.6)	1.6 (0.6)
BMI (N = 1,110)	30.0 (7.1)	29.5 (6.8)	30.2 (6.8)	30.2 (7.6)	30.5 (7.1)	30.0 (7.1)
	Perphenazine N = 213 M (SD)	Olanzapine N = 273 M (SD)	Quetiapine N = 244 M (SD)	Risperidone N = 258 M (SD)	Ziprasidone N = 133 M (SD)	Total N = 1,121 M (SD)
Heinrichs-Carpenter QOL total (N = 1,118)	2.8 (1.3)	2.7 (1.1)	2.7 (1.2)	2.7 (1.0)	2.6 (1.0)	2.7 (1.1)
Neurocognition Composite	0.00 (0.63)	−0.02 (0.62)	−0.02 (0.65)	−0.05 (0.61)	−0.04 (0.66)	−0.02 (0.65)
Lehman QOL Total (N = 1,117)	2.8 (1.1)	2.8 (1.1)	2.8 (1.1)	2.7 (1.0)	2.7 (1.1)	2.8 (1.1)

Notes: [1] p = 0.05.
[2]Excludes those with tardive dyskinesia.

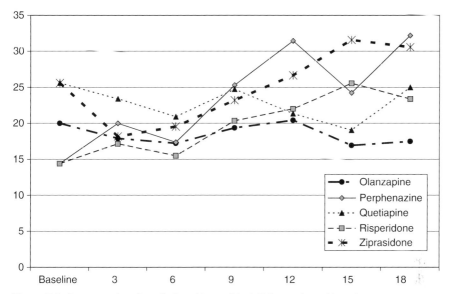

Figure 7.1. Percentage (unadjusted) of participants (N = 1,121) reporting paid employment in the past month.

longer; 41% remained on initial study medication for at least 12 months, although this percentage had decreased to 30% by 18 months.

Across Phase 1, 201 (17.9%) participants reported at least 1 month with 1 day of employment. Rates of employment varied considerably throughout the trial, with a low of approximately 15% at baseline for those assigned to perphenazine and risperidone, to a high of slightly over 30% for those on ziprasidone and perphenazine at 18 months (Figure 7.1). For those who worked, the mean number of days worked in the past 30 days was 14.2 (SD = 7.2). A somewhat greater number (N = 282, 25.2%) reported at least one visit involving PSR services. There was a moderate but significant relationship between employment status and participation in PSR ($\Phi = 0.21$; $p < 0.0001$), suggesting that participation in PSR is associated weakly but significantly with current employment.

Primary analyses

Four separate analyses on the four data sets described above were conducted in order to examine the relationship between medication assignment and the two dependent variables, adjusting for co-morbid depressive disorder. None of the models yielded significant differences between treatment groups on employment at $p < 0.05$ (i.e., even without adjustment for multiple comparisons (Table 7.2; Figure 7.1)). There were also no significant relationships between medication assignment and likelihood of participation in PSR.

Exploratory analyses

The bivariate and multivariate relationships between potential baseline predictors with both employment measures and participation in PSR were examined next. Bivariate comparisons on baseline values indicated that the group of individuals who had worked at any time during the study period was younger, more likely to be White, had lower levels

Table 7.2. Relationships between antipsychotic medication, paid employment, and PSR services in Phase I (N = 1,121)

Data Set	Any paid employment			Any PSR		
	OR	95% CI		OR	95% CI	
I. [1,2]Perphenazine (reference)						
Olanzapine	1.00	0.94	1.06	1.00	0.96	1.04
Quetiapine	1.01	0.95	1.07	1.01	0.97	1.06
Risperidone	0.98	0.93	1.03	1.01	0.96	1.05
II. Risperidone (reference)						
Olanzapine	1.01	0.96	1.06	0.98	0.94	1.02
Quetiapine	1.03	0.98	1.08	1.00	0.95	1.04
III. [1]Perphenazine (reference)						
Ziprasidone	1.02	0.95	1.11	0.98	0.93	1.03
IV. Ziprasidone (reference)						
Olanzapine	0.98	0.91	1.05	0.98	0.93	1.03
Quetiapine	0.96	0.89	1.03	1.01	0.95	1.07
Risperidone	0.97	0.91	1.05	1.01	0.95	1.07

Notes: All comparisons are not significant.
[1]Excludes participants with tardive dyskinesia.
[2]Excludes participants on ziprasidone.

of public support income, greater years of education, lower Positive and Negative Syndrome Scale (PANSS) total scores, less severe tardive dyskinesia and greater quality of life as assessed by both the Heinrichs-Carpenter and the Lehman Quality of Life Scale, and more positive neurocognitive status than those who had not worked during the course of the study (Table 7.3).

These variables were then entered into three multivariate models to examine the relationship between these potential predictors from the bivariate analyses with the three dependent measures (both employment measures and participation in PSR). Greater age was associated with a decreased likelihood of both employment (odds ratio [OR] = 0.96; 95% confidence interval [CI] = 0.96 to 0.96) and participation in PSR (OR = 0.98; 95% CI = 0.98 to 0.99), but not earned income. Higher baseline public support income was associated with a decreased likelihood of employment (OR = 0.95; 95% CI = 0.94 to 0.97) and decreased earned income ($F = 5.72$; $p = 0.02$) but with a small but significantly increased likelihood of participation in PSR services (OR = 1.04; 95% CI = 1.02 to 1.06). No other variables were significantly associated with any outcome.

The last set of analyses repeated the two models exploring employment outcomes with the addition of a time-varying measure of PSR participation, that is, the relationship between participation in PSR and employment at the subsequent assessment point. Participation in PSR was associated with a small but significantly increased likelihood of employment

Table 7.3. Baseline bivariate comparisons between those who worked at any time during the study period (N = 201) and those who did not work (n = 920)[1]

	No work		Some work		Test of significance
	N	%	N	%	
Marital status					
Never married	380	41.3%	80	39.8%	$\chi^2(1)=0.15$, ns
Ever married	540	58.7%	121	60.2%	
Gender					
Male	672	73.0%	155	77.1%	$\chi^2(1)=1.41$, ns
Female	248	27.7%	46	22.9%	
Race (n = 1,121)					
White	548	59.6%	139	69.2%	$\chi^2(2)=6.86$, p=0.03
Black	325	35.4%	52	25.9%	
Other	46	5.0%	10	5.0%	
Hispanic					
No	812	88.3%	181	90.1%	$\chi^2(1)=0.52$, ns
Yes	108	11.7%	20	10.0%	
	No work		Some work		Test of significance
	N	%	N	%	
Public support income					
None	288	31.3%	104	51.7%	$\chi^2(2)=32.7$, p<0.0001
$1–$650	324	35.2%	59	29.4%	
>$650	308	33.5%	38	18.9%	
Current alcohol use disorder					
No	860	93.5%	188	93.5%	$\chi^2(1)=0.00$, ns
Yes	60	6.5%	13	6.5%	
Current drug use disorder					
No	827	89.9%	182	90.6%	$\chi^2(1)=0.08$, ns
Yes	93	10.1%	19	9.5%	
Current major depression diagnosis					
No	815	88.6%	184	91.5%	$\chi^2(1)=1.5$, ns
Yes	105	11.4%	17	8%	
	M	SD	M	SD	
Age	41.5	11.2	38.8	9.9	$t(320)=3.31$, p=0.001

Table 7.3. (*cont.*)

	No work		Some work		Test of significance
	N	%	N	%	
Years education (N = 116)	12.0	2.2	12.6	2.6	$t(267) = -3.15, p = 0.0018$
PANSS Total (N = 1,120)	76.5	17.3	70.6	18.4	$t(1,118) = 4.33, p < 0.0001$
PANSS Positive	18.5	5.5	17.4	6.0	$t(1,118) = 2.58, p < 0.01$
PANSS Negative	20.6	6.4	18.5	6.1	$t(1,118) = 4.28, p < 0.0001$
PANSS General	37.4	9.2	34.7	9.6	$t(1,118) = 3.67, p = 0.0003$
Depression (Calgary Scale) (N = 1,120)					
Movement Side effects	1.6	0.6	1.5	0.5	$t(1,119) = 1.39$, ns
AIMS severity (TD) total	0.27	0.47	0.19	0.34	$t(381) = 2.95, p < 0.003$
Barnes akathisia total	0.36	0.56	0.29	0.47	$t(336) = 1.74$, ns
Simpson-Angus total	0.22	0.33	0.22	0.30	$t(1,119) = 0.20$, ns
BMI (n = 1,101)	30.1	7.1	29.9	6.9	$t(1,108) = 0.33$, ns
Heinrichs-Carpenter QOL total (n = 1,118)	2.5	1.0	3.5	1.1	$t(1,116) = -12.46, p < 0.0001$
Lehman QOL Total (n = 1,117)	2.6	1.0	3.6	1.1	$t(1,115) = -12.21, p < 0.0001$
Neurocognition Composite	−.05	0.63	0.11	0.62	$t(1,119) = -3.34, p = 0.0009$

Box 1 Correlates of Employment in CATIE Phase 1

Younger age
White race
Lower levels of public income support
Greater number of years of education
Lower Positive and Negative Syndrome Scale (PANSS) Score
Less severe abnormal involuntary movements
Better quality of life (higher scores on the Heinrichs-Carpenter and Lehman Scales)
Higher neurocognitive summary score
Bolded items significant in multivariable model

---

at the following assessment point (OR = 1.06; 95% CI = 1.02 to 1.09) but not with earned income.

Conclusions

In Phase 1 of the CATIE schizophrenia trial, there were no significant relationships between randomly assigned medications and either employment outcomes or participation in PSR. Although these findings deserve replication, they provide the most methodologically rigorous examination yet conducted of the relationship of SGAs (other than clozapine) to employment outcomes.

However, because there were significant differences in time to all-cause discontinuation between the drugs evaluated in both the clozapine [17] and ziprasidone [18] substudies in the Phase 2 CATIE trials, the authors also examined these data sets for differences between drugs and employment outcomes. There were no significant differences between groups in either substudy. In contrast, Percudani et al. identified eight studies which found a positive relationship between employment and clozapine [5], although seven of eight studies were based on uncontrolled, naturalistic designs. In light of these discrepant findings, as well as the smaller samples in the clozapine component of CATIE Phase 2 (N = 99), the finding of no benefit for clozapine should be considered with caution.

Employment rates varied considerably throughout the study, suggesting that individuals with schizophrenia have a difficult time obtaining stable employment. In the current study, only 18% of study participants reported working at any time point, a rate that is consistent with the employment base rate for individuals with schizophrenia [19].

An important factor negatively associated with employment identified by this study is receipt of public support income. This relationship, consistently demonstrated in past research [12,20–22], suggests that many individuals who rely on public support income fear that employment income will jeopardize their benefits, including associated medical benefits [23–25]. In response to these disincentives, the Social Security Administration has developed work incentive programs that allow for trial work periods, although many recipients are either unaware of this program or are unclear about its requirements [23].

Although we did not observe an association between medication and employment, participation in PSR was significantly associated with subsequent employment. In general, rates of paid employment are higher for individuals participating in vocational rehabilitation [26]. However, there were low rates of participation in PSR in the CATIE sample—only 25% of participants received any PSR services during the 18-month study period.

Reasons for the low rates of both participation in PSR and employment cannot be determined from available data, but the most probable explanation is that PSR services for people with severe mental illness were simply not available. Most troubling is the low rate of participation in vocational rehabilitation, and especially evidence-based supported employment.

Supported employment is a vocational rehabilitation approach that focuses on individualized and rapid search for competitive jobs in the community. Supported employment is considered to be an evidence-based practice, with 11 methodologically sound randomized controlled trials indicating higher rates of competitive employment for those participating in supported employment when compared to control groups of other types of vocational rehabilitation [27]. Supported employment has not been widely implemented [28], even though it has been identified as a "best practice" in recent reviews [29], and increasingly considered to be part of a "recovery" based mental health system [30–32]. Two large dissemination projects are currently in progress designed to increase the number of evidence-based supported employment programs in the United States, one in the public sector [30] and the other in the Veterans Health Administration [33]. These projects should not only increase the availability of supported employment services, but should also help to identify facilitators and barriers to implementation which will aid in future efforts.

Several limitations should be noted. The relationship between medication assignment and employment may be significant with regard to some types of employment; however, this cannot be determined from the available data. Similarly, participants were asked about participation in various services, including PSR, vocational rehabilitation, and supported employment. Participants may have not known formal labels for services, and thus may have under-reported such participation. The definition of employment used here was based on self-report, and did not discriminate between competitive, transitional, or sheltered employment. However, the rate of overall employment in this sample is similar to published rates of competitive employment for individuals with severe mental illness not participating in vocational rehabilitation, which range from 10% to 23% [19,34].

Another potential limitation is from data loss due to attrition, which has been addressed in previous reports on CATIE [15,35]. While overall attrition was substantial because CATIE was an 18-month trial, dropout rates were similar, and mostly lower, than those in other SGA trials when comparisons are made at similar time points [35]. Differences between pairs of treatments in 18-month attrition were modest, ranging from 1% to 15%. The largest difference in attrition was between olanzapine and ziprasidone (15%). To the extent that this difference introduces selection bias, it would favor olanzapine since patients tend to do better at later assessments, but no significant differences were observed in employment between these two medications. Nevertheless, these results cannot be considered definitive in view of the substantial losses to follow-up in the later months of the trial.

Although the CATIE study is notable for the diversity of geographic locations and mental health settings from which the sample was recruited, the generalizability of these findings is uncertain. These findings may not apply to individuals with current TD, as individuals with TD were not randomized to perphenazine, or to individuals who are satisfied with their current medication. In addition, the follow-up period was shorter than the 18-month duration of the trial due to medication changes and study discontinuation. However, studies of supported employment have shown short-term divergence between treatment groups, with significant differences noted as early as the second study month [36], and participation in CATIE ranged from 3.5 to 9.2 months across treatments [13]. As such, a treatment that positively influences employment outcomes could show this effect rapidly.

Employment in the competitive economy is a primary goal of recovery-oriented behavioral health services. This study suggests that SGAs are no more likely to facilitate achievement of that goal than FGAs, at least intermediate or low potency FGAs like perphenazine. While antipsychotic medication is an important component of treatment for schizophrenia, psychiatric rehabilitation services such as supported employment are clearly essential to achieving recovery goals.

References

1. Hunt MG. *We Are What We Do: Examining Social Roles of People With Serious Mental Illness and Their Parents.* Bowling Green, OH: Bowling Green State University; 2005.

2. Thoits PA. On merging identity theory and stress research. *Social Psychology Quarterly* 1991;54:101–12.

3. Bond GR, Resnick SG, Drake RE, Xie H, McHugo GJ and Bebout RR. Does competitive employment improve nonvocational outcomes for people with severe mental illness? *Journal of Consulting and Clinical Psychology* 2001;69:489–501.

4. Wolfensberger W. A brief overview of Social Role Valorization. *Mental Retardation* 2000;38:105–23.

5. Percudani M, Barbui C and Tansella M. Effect of second-generation antipsychotics on employment and productivity in individuals with schizophrenia. *Pharmacoeconomics* 2004;**22**:701–18.

6. Salkever D, Slade E and Karakus M. Differential effects of atypical versus typical antipsychotic medication on earnings of schizophrenia patients: Estimates from a prospective naturalistic study. *Pharmacoeconomics* 2006;**24**:123–39.

7. Malla AK, Norman RM, Scholten DJ, Zirul S and Kotteda V. A comparison of long-term outcome in first-episode schizophrenia following treatment with risperidone or a typical antipsychotic. *Journal of Clinical Psychiatry* 2001;**62**:179–84.

8. Hamilton SH, Edgell ET and Revicki DA. Functional outcomes in schizophrenia: A comparison of olanzapine and haloperidol in a European sample. *International Clinical Psychopharmacology* 2000;**15**:245–55.

9. Bond GR, Kim HW, Meyer PS, *et al.* Response to vocational rehabilitation during treatment with first- or second- generation antipsychotics. *Psychiatric Services* 2004;**55**:59–66.

10. Meyer PS, Bond GR and Tunis SL. Comparison between the effects of atypical and traditional antipsychotics on work status for clients in a psychiatric rehabilitation program. *Journal of Clinical Psychiatry* 2002;**63**:108–16.

11. Voruganti L, Cortese L, Oyewumi L, Cernovsky Z, Zirul S and Awad A. Comparative evaluation of conventional and novel antipsychotic drugs with reference to their subjective tolerability, side-effect profile and impact on quality of life. *Schizophrenia Research* 2000;**43**:135–45.

12. Rosenheck R, Leslie D, Keefe R, *et al.* Barriers to employment for people with schizophrenia. *American Journal of Psychiatry* 2006;**163**:411–7.

13. Lieberman JA, Stroup TS, McEvoy JP, *et al.* Effectiveness of antipsychotic drugs in patients with chronic schizophrenia. *New England Journal of Medicine* 2005;**353**:1209–23.

14. Liang K and Zeger S. Regression analysis for correlated data. *Annual Review of Public Health* 1993;**14**:43–68.

15. Rosenheck RA, Leslie DL, Sindelar J, *et al.*, Cost-effectiveness of second generation antipsychotics and perphenazine in the treatment of chronic schizophrenia. *American Journal of Psychiatry* 2006;**163**:2080–9.

16. Hochberg YA. A sharper Bonferroni procedure for multiple tests of significance. *Biometrika* 1988;**75**:800–2.

17. McEvoy JP, Lieberman JA, Stroup TS, *et al.* Effectiveness of clozapine versus olanzapine, quetiapine, and risperidone in patients with chronic schizophrenia who did not respond to prior atypical antipsychotic treatment. *American Journal of Psychiatry* 2006;**163**:600–10.

18. Stroup TS, Lieberman JA, McEvoy JP, *et al.*, Effectiveness of olanzapine, quetiapine, risperidone, and ziprasidone in patients with chronic schizophrenia following discontinuation of a previous atypical antipsychotic. *American Journal of Psychiatry* 2006;**163**:611–22.

19. Mueser K, Salyers M and Mueser P. A prospective analysis of work in schizophrenia. *Schizophrenia Bulletin* 2001;**27**:281–96.

20. Drew D, Drebing CE, Van Ormer A, *et al.* Effects of disability compensation on participation in and outcomes of vocational rehabilitation. *Psychiatric Services* 2001;**52**:1479–84.

21. Resnick SG, Rosenheck RA and Drebing CE. What makes vocational rehabilitation effective?: Program characteristics versus employment outcomes nationally in VA. *Psychological Services* 2006;**3**:239–48.

22. Rosenheck R, Frisman L and Sindelar J. Disability compensation and work among veterans with psychiatric and nonpsychiatric impairments. *Psychiatric Services* 1995;**46**:359–65.

23. O'Day B and Killeen M. Does U.S. federal policy support employment and recovery for people with psychiatric disabilities. *Behavioral Science and the Law* 2002;**20**:559–83.

24. MacDonald-Wilson KL, Rogers ES, Ellison ML, *et al.* A study of the social security work incentives and their relation to perceived barriers to work among persons with psychiatric disability. *Rehabilitation Psychology* 2003;**48**:301–9.

25. Polak P and Warner R. The economic life of seriously mentally ill people in the community. *Psychiatric Services* 1996;**47**:270–4.

26. Bond GR. Supported employment: Evidence for an evidence-based practice. *Psychiatric Rehabilitation Journal* 2004;**27**:345–58.

27. Bond GR, Drake RE, Becker DR. An update on randomized controlled trials of evidence-based supported employment. *Psychiatric Services* 2008;**31**:280–90.

28. Lehman AF, Steinwachs DM and the Survey Co-investigators of the PORT Project. Patterns of usual care for schizophrenia: Initial results from the Schizophrenia Patient Outcomes Research Team (PORT) Client Survey. *Schizophrenia Bulletin* 1998;**24**:11–20.

29. Lehman AF, Kreyenbuhl J, Buchanan RW, *et al.* The Schizophrenia Patient Outcomes Research Team (PORT): Updated treatment recommendations 2003. *Schizophrenia Bulletin* 2004;**30**:193–217.

30. Becker DR, Lynde D and Swanson SJ. Strategies for state-wide implementation of supported employment: The Johnson & Johnson – Dartmouth Community Mental Health Program. *Psychiatric Rehabilitation Journal* 2008;**31**:296–9.

31. President's New Freedom Commission on Mental Health. *Achieving the Promise: Transforming Mental Health Care in America. 2003*: Washington, DC: President's New Freedom Commission on Mental Health; 2003. p. 98.

32. Resnick SG, Rosenheck RA and Lehman AF. An exploratory analysis of recovery and its correlates in people with schizophrenia. *Psychiatric Services* 2004;**55**:540–7.

33. Resnick SG and Rosenheck RA. Dissemination of supported employment in VHA. *Journal of Rehabilitation Research and Development* 2007;**44**:867–77.

34. Anthony WA and Blanch A. Supported employment for persons who are psychiatrically disabled: An historical and conceptual perspective. *Psychosocial Rehabilitation Journal* 1987;**XI**:5–23.

35. Rosenheck RA, Swartz M, McEvoy J, *et al.* Changing perspectives on second generation antipsychotics: Reviewing the cost-effectiveness component of the CATIE trial. *Expert Review of Pharmacoeconomics and Outcomes Research* 2007;**7**:103–11.

36. Drake RE, McHugo GJ, Becker DR, Anthony WA and Clark RE. The New Hampshire study of supported employment for people with severe mental illness. *Journal of Consulting and Clinical Psychology* 1996;**2**:391–9.

Chapter 8

Family outcomes

Deborah A. Perlick, Richard Kaczynski, and Robert A. Rosenheck

Despite advances in pharmacotherapy and psychosocial treatments, schizophrenia remains a disabling, lifelong illness which greatly alters the life experience not only of those afflicted, but also the experience of the family members who live with them, support them, and must negotiate through illness exacerbations as well as periods of remission and relative stability. Research has documented that up to 83% [1] of the friends and family members of people diagnosed with schizophrenia experience financial, emotional, and practical burdens. They report time lost from work, unreimbursed medical and other patient-related expenses, limited time for leisure and socializing, elevated symptoms of psychological distress, and disturbed sleep [1–6]. For example, between 30–40% of caregivers of people with schizophrenia score above the standard cut-off for depression (i.e., > 16) on a common survey instrument, the Center for Epidemiological Study of Depression (CES-D) [7,8].

Another problem affecting caregivers is stress related to the stigma of mental illness. Studies have demonstrated that from 40% to 79% of caregivers feel that "most people" devalue caregivers of people with schizophrenia. Specifically, 79% felt that family members were viewed as incompetent and 62% felt that they were blamed for their relative's illness [9]. In response to such perceptions, family members practice social withdrawal and/or secrecy about the relatives' illness in order to avoid embarrassment and anticipated rejection [10]. However, such avoidance limits their access to social support which might serve as a buffer to depressive symptoms.

In addition to its impact on caregiver quality of life, caregiving strain has been associated with other adverse effects for caregivers, including poorer self-rated health and/or chronic medical conditions [11–16], increased primary care physician visits [12,17–19], greater use of psychotropic drugs such as tranquilizers and antidepressants [20–23], and increased risk of medical hospitalization [12]. Thus, prior studies have shown that the caregiving tasks and strains experienced by family members of people with schizophrenia have serious repercussions for their physical and mental health, financial status, and general quality of life. These costs for the individual caregiver in turn have costs for society [24].

Family burden as an outcome variable in clinical trials

The findings from studies of caregiving cited above suggest that it is important to examine caregiving strain as a treatment outcome variable. Studies of psychosocial treatment for schizophrenia and related mental disorders have increasingly done so. In their pioneering study of family psychoeducation, Falloon and colleagues found that reductions in family

Antipsychotic Trials in Schizophrenia, ed. T. Scott Stroup and Jeffrey A. Lieberman. Published by Cambridge University Press. © Cambridge University Press 2010.

133

burden associated with family psychoeducation were associated with improvements in patient clinical status and reductions in relapse over time [25,26]. More recently a meta-analysis of 18 studies found that family intervention of at least 6 weeks' duration was effective in reducing family burden [27]. To our knowledge, however, only one prior study comparing different pharmacotherapies has included family burden as an outcome variable. Rosenheck *et al.* [28] compared the effectiveness of clozapine vs. haloperidol in reducing the burden experienced by family members of veterans with treatment-resistant schizophrenia and found a reduction in some but not all burden factors with treatment with clozapine over 12 months.

Evaluation of family burden in CATIE

The design of CATIE permitted investigation of the impact of random assignment to the first-generation antipsychotic perphenazine and four second-generation drugs (olanzapine, quetiapine, risperidone, or ziprasidone) on family outcomes as measured by four factors: *problem behavior, resource demands and disruption, impairment in activities of daily living*, and *patient helpfulness* over an 18-month study period. Consistent with the results of prior studies [28], we hypothesized that the family caregivers of patients assigned to second-generation antipsychotics would report less burden overall over 18 months than the caregivers of patients assigned to perphenazine.

Methods

Participants

CATIE was conducted between January 2001 and December 2004 at 57 US sites. Participants in the present study were 623 of the 1,460 (42.7%) patients enrolled in CATIE with a diagnosis of schizophrenia who identified caregivers who agreed to be interviewed about their life situation and experiences with the patient. Inclusion and exclusion criteria for patients are described in Chapter 1 and led to the inclusion of a group with chronic schizophrenia meant to represent those in typical treatment settings; individuals experiencing a first episode of psychosis and those with treatment-refractory schizophrenia were excluded. Caregivers were identified by the patient as the family member or friend most directly involved in his/her care.

Bivariate-level comparisons revealed that CATIE participants who identified a caregiver were younger, more often Caucasian, less often Black, less often married, had fewer years in treatment, more years of education, and received less public support and more earned income than those who did not identify a caregiver (Table 8.1).

Patients who identified a caregiver for study also had lower total and negative symptom scores on the Positive and Negative Syndromes Scale (PANSS), but more serious tardive dyskinesia (TD) symptoms as rated on the AIMS, and overall lower neurocognitive functioning, although the effect sizes associated with all comparisons reported were relatively small [29]. All patients and caregivers gave written informed consent to participate in protocols approved by local institutional review boards.

Study procedures

Study procedures are described in detail in Chapter 1 and in previous publications [30,31]. Briefly, patients were initially randomized to olanzapine, perphenazine, quetiapine, risperidone, or ziprasidone under double-blind conditions. Patients who discontinued their first treatment were invited to receive other second-generation antipsychotics, including clozapine if they so desired, with random assignment to specific agents (Phase 2). Open treatment was

Table 8.1. Comparison of patients with/without family interviews [29]

Patient demographics	No family interview (N = 837)		Family interview (N = 623)		t/χ^2	p value	Effect size
	N or mean	SD or %	N or mean	SD or %			
Age	41.83	10.41	38.84	11.75	5.05	<0.001	0.27
Race							
White race	468	56	422	68	20.48[1]	<0.001	0.24
Black race	348	42	178	29	25.65[1]	<0.001	0.27
Hispanic	107	13	63	10	2.23[1]	0.14	0.08
Other	37	4	34	6	0.61[1]	0.44	0.04
Years of education	12.00	2.19	12.24	2.32	−1.98	0.05	0.10
Marital status					39.15[1]	<0.001	0.33
Married	74	9	93	15			
Divorced/separated	269	32	121	19			
Never married	472	57	396	64			
Widowed	21	3	13	2			
Income							
Earned income	87.05	330.42	156.04	582.42	−2.65	0.008	0.14
Public support[2]	612.52	599.12	528.64	585.14	2.67	0.008	0.14
Symptoms/deficits							
PANSS total	74.75	16.68	76.87	18.61	−2.28	0.02	0.12
PANSS positive	18.41	5.50	18.55	5.81	−0.47	0.64	0.02
PANSS negative	19.75	6.13	20.74	6.73	−2.92	0.004	0.15
Depression (Calgary)	1.59	0.57	1.54	0.53	1.48	0.14	0.08
Drug use	1.35	0.72	1.37	0.73	−0.50	0.62	0.03
Alcohol use	1.44	0.74	1.48	0.68	−1.08	0.28	0.06
Cognitive deficits	−0.07	0.63	0.06	0.67	−3.38	0.001	0.19
Side effects							
Tardive dyskinesia (AIMS)	0.31	0.51	0.19	0.36	5.32	<0.001	0.28
Akathisia (Barnes)	0.37	0.55	0.32	0.53	1.51	0.13	0.08
EPS (Simpson Angus)	0.23	0.35	0.20	0.29	1.72	0.09	0.09

Table 8.1. (*cont.*)

Patient demographics	No family interview (N = 837)		Family interview (N = 623)		t/χ^2	p value	Effect size
	N or mean	SD or %	N or mean	SD or %			
Service Use Years in treatment							
Quality of Life	17.53	10.53	15.23	11.39	3.92	<0.001	0.21
Quality of Life	2.66	1.06	2.67	1.08	−0.13	0.90	0.01

Notes: [1]χ^2.
[2]Average monthly payment.
Reprinted with permission from Psychiatric Services, (Copyright 2006). American Psychiatric Association.

also offered to patients who refused or whose treatment failed after further randomization (Phase 3), but only a small number chose first-generation antipsychotics (FGAs).

Measures
Patient measures

The diagnosis of schizophrenia was confirmed by the SCID in all participants [32]. Symptoms of schizophrenia were assessed with the rater-administered PANSS, which yields a total average symptom score, based on 31 items rated from 1 to 7 (with higher scores indicating more severe symptoms), as well as subscales reflecting positive and negative symptoms [33]. Depression was measured with the Calgary Depression Rating Scale [34]. Co-morbid use of drugs and alcohol over the past 3 months was evaluated on a 5-point scale (with 1 = abstinent and 5 = dependence) using the clinician-rated Alcohol Use and Drug Use Scale (AUS/DUS) [35]. Severity of antisocial behavior prior to age 15 was assessed using the sum of six items taken from the SCID including violation of rules (e.g., school truancy or expulsion), running away from home, destruction of property, aggression (initiation of physical fights), and trouble with the law (e.g., getting arrested).

Quality of life was evaluated by the Heinrichs-Carpenter Quality of Life Scale (QLS) [36], a 22-item rater-administered scale assessing overall quality of life and functioning in four areas: a) intrapsychic foundations (e.g., motivation, curiosity, empathy), b) interpersonal relations, c) instrumental role, and 4) common objects and activities. Items were rated from 0–6, with higher scores reflecting better quality of life. In addition, questions from the Lehman Quality of Life Interview (QOLI) [37] were used to evaluate the adequacy of the patient's finances over the past six months and the total number of hours of employment per week.

Medication side effects were evaluated using the Barnes scale for akathisia (range 0–14) [38], the Abnormal Involuntary Movement Scale (AIMS for tardive dyskinesia (range 0–40) [39] and the Simpson-Angus scale for extrapyramidal side effects (EPS) (range 0–40) [40].

Service use variables represented use of mental health outpatient services and/or residential treatment in the past month, occurrence of an exacerbation of mental symptoms requiring psychiatric hospitalization or crisis stabilization during the past 3 months, use of any type of hospitalization for any reason in the past month (all coded as yes/no), total number of years in mental health treatment, and the patient's subjective response to medications, evaluated by the Drug Attitude Inventory (DAI) [41], a 10-item "true"/"false" scale, where higher numbers indicate more positive views toward medication.

Caregiver measures

Family burden was evaluated using an adapted version of the Family Experience Interview Schedule (FEIS) [42], which evaluates patient problem behavior, activities of daily living, role functioning, disruption of household routine, caregiver contributions in time and money to the patient's general support and treatment, and the amount of practical and emotional support provided to the caregiver by the patient. Because the FEIS is comprised of scales and items selected conceptually based on the findings of prior studies of family burden [42], we used factor analysis to reduce the FEIS to dimensions that were statistically as well as conceptually meaningful for CATIE participants. The pool of 44 variables and scales derived from the FEIS were subjected to an exploratory principal components factor analysis with orthogonal (Varimax) rotation. Data were randomly divided into two approximately equal samples using the SPSS "Sample" procedure [43] for use in exploratory (N = 304) and confirmatory (N = 319) analyses.

Exploratory analysis

Examination of the skree plot of Eigenvalues indicated a four-factor solution, eliminating six items which failed to load on any factor. Factor 1 (problem behavior) (Table 8.2) represented illness-related behaviors problematic to caregivers (e.g., violent outbursts, referential thinking, excessive use of drugs and alcohol). Factor 2 (resource demands and routine disruption) captured demands on the caregiver and household (e.g., financial costs, social limitations, strained relations). Items loading on factor 3 (impairment in activities of daily living) related to patients' functional ability or activities of daily living, (e.g., meal preparation, hygiene). The fourth factor (perceived patient helpfulness), assessed the degree to which the patient helped the caregiver emotionally, financially, and practically (e.g., participated in household chores).

Confirmatory analysis

Results of the confirmatory model indicated a good fit for this factor structure, with a χ^2/df ratio of 2.26, Goodness of Fit Index (GFI) of 0.82, and Root Mean Square Error of Approximation (RMSEA) of 0.06. Given agreement in both samples on the underlying factor structure of family burden, the samples were combined in subsequent analyses.

Table 8.2. Four-factor solution for CATIE data [29]

Burden item	Factor loading
Factor 1: Problem behavior	
1. Violent/threatening behavior	0.702
2. Verbally abusive	0.690
3. Temper tantrum	0.680
4. Run away	0.618
5. Destroy property	0.609

Table 8.2. *(cont.)*

Burden item	Factor loading
6. Think people are talking about him/her	0.547
7. Socially inappropriate (tantrums/embarrassing behavior)	0.526
8. Excessive use of drugs	0.461
9. Hallucinations/delusions	0.458
10. Careless with safety (cigarettes, etc)	0.453
11. Socially withdrawn	0.449
12. Excessive use of alcohol	0.442
13. Pace aimlessly	0.441
14. Disturbing behaviors at night (pacing, listening to loud TV, etc)	0.425
15. Threatens/talks of suicide	0.419
Factor 2: Resource demands/routine disruption	
1. No. of areas where financial support was provided	0.716
2. How burdened in past month by financial support provided	0.635
3. Total dollars spent in the past month on patient	0.626
4. Limited social activities of household members	0.612
5. Other household members feel neglected	0.585
6. Household relations strained	0.535
7. Time lost (days of work or household responsibilities)	0.530
8. Disruption of household routine	0.517
9. Worry	0.471
10. Lost job opportunities for adult household members	0.465
11. Total hours/week spent providing care	0.416
Factor 3: Impairment in activities of daily living	
1. Problems preparing meals	0.685
2. Problems doing household chores	0.679
3. Problems maintaining personal hygiene	0.642
4. Problems getting up and dressed	0.632
5. Problems making use of leisure time	0.547
6. Problems taking medication	0.466
Factor 4: Perceived patient helpfulness	
1. Provides emotional support	0.798
2. Helps w/household chores	0.762
3. Provides financial assistance	0.668

Reprinted with permission from Psychiatric Services, (Copyright 2006). American Psychiatric Association.

Analytic strategy
Preliminary analyses

First, participants with follow-up family interview data were compared with those who had baseline family interviews only, in order to evaluate potential limitations in generalizability due to attrition associated with either the dependent (i.e., burden measures) or other baseline patient or caregiver characteristics. Second, we compared the percentage of participants randomized to each of the five treatment conditions with and without follow-up data, to determine whether there was differential attrition across treatment groups. Participants with follow-up data on family burden were compared both to those who had a baseline family interview but no follow-up data and to the larger group of CATIE participants including those without a baseline family interview. Third, preliminary bivariate level analyses were conducted to identify patient and family sociodemographic, and patient baseline clinical variables associated with the dependent variables, and one-way analyses of variance were conducted to check for baseline differences between treatment groups resulting from failure of the randomization procedure.

Multivariate models

Because 231 patients with TD were excluded from assignment to perphenazine, and ziprasidone was added to the trial after 40% of the patients had been enrolled, randomization took place under four separate regimens: including and excluding patients with TD, and including and excluding ziprasidone. To ensure that each data set only included patients with an equal chance of being randomly assigned to the treatments under comparison, the primary analyses were conducted on four different data sets with overlapping membership. For example, perphenazine patients were only compared to equivalent patients who did not have TD at baseline, and ziprasidone patients were only compared to patients enrolled after ziprasidone was added to the trial.

The primary comparison between the four treatments available at the beginning of the trial was an overall 3 degree of freedom test. This test was performed on Analytic Set I, excluding patients with TD and those randomized to ziprasidone. (See Chapter 2 for a detailed description of all four Analytic Sets.) If the overall test was significant at $p < 0.05$, the three second-generation drugs were compared with perphenazine with a Hochberg adjustment for multiple comparisons [29] in which the smallest p-value was compared to $0.05/3 = 0.017$ and the largest to $p = 0.05$. Next, using Analytic Set II, which excludes perphenazine and includes TD patients, the three second-generation drugs were compared to each other via step-down testing. If the overall 2 degree of freedom test was significant at $p < 0.05$, an alpha of $p < 0.05$ was applied for all comparisons.

Analytic Sets III and IV were used to compare ziprasidone to the other four drugs among patients randomized after ziprasidone became available, but with TD patients excluded from the perphenazine comparison. Hochberg adjustment for four pair-wise comparisons was used to compare ziprasidone and perphenazine in Analytic Set III, and ziprasidone to the other three drugs using Analytic Set IV. The smallest p-value was considered significant if $p = 0.05/4 = 0.013$.

The central analysis was a paired comparison between treatment groups of the degree of burden identified by each of the four FEIS factors using a mixed model including terms representing treatment group, the baseline value of the dependent burden value, time (treated as a classification variable for months 1–18), site, a history of recent clinical exacerbation, and an interaction term representing the baseline value of the dependent variable by time. The baseline-by-time term adjusts for baseline differences in characteristics of patients who dropped out early and thus are less well represented at later time points. Group-by-time interactions to evaluate differences in time trends between groups were also tested. A random subject effect and a first-order autoregressive covariance structure were used to adjust standard errors for the correlation of observations from the same individual using standard mixed model procedures.

Results
Attrition

The family caregivers of 449 or 72.8% of the original 623 patient participants were able to be followed and were included in the intent-to-treat analysis using all available follow-up data. Table 8.3 demonstrates that, on sociodemographic variables, patient participants who were followed had a higher level of education, were more often employed, and earned more income in the past 30 days than those who did not have any follow-up data. Family caregiver participants were older and more educated than those who were not followed up. Both patient and family participants were less often of African-American descent than those lost to follow-up. Additional comparisons between participants with follow-up data vs. those with baseline data alone on 15 clinical and other baseline variables demonstrated that those followed were rated lower on the PANSS total and positive symptom scales and higher in antisocial behavior and drug use. They also had more severe tardive dyskinesia symptoms, were less likely to have experienced an exacerbation within the past 3 months, and had less favorable attitudes toward medication.

Among burden factors, patients who were followed were rated lower at baseline in *problem behavior*; however those followed vs. those who were not did not differ significantly on any of the other three burden factors (Table 8.3). These data suggest that those followed were less symptomatic, more functional, and of higher socioeconomic status than those who were not. They also had fewer problem behaviors as rated by their family members.

There were no significant differences in the proportion of participants with follow-up family burden interviews across randomized treatments, as compared both to those with family burden interviews at baseline only and to the entire CATIE sample, including those without family burden baseline interviews. Because differential attrition between randomized treatment groups was not observed, the slight under-representation of the most symptomatic and burdensome patients in the follow-up sample is not likely to serious bias findings on level of burden over time between treatment groups. Moreover, no significant differences in baseline sociodemographic or clinical variables associated with any of the burden factors were observed.

Table 8.4 presents data on the mixed model intent-to-treat analysis from each of the four data sets described above, and Table 8.5 presents the results of mixed effects models for the same four data sets with crossovers (i.e., all observations after the first medication change) excluded, i.e., only considering treatment on initially assigned medication. Although there was a significant reduction in burden over 18 months on all burden factors, there were no significant differences in any measure of family burden in paired

Table 8.3. Comparison of participants with and without family follow up data

Patient demographics	Follow-up data N = 449 (mean ± SD or %)	No follow-up data N = 168 (mean ± SD or %)	t/x²	p value
Age	38.98 ± 11.55	38.30 ± 12.38	0.64	0.525
Race			12.44	0.002
White race	70.4	55.4		
Black race	24.9	36.9		
Hispanic	10.07	10.7	0.11	0.918
Other	4.7	7.7		.
Gender (% male)	76.20	73.20	0.51	0.463
Years of education	12.36 ± 2.37	11.88 ± 2.18	2.30	0.022
Marital status			6.77	0.149
Married	15.8	13.1		
Divorced/separated	18.0	23.2		
Never married	64.6	60.7		
Widowed	1.6	3.0		
Income/employment				
Earned income (past 30 days)	$188.67 ± 665.73	$74.80 ± 255.71	3.07	0.002
Public support[1]	$534.47 ± 568.20	$492.88 ± 599.06	0.80	0.426
Percent employed	81.30	88.0	3.91	0.141
Hours worked/week	5.73 ± 13.05	3.27 ± 9.65	2.54	.012
Caregiver Demographics				
Age	52.99 ± 13.78	49.37 ± 15.89	2.67	0.008
Race			14.73	<0.001
White race	65.3	49.1		
Black race	23.4	37.7		
Other	11.7	12.2		
Hispanic	11.0	10.8	0.000	1.00
Years of education	13.49 ± 3.07	12.90 ± 3.47	1.99	0.047
Marital status			8.69	0.069
Married	61.4	62.5		
Divorced/separated	17.8	14.4		
Never married	7.9	14.4		
Widowed	12.9	8.8		

Table 8.3. (cont.)

Patient demographics	Follow-up data N = 449 (mean ± SD or %)	No follow-up data N = 168 (mean ± SD or %)	t/x²	p value
Income/employment				
Employed (yes/no)	55.1	51.8	0.39	0.532
Patient Symptoms/Substance Use				
PANSS Total	75.89 ± 18.66	79.33 ± 18.34	−2.05	0.041
PANSS Positive	18.19 ± 5.78	19.36 ± 5.78	2.23	0.026
PANSS Negative	20.62 ± 6.74	21.08 ± 6.72	−0.75	0.451
Depression (Calgary)	1.53 ± 0.52	1.59 ± 0.57	−1.27	0.203
Drug use	1.32 ± 0.54	1.51 ± 0.88	−2.93	0.004
Alcohol use	1.46 ± 0.68	1.52 ± 0.67	−1.08	0.280
Antisocial behavior	0.15 ± 0.19	0.26 ± 0.26	−5.91	0.000
Patient side effects				
Tardive dyskinesia (AIMS)	0.31 ± 0.51	0.19 ± 0.36	5.32	<0.001
Akathisia (Barnes)	0.37 ± 0.55	0.32 ± 0.53	1.51	0.13
EPS (Simpson Angus)	0.23 ± 0.35	0.20 ± 0.29	1.72	0.09
Patient Service Use				
Favors medication	0.01 ± 0.48	0.11 ± 0.54	−2.71	0.007
Years in treatment	14.82 ± 11.31	16.29 ± 12.07	−1.41	0.160
Recent exacerbation (90 days)	26.10	36.9	6.98	0.010
Patient Quality of Life				
Quality of Life (Heinrichs- Carpenter total)	2.69 ± 1.10	2.61 ± 1.08	0.84	0.400
Crime (victim/agent)	0.23 ± 0.61	0.24 ± 0.64	−0.22	0.824
Burden factors				
F 1: Problem Behavior	0.65 ± 0.51	0.87 ± 0.58	−4.35	0.000
F 2: Resource Demands/Routine Disruption	0.01 ± 0.61	0.08 ± 0.63	−1.58	0.114
F 3: Perceived Functional Impairment	0.97 ± 0.78	1.01 ± 0.80	−0.49	0.625
F 4: Perceived Client Helpfulness	1.50 ± 0.63	1.53 ± 0.64	−0.39	0.700

Note: [1]Average monthly payment.

Reprinted from Schizophrenia Research, epublication before print, Perlick DA, Rosenheck RA, Kaczynski R, Swartz MS, Canive JM, Lieberman JA. Impact of antipsychotic medication on family burden in schizophrenia: Longitudinal results of CATIE trial. Copyright 2009, with permission of Elsevier.

Table 8.4. Comparison of effectiveness: mixed model analyses of monthly family burden values by group[1,2]: Intention-to-treat Analysis

	Olanzapine (O)	Perphenazine (P)	Quetiapine (Q)	Risperidone (R)	Ziprasidone (Z)	F	p value	Paired comparisons[7]
Total (N=)	115	118	111	126	54			
Data Set I (do=3): P vs. O, Q and R Excluding patients with TD and patients on ziprasidone (N=)	101	118	97	106	–			
Problem behavior[3]	0.426	0.480	0.477	0.472	–	0.47	0.702	ns
Resource demands[4]	–0.185	–0.235	–0.238	–0.229	–	0.33	0.803	ns
ADL impairment[5]	0.758	0.804	0.820	0.947	–	1.14	0.332	ns
Perceived patient helpfulness[6]	1.493	1.606	1.643	1.484	–	0.83	0.478	ns
Data Set II (df=2): O vs. Q vs. R Including Patients with TD but excluding those on zipr. or perph. (N=)	115	–	111	126	–			
Problem behavior[3]	0.426	–	0.505	0.474	–	1.10	0.336	ns
Resource demands[4]	–0.190	–	–0.195	–0.205	–	0.03	0.973	ns
ADL impairment[5]	0.861	–	0.869	0.968	–	0.63	0.533	ns
Perceived patient helpfulness[6]	1.478	–	1.608	1.443	–	1.13	0.329	ns

Table 8.4. (cont.)

	Olanzapine (O)	Perphenazine (P)	Quetiapine (Q)	Risperidone (R)	Ziprasidone (Z)	F	p value	Paired comparisons[7]
Data Set III: Z vs. P								
Excluding Patients with TD but including those on Ziprasidone (N=)	–	65	–	–	46			
Problem behavior[3]	–	0.513	–	–	0.457	Not applicable	Not applicable	ns
Resource demands[4]	–	–0.255	–	–	–0.194	Not applicable	Not applicable	ns
ADL impairment[5]	–	0.897	–	–	0.739	Not applicable	Not applicable	ns
Perceived patient helpfulness[6]	–	1.541	–	–	1.411	Not applicable	Not applicable	ns
Data Set IV: Z vs. O, Q and R								
Including Patients with TD and those on Ziprasidone (N=)	56	–	50	56	54			
Problem behavior[3]	0.441	–	0.470	0.505	**0.425**	Not applicable	Not applicable	ns
Resource demands[4]	–0.162	–	–0.219	–0.202	**–0.189**	Not applicable	Not applicable	ns
ADL impairment[5]	0.838	–	0.776	0.887	**0.652**	Not applicable	Not applicable	ns
Perceived patient helpfulness[6]	1.548	–	1.752	1.429	**1.408**	Not applicable	Not applicable	ns

Notes: [1]Bolded values highlight treatment conditions of primary interest in each data set.
[2]All pairwise p values < 0.05 are presented. * = statistically significant using criteria for multiple comparisons.
[3]Least square means of Problem Behavior scores from months 1, 3, 6, 9, 12, 15, 18 (N = 580 patient-month observations for Data Set I; 491 for Data Set II; 361 for Data Set III; and 322 for Data Set IV).
[4]Least squared means of Resource Demands scores from months 1, 3, 6 9, 12, 15, 18 (N = 518 patient-month observations for Data Set I; 418 for Data Set II; 309 for Data Set III; and 257 for Data Set IV).
[5]Least square means of ADL Impairments from months 6, 12, and 18 (N = 560 patient-month observations for Data Set I; 472 for Data Set II; 342 for Data Set III; and 304 for Data Set IV).
[6]Least square means of Perceived Patient Helpfulness Scores from months 6, 12, and 18 (N = 253 patient-month observations for Data Set I; 213 for Data Set III; 174 for Data Set III; and 152 for Data Set IV).
[7]ns = paired comparisons examined with this data set were not significantly different.

Reprinted from Schizophrenia Research, epublication before print, Perlick DA, Rosenheck RA, Kaczynski R, Swartz MS, Canive JM, Lieberman JA. Impact of antipsychotic medication on family burden in schizophrenia: Longitudinal results of CATIE trial. Copyright 2009, with permission of Elsevier.

Table 8.5. Comparison of effectiveness during CATIE Phase 1 (i.e., with treatment crossovers excluded): mixed model analyses of monthly family burden values by group[1,2]

	Olanzapine (O)	Perphenazine (P)	Quetiapine (Q)	Risperidone (R)	Ziprasidone (Z)	F	p value	Paired comparisons[7]
Total (N=)	101	102	98	113	51			
Data Set I (df = 3): P vs. O, Q and R Excluding patients with TD and patients on ziprasidone (N=)	90	102	85	98	—			
Problem behavior[3]	0.397	0.508	0.536	0.455	—	1.43	0.236	ns
Resource demands[4]	−0.210	−0.264	−0.186	−0.300	—	0.73	0.535	ns
ADL impairment[5]	0.771	0.843	0.853	0.987	—	0.87	0.458	ns
Perceived patient helpfulness[6]	1.556	1.756	1.846	1.360	—	3.05	0.040	P > R (p = 0.013)
Data Set II (df = 2): O vs. Q vs. R Including patients with TD but excluding those on zipr. or perph. (N=)	101	—	98	113				
Problem behavior[3]	0.374	—	0.526	0.442		2.07	0.130	ns
Resource demands[4]	−0.252	—	−0.181	−0.309		0.96	0.386	ns
ADL impairment[5]	0.827	—	0.839	0.918		0.22	0.804	ns
Perceived patient helpfulness[6]	1.563	—	1.927	1.350		4.75	0.100	O < Q p = 0.045; R < Q p = 0.004

Table 8.5. (cont.)

	Olanzapine (O)	Perphenazine (P)	Quetiapine (Q)	Risperidone (R)	Ziprasidone (Z)	F	p value	Paired comparisons[7]
Data Set III: Z vs. P Excluding patients with TD but including those on ziprasidone (N=)	–	55	–	–	44			
Problem behavior[3]	–	0.521	–	–	0.340	Not applicable		ns
Resource demands[4]	–	-0.268	–	–	-0.381	Not applicable		ns
ADL impairment[5]	–	0.890	–	–	0.710	Not applicable		ns
Perceived patient helpfulness[6]	–	1.557	–	–	1.226	Not applicable		ns
Data Set IV: Z vs. O, Q and R Including patients with TD and those on ziprasidone (N=)	50	–	45	51	51			
Problem behavior[3]	0.381	–	0.552	0.494	**0.291**	Not applicable		ns
Resource demands[4]	-0.220	–	-0.235	-0.240	**-0.395**	Not applicable		ns
ADL impairment[5]	0.989	–	0.870	0.999	**0.551**	Not applicable		ns
Perceived patient helpfulness[6]	1.576	–	N/A	1.272	**1.239**	Not applicable		O > Z $p = 0.023$

Notes: [1] Bolded values highlight treatment conditions of primary interest in each data set.
[2] All pairwise p values <.05 are presented. * = statistically significant using criteria for multiple comparisons.
[3] Least square means of Problem Behavior scores from months 1, 3, 6, 9, 12, 15, 18 (N = 340 patient-month observations for Data Set I; 296 for Data Set II; 191 for Data Set III; and 177 for Data Set IV).
[4] Least square means of Resource Demands scores from months 1, 3, 6, 9, 12, 15, 18 (N = 314 patient-month observations for Data Set I; 257 for Data Set II; 176 for Data Set III; and 148 for Data Set IV).
[5] Least square means of ADL Impairments from months 6, 12, and 18 (N = 331 patient-month observations for Data Set I; 283 for Data Set II; 183 for Data Set III; and 164 for Data Set IV).
[6] Least square means of Perceived Patient Helpfulness scores from months 6, 12, and 18 (N = 133 patient-month observations for Data Set I; 117 for Data Set II; 88 for Data Set III; and 86 for Data Set IV).
[7] ns = paired comparisons examined with this data set were not significantly different.
Reprinted from Schizophrenia Research, epublication before print, Pe-lick DA, Rosenheck RA, Kaczynski R, Swartz MS, Canive JM, Lieberman JA. Impact of antipsychotic medication on family burden in schizophrenia: Longitudinal results of CATIE trial. Copyright 2009, with permission of Elsevier. ADL, activities of daily living; TD, tardive dyskinesia.

comparisons of medications, including between perphenazine and any second-generation antipsychotic or between pairs of second-generation antipsychotics. There were also no significant interactions of time with treatment group.

When only observations limited to treatment with the first, randomized medication were included, patients assigned to perphenazine showed higher scores on the Perceived Patient Helpfulness factor ($p = 0.013$) than patients assigned to risperidone (Table 8.5). In Data Set II, which included patients with tardive dyskinesia but excluded those on ziprasidone or perphenazine, patients on quetiapine showed greater helpfulness (i.e., lower burden) than those treated with risperidone or olanzapine on the Perceived Patient Helpfulness scale (Table 8.5). Finally in Data Set IV patients assigned to olanzapine were more helpful (i.e., lower burden ratings) as compared to ziprasidone ($p = 0.023$). These findings should be regarded as descriptive since we examined four outcomes. Further adjustment of the alpha level for the number of measures would have rendered these findings statistically not significant.

Changes in burden over time

Although burden did not vary with treatment assignment over time, family members reported less burden over time across all treatments. Analysis of covariance, controlling for the level of burden at baseline demonstrated a significant reduction in burden for Problem Behavior Burden ($F6,1047 = 10.42$; $p < 0.001$) and Resource Demands and Routine Disruption Burden ($F6,930 = 4.21$), but not for the other two burden factors. Figures 8.1 and 8.2 display the levels of perceived burden over time for these two factors for each treatment group. While the reduction in burden observed for Problem Behavior Burden and Resource Demands/Routine Disruption Burden may simply reflect initial high levels of burden among family members agreeing to be interviewed (and a consequent regression to the mean), this interpretation does not explain the relatively stable levels of

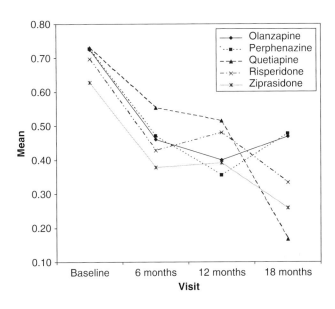

Figure 8.1. Problem behavior burden by treatment group over time. Values on the abscissa represent mean standardized scores for the Problem Behavior factor.

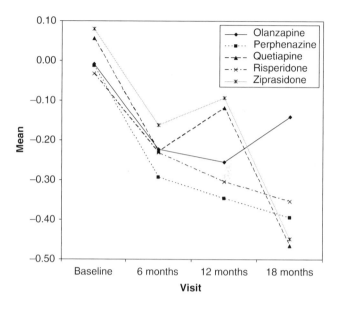

Figure 8.2. Resource demands and routine disruption burden by treatment group over time. Values on the abscissa represent mean standardized scores for the Resource Demands and Routine Disruption factor.

burden observed for the other two burden factors. Another possible explanation is that the reduced burden reports over time in Problem Behavior and Resources Demands/Routine Disruption reflect the cumulative benefits to families of knowing their relative is engaged in a stable treatment with a competent practitioner and predictable clinic visits, such as that provided by the CATIE protocol. Clinical observation shows that family members' primary concerns for their relative with schizophrenia and other serious mental illnesses most consistently relate to the quality and appropriateness of the treatment their relative is receiving, i.e., is the relative seeing the "best" doctor and on the "best" medication for him or her. Available research on family members' needs regarding their relative supports this impression [44].

Predictors of level of burden

The findings that different antipsychotics are equally beneficial overall, not only for patients with schizophrenia [45], but also for the family members who help care for them, is an important finding. However, given that the majority of family members report experiencing burden in their caregiving role, the question of what patient or caregiver-related attributes contribute to the level of burden experienced is an equally important one. Gaining a better understanding of factors associated with high levels of burden may be helpful in both identifying and intervening with family members who are at risk for high levels of perceived burden and associated health and mental health risks. To address this important question, we used CATIE baseline data to evaluate the relationships between patient symptoms, quality of life, service use, and caregiver burden, controlling for patient and caregiver sociodemographic variables. Preliminary bivariate level analyses identified patient and caregiver variables for inclusion in the multivariate analyses: Measures that had significant bivariate associations at the 0.05 level or better with at least one of the four burden factors were entered into four separate hierarchical regression analyses to identify correlates of each burden factor. Variables were grouped conceptually, and each group was entered in a single step, in order to evaluate the total impact (change in r square) of that domain as a whole, in addition to the significance of individual measures. Patient demographic variables were entered in Step 1, and caregiver demographics in Step 2. Symptom measures were entered in Step 3, and quality of life and service use measures were entered in Steps 4 and 5, respectively [29]. The results of these analyses are presented in Table 8.6. For ease of explication, only the fifth step, which controls for the effects of all other variables, is presented. We anticipated that caregivers would experience less burden from patients who had lower symptom levels, a higher quality of life, superior cognitive functioning, fewer medication side effects, positive attitudes toward medication, more years in treatment, and less intensive current treatment.

The model for each of the four burden factors was highly significant, with R squares ranging from 0.38 for perceived patient helpfulness to 0.21 for impairment in activities of daily living. A pattern of results emerged in which the conceptually defined categories of "predictor" variables were differentially related to the burden factors. For example caregiver and patient demographic variables explained a relatively large amount of variance for perceived patient helpfulness (30%) and resource demands/routine disruption (19%) (Table 8.6), but contributed relatively little explanatory power to the models for problem behavior and impairment in activities of daily living (6% each). Living with and being married to the caregiver were both associated with greater perceived helpfulness, while caregiver age and employment status were both inversely related to perceived helpfulness: older, employed caregivers viewed the patient as less helpful. Younger patient age and residing with the caregiver were associated with greater resource (i.e., financial) demands or disruption of routine, while Black race of caregiver (vs. White or other) was associated with lower levels of resource demands.

Patient symptomatology explained modest additional variance in patient helpfulness and resource demands (4% and 8%, respectively) but explained 20% additional variance in problem behavior burden and 9% more variance for impairment in activities of daily living. After demographics, symptoms were the strongest predictor of burden across all four measures. Interestingly, the four burden factors were differentially related to the PANSS negative and positive symptoms dimensions. The impairment in activities of daily living was positively associated with negative but not positive symptoms, while the reverse was true for the problem behavior factor which was positively associated with positive but not negative symptoms. Perceptions of patient helpfulness were not significantly related to either symptom scale; by contrast, the resource demands and disruption of routine factor was positively and significantly related with both positive and negative symptoms.

Higher quality of life among patients was associated with higher caregiver reports of patient helpfulness and lower reports of impairment in activities of daily living. The problem behavior and resource demands factors were strongly associated with the number of hours worked each week but not with patient quality of life: caregivers of patients who worked more hours reported less burden. Altogether, quality of life contributed modestly (2–5% additional variance) to the models for the four burden factors, after controlling for patient symptoms and patient and caregiver demographics.

Treatment in residential settings was negatively correlated with reports of problem behavior burden, but inpatient treatment was positively associated with the problem behavior and resource demands factors, most likely reflecting the short duration of inpatient episodes relative to residential treatment. Service use measures explained only an additional 5% of variance for problem behavior and resource demands, but did not contribute significantly to the other models.

Conclusions and implications of study findings

This study represents one of the largest longitudinal studies of family members of people with schizophrenia to date, and the only study to systematically evaluate the effects of a controlled medication regimen on family burden. We used factor analysis to identify three unique domains in which CATIE family members reported experiencing caregiving strain: 1) coping with problem behaviors (Problem Behavior Burden), 2) managing the demands on personal finances and time (Resource Demands and Routine Disruption), and 3) making adjustments to accommodate functional impairment (Perceived Functional Impairment Burden). The adverse impact of these stressors may be partially countered by a fourth domain identified related to the perceived helpfulness of the relative with schizophrenia. The level of burden reported was additionally related to patient and caregiver demographic characteristics, patient symptoms, patient quality of life, and patient service use. Moreover, the pattern of inter-relationships varied between domains. Of particular interest is the finding that burden associated with patient problem behaviors was positively associated with positive but not with negative symptoms, while perceived functional impairment was related to negative but not positive symptoms and resource demands and routine disruption were related to both. Other characteristics were more uniformly related to burden level. Older patients were rated as significantly less burdensome on all three burden factors (Problem Behaviors, Perceived Functional Impairment, Resource Demands/Routine Disruption), and caregivers who were Black reported significantly less burden in two of the three domains. Perceived patient helpfulness was highest when the patient resided with the caregivers and was employed.

Table 8.6. Hierarchical regression analyses on CATIE burden factors: standardized (Beta) weights and R^2

	Problem Behavior	Resource Demands/ Routine Disruption	Perceived Functional Impairment	Perceived Patient Helpfulness
Patient demographics				
Age	−0.12*	−0.28***	−0.24***	0.08
Male gender	−0.03	−0.02	0.02	−0.01
Years of education	−0.11*	0.00	−0.02	−0.01
Lives with caregiver	0.01	0.12*	0.04	0.38***
Married to caregiver	0.01	0.05	0.03	0.12**
Caregiver demographics				
Age	−0.09	−0.05	0.08	−0.11*
Male gender	0.02	0.01	0.01	0.04
Black race (vs. White/other)	−0.12**	−0.21***	−0.09	0.03
Hispanic	0.00	0.06	−0.04	0.03

Table 8.6. (cont.)

	Problem Behavior	Resource Routine	Demands/ Disruption	Perceived Functional Impairment	Perceived Patient Helpfulness
Years of education	0.01	0.05		0.01	−0.07
Employed	−0.01	0.00		0.02	−0.17***
Income	−0.09*	−0.07		−0.05	−0.06
Symptoms					
PANSS positive	0.26***	0.13**		0.05	−0.07
PANSS negative	0.08	0.12*		0.16**	−0.08
Depression (Calgary)	−0.01	−0.07		−0.01	0.09*
Drug use	0.09*	0.04		0.05	0.02
Alcohol use	0.15**	0.02		0.05	−0.04
Antisocial	−0.03	−0.13**		−0.05	0.08
Quality of Life					
Quality of Life	−0.06	−0.05		−0.18***	0.14**
Crime (victim/agent)	0.06	−0.01		−0.05	0.01
Finances sufficient	−0.01	−0.03		−0.09	0.07
Hours worked/week	−0.13**	−0.13**		−0.06	0.07
Service use					
Favors medication	0.08	0.11*		0.00	−0.01
Years in treatment	0.11	0.03		0.10	0.01
Recent exacerbation	0.04	0.10		0.05	−0.08
MH OP visits (Y/N)	0.04	0.04		0.05	−0.03
Residential treatment	−0.16***	−0.05		0.09	−0.07
Inpatient treatment	0.18**	0.12*		0.01	0.03
R^2 by step[†]					
Patient demographics	0.05***	0.14***		0.04***	0.25***
Caregiver demographics	0.01	0.05**		0.02	0.05***
Symptoms	0.20***	0.08***		0.09***	0.04***
Quality of Life	0.03**	0.02**		0.05***	0.03***
Service Use	0.05***	0.05***		0.02	0.01
Model Summary					
Adjusted R^2	0.30	0.29		0.16	0.34
R^2	0.34***	0.34***		0.21***	0.38***

Our findings suggest that the different burden factors identified represent different aspects of caregiving strain related to different patient and caregiver profiles.

Contrary to our prediction, level of burden was not related to treatment with first vs. second-generation antipsychotics. There was a tendency for burden levels to decline over time, but this effect was uniform across treatment groups: a significant time by group interaction was not observed. Because the first-generation antipsychotic, perphenazine, was not less effective when compared to second-generation antipsychotics on symptom or quality of life measures, the failure to find treatment group differences for burden is not surprising. Because perphenazine was consistently significantly less costly as compared to the second-generation drugs studied [45], the finding that it is both no less effective in reducing symptoms nor in ameliorating caregiving strain is important information for family members who must shoulder the financial burdens of medication that are not covered by insurance.

There are several implications to the study findings. First, because family caregivers do report caregiving strain in relation to patient illness characteristics, it would be helpful to offer them services that help reduce caregiving strain, both through education in more effective methods of illness management, and in stress management/self-care. There are a number of evidence-based options available to family members, ranging from Family Psychoeducation, a clinician-led course of 20+ sessions involving both the patient and family member, focusing on illness education, problem solving, and communication skills, to the Family to Family Program developed by the National Alliance on Mental Illness (NAMI), a peer-facilitated, 12-session group intervention for caregivers alone that teaches survival skills. Family Psychoeducation has demonstrated efficacy in both reducing patient relapse rates and family burden [22] in meta-analytic studies, while the Family to Family program has been shown to reduce subjective family burden and increase family empowerment [46,47]. Despite its effectiveness, Family Psychoeducation is not widely offered, due to challenges in implementation, but alternate, more accessible formats are being developed [48].

Finally, the findings of the CATIE study underscore the importance of involving family caregivers in treatment planning for their relative with schizophrenia. Because no one medication emerged as the "gold standard", clinicians must rely on feedback from patients to a large extent, as well as on clinical observation to guide their choice and dose of antipsychotic. Family members often have more detailed and objective information about clinical response over a broader time frame than either the patient or clinician. In addition, family members frequently take an active role in helping patients manage their medication and in other aspects of preventing relapse and promoting recovery. It is therefore a potential benefit to the clinician as well as to the family member and relative with schizophrenia to enlist their support.

References

1. Magliano L, Marasco C, Fiorillo A, *et al.* The impact of professional and social network support on the burden of families of patients with schizophrenia in Italy. *Acta Psychiatrica Scandinavica* 2002;**106**:291–8.

2. Lowyck B, De Hert M, Peeters E, *et al.* Burden on the family: A study of 120 relatives of schizophrenic patients in Belgium. *Tijdschrift Voor Psychiatrie* 2002;**44**:151–8.

3. Schene AH, Van Wijngaarden B and Koeter MWJ. Family caregiving in schizophrenia: Domains and distress. *Schizophrenia Bulletin* 1998;**4**:609–18.

4. McDonell MG, Short RA, Berry CM, *et al.* Burden in schizophrenia caregivers: Impact of family psychoeducation and awareness of patient suicidality. *Family Practice* 2003;**42**:91–103.

5. Angermeyer MC, Liebelt P and Matschinger H. Distress in parents of

patients suffering from schizophrenia or affective disorders. *Psychotherapie, Psychosomatik, Medizinische Psychologie* 2001;**51**:255–60.

6. Ohaeri JU. Caregiver burden and psychotic patients' perception of social support in a Nigerian setting. *Social Psychiatry and Psychiatric Epidemiology* 2001;**36**:86–93.

7. Struening EL, Stueve A, Vine P, *et al.* Factors associated with grief and depressive symptoms in caregivers of people with serious mental illness. In: Greenley JR, ed. *Research in Community Mental Health.* Greenwich, CT: JAI Press Inc; 1995. pp 91–124.

8. Dyck DG, Short R, and Vitaliano PP. Predictors of burden and infectious illness in schizophrenia caregivers. *Psychosomatic Medicine* 1999;**61**:411–9.

9. Struening EL, Perlick DA, Link BG, Hellman F, Herman D and Sirey JA. The extent to which caregivers believe most people devalue consumers and their families. *Psychiatric Services* 2001;**52**:1633–8.

10. Link BG, Cullen FT, Struening EL, Shrout PE and Dohrenwend BP. A modified labeling theory approach to mental disorders: An empirical assessment. *American Sociological Review* 1989;**54**:400–23.

11. Perlick DA, Rosenheck RA, Miklowitz DJ, *et al.* Prevalence and correlates of burden among caregivers of patients with bipolar disorder enrolled in the Systematic Treatment Enhancement Program for Bipolar Disorder (STEP-BD). *Bipolar Disorders* 2007;**9**:262–73.

12. Gallagher SK and Mechanic D. Living with the mentally ill: Effects on the health and functioning of other household members. *Social Science & Medicine* 1996;**42**:1691–701.

13. Mui AC. Perceived health and functional status among spouse caregivers of frail older persons. *Journal of Aging and Health* 1995;**7**:283–300.

14. Beach SR, Schulz R, Yee JL, *et al.* Negative and positive health effects of caring for a disabled spouse: Longitudinal findings from the caregiver health effects study. *Psychology and Aging* 2000;**15**:259–71.

15. Lieberman MA and Fisher L. The impact of chronic illness on the health and well-being of family members. *Gerontologist* 1995;**35**:94–102.

16. Sparks MB, Farran CJ, Donner E, *et al.* Wives, husbands, and daughters of dementia patients: Predictors of caregivers' mental and physical health. *Scholarly Inquiry for Nursing Practice* 1998;**12**:221–35.

17. Esterling BA, Kiecolt-Glaser JK, Bodnar JC, *et al.* Chronic stress, social support, and persistent alterations in the natural killer cell response to cytokines in older adults. *Health Psychology* 1994;**13**:291–8.

18. Haley WE, Levine EG, Brown SL, *et al.* Psychological, social, and health consequences of caring for a relative with senile dementia. *Journal of the American Geriatrics Society* 1987;**35**:405–11.

19. Kiecolt-Glaser JK, Marucha PT, Malarkey WB, *et al.* Slowing of wound healing by psychological stress. *Lancet* 1995;**346**:1194–6.

20. O'Reilly F, Finnan F, Allwright S, *et al.* The effects of caring for a spouse with Parkinson's disease on social, psychological and physical well-being. *British Journal of General Practice* 1996;**46**:507–12.

21. Pruchno RA and Potashnik SL. Caregiving spouses: Physical and mental health in perspective. *Journal of the American Geriatrics Society* 1989;**37**:697–705.

22. George LK and Gwyther LP. Caregiver well-being: A multidimensional examination of family caregivers of demented adults. *Gerontologist* 1986;**26**:253–9.

23. Dyck DG, Short R and Vitaliano PP. Predictors of burden and infectious illness in schizophrenia caregivers. *Psychosomatic Medicine* 1999;**61**:411–9.

24. Wolff N, Helminiak TW and Diamond RJ. Estimated societal costs of assertive community mental health care. *Psychiatric Services* 1995;**46**:898–906.

25. Falloon I, Boyd JL, McGill CW, *et al.* Family management in the prevention of morbidity of schizophrenia: Clinical outcome of a two-year longitudinal study. *Archives of General Psychiatry* 1985;**42**:887–96.

26. Falloon IR and Pederson J. Family management and the prevention of morbidity in schizophrenia: The adjustment of the family unit. *British Journal of Psychiatry* 1985; **147**:156–63.

27. Pilling S, Bebbington P, Kuipers E, *et al.* Psychological treatments in schizophrenia: I. Meta-analysis of family intervention and cognitive behaviour therapy. *Psychological Medicine* 2002;**32**:763–82.

28. Rosenheck RA, Cramer J, Jurgis G, *et al.* Clinical and psychopharmacological factors influencing family burden in refractory schizophrenia. *Journal of Clinical Psychiatry* 2000;**61**:671–6.

29. Perlick DA, Rosenheck R, Kaczynski R, Swartz MA, Canive JM, and Lieberman JA. Components and correlates of family burden in schizophrenia. *Psychiatric Services* 2006;**57**:1117–25.

30. Lieberman JA, Stroup TS, McEvoy JP, *et al.* Effectiveness of antipsychotic drugs in patients with chronic schizophrenia. *New England Journal of Medicine* 2005;**353**:1209–23.

31. Stroup TS, McEvoy JP, Swartz MS, *et al.* The National Institute of Mental Health Clinical Antipsychotic Trials of Intervention Effectiveness (CATIE) project: Schizophrenia trial design and protocol development. *Schizophrenia Bulletin* 2003;**29**:15–31.

32. First MB, Gibbon M, Spitzer RL, and Williams JBW. *Structured Clinical Interview for DSM-IV Axis I Disorders—Research Version (SCID-I).* New York: Biometrics Research; 1996.

33. Kay SR, Fiszbein A and Opler LA. The Positive and Negative Syndrome Scale (PANSS) for schizophrenia. *Schizophrenia Bulletin* 1987;**13**:261–76.

34. Addington D, Addington J and Maticka-Tyndale E. A depression rating scale for schizophrenics. *Schizophrenia Research* 1996;**3**:247–51.

35. Drake RE, Osher FC, Noordsy DL, *et al.* Diagnosis of alcohol use disorders in schizophrenia. *Schizophrenia Bulletin* 1990;**16**:57–67.

36. Heinrichs DW, Hanlon ET and Carpenter WT. The Quality of Life Scale: An instrument for rating the schizophrenic deficit syndrome. *Schizophrenia Bulletin* 1984;**10**:388–98.

37. Lehman A. A quality of life interview for the chronically mentally ill. *Evaluation and Program Planning* 1988;**11**:51–62.

38. Barnes TR. A rating scale for drug induced akathisia. *British Journal of Psychiatry* 1989;**154**:672–6.

39. Guy W. *ECDEU Assessment Manual for Psychopharmacology.* Washington, DC: US Department of Health, Education, and Welfare; 1976.

40. Simpson GM and Angus JWS. A rating scale for extrapyramidal side effects. *Acta Psychiatrica Scandinavica* 1970;**212**:S11–S19.

41. Hogan TP, Awad AG and Eastwood MR. A self-report scale predictive of drug compliance in schizophrenics: Reliability and discriminative validity. *Psychological Medicine* 1983;**13**:177–83.

42. Tessler RT and Gamache G. *Toolkit for Evaluating Family Experiences With Severe Mental Illness.* Cambridge, MA: Health Services Research Institute Evaluation Center; 1995.

43. SPSS for Windows, version 12.0. Chicago: SPSS; 2003.

44. Perlick DA, Wolff N, Miklowitz DJ, Menard K, Rosenheck RR; STEP-BD Family Experience Collaborative Study Group. Development of an integrated model of family burden in bipolar illness. *The Journal of Mental Health Policy and Economics* 2003;**6**.

45. Rosenheck R, Leslie D, Sindelar J, *et al.* Cost-effectiveness of second generation antipsychotics and perphenazine in a randomized trial of treatment for chronic schizophrenia. *American Journal of Psychiatry* 2006;**163**:2080–9.

46. Dixon L, Stewart B, Burland J, Delahanty J, Lucksted A and Hoffman M. Pilot study of the effectiveness of the family-to family education program. *Psychiatric Services* 2001;**52**:965–67.

47. Dixon L, Lucksted A, Stewart B, *et al.* Outcomes of the peer-taught 12-week Family-to-Family Education Program for

severe mental illness. *Acta Psychiatrica Scandinavica* 2004;**109**:207–15.

48. Cohen AN, Glynn SM, Murray-Swank AB, *et al.* The family forum: Directions for the implementation of family psychoeducation for severe mental illness. *Psychiatric Services* 2008; **59**:40–8.

Extrapyramidal side effects

Stanley N. Caroff, Del D. Miller, and Robert A. Rosenheck

From the beginning of the use of chlorpromazine and other neuroleptic drugs, signs of parkinsonism (e.g., tremor, rigidity, and bradykinesia) were observed as frequent side effects and, despite numerous studies to the contrary, were considered to be inextricably linked to therapeutic antipsychotic effects [1,2]. Within a few years, investigators also observed an association between these drugs and abnormal involuntary movements that came to be known as tardive dyskinesia (TD) [3,4]. These and other drug-induced extra-pyramidal side effects (EPS) can be mistaken for or worsen primary psychotic symptoms, are sometimes irreversible or lethal, often necessitate additional burdensome side effects from antiparkinsonian agents, can be disfiguring and stigmatizing, and have been shown to influence compliance, relapse, and rehospitalization [1,5,6]. As a result, EPS dominated concerns about tolerability of antipsychotic drugs for decades, and their elimination served as a major impetus for new drug research and development.

In 1988, clozapine was found to have broader efficacy in schizophrenia with negligible EPS, stimulating the search for other antipsychotics with improved tolerability [7]. The drugs that were introduced after clozapine came to be known as atypical or second-generation antipsychotics (SGAs) while the earlier drugs were now called typical or first-generation antipsychotics (FGAs). Industry-sponsored clinical trials suggested that SGAs were superior to FGAs in the treatment of schizophrenia, reducing psychotic symptoms and causing fewer EPS [8–20]. Cumulative evidence supporting reduced liability for EPS with SGAs contributed to the widespread dominance of these drugs in the marketplace and fostered the concept of "atypicality" in the mechanism of action of the new drugs [21–25].

Further studies mostly confirmed a reduced risk of EPS with SGAs but also raised questions about the degree or significance of the advantages of SGAs seen in earlier trials. Although haloperidol, as the most widely prescribed FGA, was a reasonable choice as a comparator in industry-sponsored trials because of its widespread use, several reviews and meta-analyses suggested that the relative advantages of SGAs in reducing EPS liability were diminished when lower doses or lower-potency FGAs are used, or if prophylactic anti-parkinsonian drugs are administered [21,26–33]. In view of these conflicting findings, the CATIE schizophrenia trial offered an opportunity to address the lingering controversy over the significance of the relative liability for EPS between first- and second-generation antipsychotics.

Antipsychotic Trials in Schizophrenia, ed. T. Scott Stroup and Jeffrey A. Lieberman. Published by Cambridge University Press. © Cambridge University Press 2010.

Initial analysis of EPS in the CATIE schizophrenia trial

The rationale, design, methods, and statistical analysis of the CATIE trial have been described previously and in Chapters 1 and 2 [34–36]. Here, only features of CATIE that are relevant to interpretation of EPS findings are briefly summarized. CATIE was designed to address the overall effectiveness of SGAs versus a mid-potency FGA, perphenazine, based on treatment discontinuation for any cause. The key secondary outcomes were the specific reasons for discontinuation including inefficacy or intolerability. Among the latter was the influence of EPS on tolerability and effectiveness.

Patients were initially assigned randomly to receive olanzapine, perphenazine, quetiapine, risperidone, or ziprasidone under double-blind conditions (Phase 1). The daily mean modal doses were 20.1 mg for olanzapine, 20.8 mg for perphenazine, 543.4 mg for quetiapine, 3.9 mg for risperidone, and 112.8 mg for ziprasidone. Patients with TD (n = 231, 15% of the sample) were excluded from randomization to perphenazine and were assigned to one of the four SGAs (Phase 1A). Ziprasidone was added to the trial after 40% of the patients had been enrolled. Comparisons involving perphenazine were limited to patients without TD and comparisons involving ziprasidone limited to patients randomized after ziprasidone was added. Patients who discontinued their first treatment were invited to participate in subsequent phases of the trial, which will be discussed in a later section of this chapter. The data presented in this and the following section on the initial and second analyses of EPS deal only with Phases 1 and 1A.

Baseline data revealed that the CATIE sample represents a chronic and moderately symptomatic population of middle-aged patients with schizophrenia who have experienced long-term treatment with antipsychotics, which are important considerations in interpreting EPS findings and generalizability to other patient samples. Patients had received antipsychotic drugs for a mean of 14.4 years, starting at a mean age of 24 years. A total of 72% of patients were receiving antipsychotics at baseline, and 56% were on SGAs.

There were significant differences among drugs in time to discontinuation for any cause, time to discontinuation for inefficacy, and duration of successful treatment, with median time on drug of 9.2 months for olanzapine, 4.6 months for quetiapine, 4.8 months for risperidone, 5.6 months for perphenazine, and 3.5 months for ziprasidone.

The study showed no significant difference between treatment groups in time to discontinuation due to intolerable side effects overall ($p = 0.054$). However, the rates of discontinuation due to side effects differed significantly ($p = 0.04$), with risperidone showing the lowest and olanzapine the highest due to metabolic effects of the latter drug. In contrast, more patients discontinued perphenazine owing to EPS (8% versus 2% to 4% for the SGAs, $p = 0.002$) (Table 9.1). Quetiapine was associated with a higher rate of anticholinergic effects (31% versus 20% to 25%, $p < 0.001$), and conversely, quetiapine had the lowest and perphenazine the highest rate of concomitant use of anticholinergic drugs (3% versus 10%, $p = 0.01$).

There were no significant differences among groups in the incidence of parkinsonism, akathisia, or TD assessed by rating scale measures of severity (Table 9.1). Parkinsonism was defined as a mean score of one or more on the Simpson-Angus Extrapyramidal Signs Scale (SAS), indicating at least mild severity of parkinsonism [37]. Scores of three or more on the global assessment of the Barnes Akathisia Rating Scale (BAS) were chosen to indicate at least moderate severity of akathisia [38]. Finally, scores of two or more on the Abnormal Involuntary Movement Scale (AIMS) global severity score were chosen to indicate at least mild severity of dyskinesia [39]. In Table 9.1, all values listed for each EPS category are for

Table 9.1. Initial analysis of CATIE outcome measures related to EPS [34]

Outcome	Olanzapine	Quetiapine	Risperidone	Perphenazine	Ziprasidone	p Value
Discontinuations due to extrapyramidal symptoms*						
	8/336 (2)	10/337 (3)	11/341 (3)	22/261 (8)	7/185 (4)	0.002
Extrapyramidal side effects*‡						
Parkinsonism	16/240 (7)	10/247 (4)	20/238 (8)	15/243 (6)	6/129 (5)	0.50
Akathisia	12/234 (5)	12/248 (5)	12/240 (6)	16/241 (7)	13/132 (10)	0.19
TD	32/236 (14)	30/236 (13)	38/238 (16)	41/237 (17)	18/126 (14)	0.23
Anticholinergic side effects*ϵ						
	79/336 (24)	105/337 (31)	84/341 (25)	57/261 (22)	37/185 (20)	<0.01
Anticholinergic medications added*						
	25/336 (7)	11/337 (3)	32/341 (9)	26/261 (10)	14/185 (8)	0.01

Notes: *Number/total number of patients (%).
‡Parkinsonism percentages = the number of patients with an SAS mean score ≥ 1, with a mean score < 1 at baseline and at least one post-baseline assessment; Akathisia percentages = the number of patients with a BAS global score ≥ 3, with a global score < 3 at baseline and at least one post-baseline assessment.
TD percentages = the number of patients with an AIMS global score ≥ 2, with a global score < 2 at baseline and at least one post-baseline assessment. Patients with TD at baseline (assigned to Phase 1A) were excluded from all EPS assessments.
ϵUrinary hesitancy, dry mouth, constipation.

patients who did not have that corresponding EPS at baseline, had at least one post-baseline assessment, and were without TD at baseline, i.e., data excludes patients from Phase 1A who were restricted from receiving perphenazine. These data differ from the original report in which SAS and BAS data included patients who had TD at baseline [34]. However, there were no significant differences observed regardless of whether or not TD patients were included in the analysis.

In summary of the initial trial analysis, there were no significant differences between perphenazine and SGAs in the proportion of patients exhibiting parkinsonism, akathisia, and TD, in contrast to previous studies using haloperidol as the representative FGA. However, more patients discontinued perphenazine (8%) than SGAs (2% to 4%) as a result of EPS, and perphenazine (10%) had a high rate of concomitant anticholinergic drug use relative to SGAs (3% to 9%).

Second analysis of EPS in the CATIE schizophrenia trial

Given the somewhat unexpected lack of significant differences in EPS found in the initial analysis, a second in-depth analysis of the CATIE schizophrenia trial data was undertaken to more rigorously assess and compare the incidence of treatment-emergent dystonia, parkinsonism, akathisia, and TD associated with SGAs and perphenazine, excluding subjects with each respective condition at baseline and using more sensitive diagnostic criteria for specific EPS symptoms [40]. Both survival analysis and mixed models were applied to each side effect.

EPS were measured using six items of the SAS for parkinsonism, the global clinical assessment item of the BAS for akathisia, and the first seven items from the AIMS as a measure of TD. Data on concomitant medications, reasons for treatment discontinuation, and reported adverse events were also used to identify the occurrence of any EPS reactions. Two of the authors (D.M. and S.C.) conducted a blind adjudication of physician reports to classify cases in which treatment was discontinued or concomitant medications were added for each of the four EPS side effect symptoms.

Dystonia was identified if it was given as the reason for adding concomitant medications or discontinuation of antipsychotic medications, or reported as an adverse event.

Patients were considered to have met criteria for parkinsonism if they scored 1 (mild) on at least two of the six SAS items or 2 (moderate) on one of the items (initial analysis required a mean score ≥ 1). Cases of parkinsonism were further identified if they were taking an antiparkinsonian medication or discontinued their antipsychotic medication due to parkinsonism. The summary score of all six SAS items was also used as a continuous measure.

Patients were considered to have met criteria for akathisia if they scored at least 2 (mild) on the BAS global item, if akathisia was specifically given as the reason for starting any medication, or if they discontinued their antipsychotic medication due to akathisia (initial analysis required a global score ≥ 3). The summary score of the BAS global item was also used as a continuous measure.

Patients were considered to have met criteria for TD if they met Schooler-Kane (S-K) criteria, i.e., if they scored 2 (mild) on at least two AIMS items or 3 (moderate) on one of the items at two or more assessments (initial analysis required a global score of ≥ 2) [41]. Analyses were also conducted using modified S-K criteria such that meeting the AIMS criteria on only one assessment was required, i.e., "probable" TD. The summary score of all seven AIMS items was also used as a continuous measure. TD was also diagnosed if it was the reason given for adding any medication or discontinuing antipsychotic medication.

Analyses of the incidence of the four EPS were conducted only on subpopulations that did not meet criteria for that side effect at the time of baseline assessment. For TD, patients were excluded from the analysis if they met modified S-K criteria at baseline, or were identified as having borderline TD, which was defined by not meeting the full modified S-K criteria but having at least one AIMS item score of mild, reporting a history of TD, taking medications for TD, or being placed in Phase 1A. A supportive analysis was repeated in which all borderline patients were included.

A second set of analyses involved repeated measures analysis of continuous measures representing change in severity of the three syndromes from baseline. Patients meeting criteria for each syndrome at baseline were not excluded from these analyses but baseline scores of the dependent measure were included as covariates in each analysis. Analyses of incidence of side effects were conducted first without adjustment for potential baseline predictors of each syndrome and then in models that included socio-demographic and other baseline measures that were significantly associated with the dependent measure. The statistical plan used for treatment group comparisons followed the same methods as in the original publication from CATIE and described in Chapter 2 [34,36,40].

Dystonia

Dystonia occurs mostly in young males and was commonly associated with FGAs in the past [42,43]. Over 95% of dystonic reactions occur within the first 5 days of treatment, with an incidence rate of 2% to 5%, although some reports suggest higher rates when more potent drugs are used parenterally. In published trials, haloperidol had up to four times greater risk of causing dystonia than SGAs [8,10,44].

By comparison, there were only six cases of acute dystonia reported in the CATIE study (6/1,460 or 0.4%) that were not present at baseline, four of which resulted in treatment discontinuation. Of these six cases of dystonia, none were receiving olanzapine, one was receiving perphenazine, one was receiving quetiapine (discontinued), one was receiving risperidone (discontinued), and three were receiving ziprasidone (two discontinued).

Parkinsonism

The risk of parkinsonism has been associated with increasing age, female gender, and increased dose and potency of antipsychotics [42,43]. It typically develops in days to weeks, with 50% to 75% of cases occurring within 1 month and 90% within 3 months. The incidence is variable depending upon risk between studies but has been estimated to occur in about 10% to 15% of patients treated in routine practice with FGAs. In randomized trials, haloperidol has been associated with two to four times the risk of parkinsonism compared with SGAs (22% to 38% versus 4% to 14%) [8,10,12,14,44–46].

In the second CATIE analysis, examination of the proportion of patients showing no evidence of parkinsonism at baseline who met at least one of the three criteria for parkinsonism during the subsequent follow-up period revealed no substantial differences between treatment groups (Table 9.2). Statistical analysis, using piecewise exponential regression of the probability of having a parkinsonian event showed no statistically significant difference between treatment groups. Covariate-adjusted 12-month event rates were notable at 37% to 44% among the four SGAs and 37% for the FGA perphenazine. The Kaplan-Meier survival plot illustrates both the substantial incidence of parkinsonian events, particularly in the first month, and the convergence of treatment groups (Figure 9.1). Finally, mixed model analysis of change in parkinsonian symptoms from baseline for all treated patients, as measured with the SAS, also showed no statistically significant group differences. Analyses of maximum change in SAS score and incidence of parkinsonism events after the first month of treatment also found no statistically significant differences.

Table 9.2. Second analysis of observed EPS events for patients without the events at baseline [40]

Extrapyramidal event	Olanzapine	Quetiapine	Risperidone	Perphenazine	Ziprasidone
Any parkinsonian event	70/201 (35)*	55/187 (29)	71/191 (37)	48/160 (30)	31/98 (32)
Any akathisia event	52/238 (22)	42/250 (17)	61/244 (25)	51/207 (25)	26/130 (20)
Tardive dyskinesia (S-K)	2/182 (1)	8/179 (5)	4/179 (2)	6/183 (3)	3/89 (3)
Tardive dyskinesia (mS-K)	20/216 (9)	19/222 (9)	21/220 (10)	26/221 (12)	10/120 (8)

Notes: *Number/total number of patients without the extrapyramidal symptom at baseline (%).
Any parkinsonian event includes meeting SAS score criteria, discontinuing treatment, or adding a medication for parkinsonism.
Any akathisia event includes meeting BAS score criteria, discontinuing treatment, or adding a medication for akathisia.
S-K = Schooler Kane criteria; mS-K = Modified Schooler Kane criteria requiring only one post-baseline assessment [41].

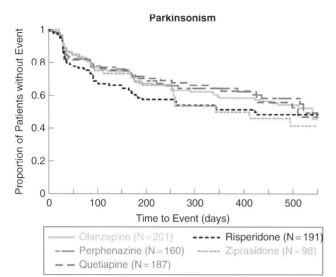

Figure 9.1. Kaplan-Meier survival curve of time until parkinsonism event for people with no parkinsonism at baseline. See plate section for color version. [40] Reprinted with permission of The British Journal of Psychiatry.

Analysis of incidence of adding medications found an overall difference ($p = 0.029$ for primary data set 1), with addition of antiparkinsonian medications most likely for risperidone patients (6.7%) and least likely for quetiapine patients (1.0%). In addition, analyses of incidence of discontinuation for parkinsonism suggested there was a lower rate of discontinuation for quetiapine and ziprasidone ($p < 0.05$ for all four data sets, although exact logistic regression methods were statistically significant only for data set 3).

Akathisia

Akathisia is another common EPS that occurs in all age groups associated with increasing dose and potency of antipsychotics [42,43]. It develops in 50% of cases within 1 month and 90% of cases within 3 months. Incidence rates vary between 5% and 50% across studies of FGAs, but it occurs in about 20% of patients in routine practice. In published trials, akathisia developed at an incidence rate of about two to seven times higher with haloperidol (15% to 40%) compared with SGAs (0% to 12%) [8,10,12,14,44–46].

In the CATIE study, examination of the proportion of patients who met at least one of the criteria for akathisia among those who had no evidence of akathisia at baseline, showed no substantial difference between treatment groups (Table 9.2). Poisson regression analysis of the probability of meeting any of the three criteria for akathisia revealed no significant difference between groups. Covariate-adjusted 12-month event rates ranged from 26% to 34% for the SGAs and 35% for perphenazine. The Kaplan-Meier plot graphically shows the close grouping of survival curves across treatment groups (Figure 9.2), and mixed model analysis of change from baseline on the BAS global rating similarly revealed no statistically significant group differences, but did suggest a general decline in akathisia over time. Analysis of maximum change in BAS global ratings found no statistically significant differences ($p = 0.071$), although perphenazine had the largest estimated change (0.44) and olanzapine had the lowest (0.22). Analyses of incidence of adding medications for

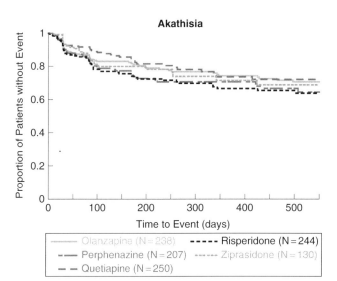

Figure 9.2. Kaplan-Meier survival curve of time until akathisia event for people with no akathisia at baseline. See plate section for color version. [40] Reprinted with permission of The British Journal of Psychiatry.

akathisia found no significant differences ($p = 0.056$), although perphenazine (8%) and risperidone (6%) had higher rates of medications added compared with quetiapine (2%). No significant differences were noted for analyses of discontinuation for akathisia.

Tardive dyskinesia

The onset of TD occurs insidiously over 3 months or more of treatment and has been associated with increasing age, possibly dose and potency as well as long-term exposure to FGAs [47,48]. Studies of FGAs have reported an incidence of 4% to 5% per year, reaching 15% to 30% in the elderly, and a prevalence of about 20% to 25% [47–49]. In contrast, studies with SGAs have suggested a significantly lower risk of TD [17,19,33,50,51].

Data from patients who had no evidence of TD at baseline show a small proportion of patients met full S-K TD criteria during Phase 1 treatment (1.1% to 4.5% receiving SGAs and 3.3% receiving perphenazine (Table 9.2). The proportion of patients who met modified S-K TD criteria ranged from 8.3% to 9.6% with SGAs and 11.8% for perphenazine. The other two measures of TD events (patient discontinuations and concomitant medications) were met by only 1% or fewer cases in all treatment groups. Poisson regression reveals no statistically significant difference between treatment groups on either TD indicator. Covariate-adjusted 12-month event rates for S-K TD ranged from 0.7% to 2.2% among the SGAs and 2.7% for perphenazine. Kaplan-Meier survival curves show both the infrequent incidence of TD and the overlapping of treatment groups (Figure 9.3), while mixed model analysis of change in TD symptoms from baseline, based on the AIMS total score, also showed no statistically significant group differences. Analyses of incidence of TD events for patients with either no or borderline TD at baseline, and maximum change in AIMS total score also found no statistically significant differences between treatment groups.

In summary, using a broad variety of more stringent measures of dystonia, parkinsonism, akathisia, and TD, the analysis of incidence rates and continuous measures from CATIE shows no significant differences between any SGA and perphenazine, or between

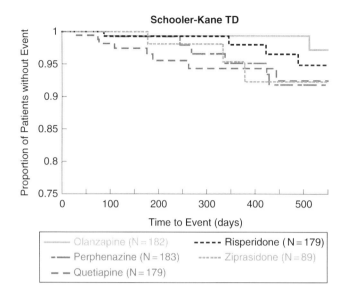

Figure 9.3. Kaplan-Meier survival curve of time until Schooler-Kane TD for people with no TD at baseline. See plate section for color version. [40] Reprinted with permission of The British Journal of Psychiatry.

any pair of SGAs. In this analysis, we utilized more sensitive criteria for parkinsonism and akathisia than in the analyses reported by Lieberman *et al.* [34], and we thus found a much higher incidence of these side effects, whereas we used more specific and standardized criteria for TD resulting in a lower incidence than in the initial analysis; in neither case did the criteria result in any significant differences in the incidence of specific EPS symptoms. However, there were differences among the secondary measures of adding concomitant medications and discontinuations for parkinsonism and less so for akathisia, with quetiapine least likely to cause either outcome, and perphenazine or risperidone more likely to do so in some instances.

Analysis of EPS in subsequent phases of the CATIE schizophrenia trial

In the CATIE trial, patients who discontinued medications assigned in Phase 1 or 1A could enter Phase 2. If the patients received perphenazine during Phase 1, they could enter Phase 1B to receive olanzapine, risperidone or quetiapine [52]. If they again discontinued treatment in Phase 1B, they could enter Phase 2. Patients entering Phase 2 from either Phase 1, 1A or 1B, could enter one of two pathways; the efficacy pathway (Phase 2E), which was designed for patients who discontinued previous treatment because of inefficacy, compared open-label clozapine to double-blind treatment with olanzapine, risperidone, or quetiapine [53]; or the tolerability pathway (Phase 2T), which was designed for patients who discontinued previous treatment due to intolerability, compared double-blind treatment with ziprasidone, olanzapine, risperidone, or quetiapine [54]. Measures of EPS based on scale scores were the same as in the initial CATIE trial analysis.

Among 444 patients who discontinued an SGA in previous phases and entered Phase 2T, olanzapine and risperidone proved more effective than quetiapine and ziprasidone based on longer time until discontinuation for any reason [54]. This ranking of relative effectiveness held true for patients who discontinued previous drugs for inefficacy. However, among patients who discontinued previous drugs for intolerability, time until discontinuation was longest for risperidone but the differences were not significant. There were no differences in the incidence of EPS between drugs based on rating scale scores or reasons for discontinuations.

Among 99 patients discontinuing SGAs in previous phases for lack of efficacy and entering Phase 2E, clozapine was more effective than olanzapine, risperidone, and quetiapine based on longer time to treatment discontinuation for any reason [53]. This was true for discontinuations for lack of efficacy, but there were no significant differences in discontinuations because of intolerable side effects. There were no significant differences in EPS, but quetiapine was associated with significantly more anticholinergic side effects.

In Phase 1B, 114 patients who previously had been randomized to perphenazine received olanzapine, risperidone, or quetiapine [52]. Although there were no differences between the drugs in the incidence of EPS based on scale scores or reasons for discontinuing treatment, quetiapine and olanzapine were more effective than risperidone as reflected in all-cause discontinuations. There were no differences between drugs for discontinuations due to inefficacy, intolerability, or patient choice considered separately. However, among patients who earlier discontinued perphenazine because of intolerability, twice as many discontinued risperidone (85%) compared with quetiapine (40%). In addition, none of these patients discontinued quetiapine because of intolerability compared with 64% receiving olanzapine and 69% receiving risperidone. Finally, among 19 patients who discontinued perphenazine specifically because of EPS, twice as many discontinued risperidone for any reason (83%) compared with quetiapine (38%) or olanzapine (40%). Therefore, in Phase 1B, among patients who had not responded well to perphenazine previously, quetiapine was more effective than in other phases, and risperidone was less effective. Stroup *et al.* speculated that patients in Phase 1B represented a subgroup of patients who were sensitive to and less tolerant of the high affinity dopamine D2 receptor mediated neurological effects of perphenazine and risperidone, and did better on quetiapine, which is least like perphenazine in this regard [52].

Clinical correlates of TD at baseline from the CATIE schizophrenia trial

As reviewed above, there were no significant differences between perphenazine and SGAs in the rate of development of TD studied prospectively in any phase of the CATIE trial. However, CATIE also afforded a unique opportunity to re-examine cross-sectional clinical correlates associated with TD at baseline in a large and well-defined population. Previous studies have suggested an association with increasing age, female gender, longer duration of antipsychotic treatment, higher ratings of negative symptoms and thought disorder, greater cognitive impairments, presence of acute EPS, and diabetes [47,48].

To re-examine these correlations, patients at baseline were divided into TD and non-TD groups [55]. Probable TD was defined by use of S-K criteria, except a history of 3 months of drug exposure was not required and the diagnosis was derived only from the AIMS ratings at baseline [41]. Patients who had no history of TD and who had no AIMS item rated greater than 1 on the baseline AIMS examination comprised the non-TD group. Patients who had a history of TD but did not meet modified S-K criteria and subjects who had one AIMS item rated 2 were considered indeterminate and were excluded from the analyses. The methods of statistical analysis were previously described [55].

Table 9.3. Clinical correlates of TD in baseline data from the CATIE schizophrenia trial [55]

	TD (N = 212) Mean ± SE	Non-TD (N = 1098) Mean ± SE	p Value
Age (years)	47.2 (0.6)	38.9 (0.3)	<0.0001
Years since first antipsychotic	21.5 (0.7)	12.8 (0.3)	<0.0001
AIMS (total)	7.6 (0.3)	0.3 (0.02)	<0.0001
SAS	0.40 (0.03)	0.16 (0.01)	<0.0001
BAS	2.06 (0.14)	0.78 (0.04)	<0.0001
Neurocognitive composite (Z-score)	−0.19 (0.05)	0.02 (0.020)	0.772
PANSS			
Total	78.2 (1.2)	75.1	0.001
Positive	19.4 (0.4)	18.3	0.058
Negative	20.2 (0.4)	20.1	0.013
General psychopathology	38.6 (0.7)	36.7	0.003
Gender (% male)	78%	74%	0.224
Current antipsychotic			0.051
None	26%	27%	
SGA only	47%	60%	
FGA (± SGA)	28%	14%	
Current anticholinergic use	28%	14%	0.009
Diabetes	13%	9%	0.682
Hypertension	41%	33%	0.405
Substance abuse	42%	37%	0.0032

Abbreviations: SAS = Simpson-Angus Extrapyramidal Signs Scale, BAS = Barnes Akathisia Rating Scale, AIMS = Abnormal Involuntary Movement Scale, PANSS = Positive and Negative Syndrome Scale; FGA = first generation antipsychotic; SGA = second-generation antipsychotic.

Of the 1,460 patients in the CATIE trial, 212 met modified S-K criteria for probable TD and 1,098 had neither a history nor current evidence of TD (Table 9.3). Sixty-eight patients who had a chart history of TD but did not currently meet modified S-K criteria, and 80 patients who had no history of TD but had one AIMS item rated 2, were considered indeterminate, and were excluded from the analyses. Patients with probable TD were found to be significantly older, and had been treated with an antipsychotic significantly longer, were more likely to be currently treated with an FGA, and to be currently treated with an anticholinergic agent. However, since these are cross-sectional data, we cannot infer that these are causal relationships. Gender, race, and ethnicity were not differentially distributed between patients with TD versus those without TD. Patients with diabetes or hypertension did not have higher rates of TD.

Having a substance abuse disorder was significantly associated with having TD after adjusting for significant covariates and when stratified by age. In addition, we also found that both alcohol ($p = 0.023$) and drug abuse/dependence ($p = 0.0032$) were significantly associated with TD in covariate-adjusted analyses. We also found that the relationship with cocaine abuse/dependence showed a trend toward being associated with TD ($p = 0.057$), stimulant abuse/dependence was significantly associated with TD ($p = 0.013$), and opiate ($p = 0.88$) and marijuana ($p = 0.33$) abuse/dependence were not associated with TD.

Although TD was associated with neurocognitive impairment in unadjusted analysis, the relationship lost significance after adjustment for covariates and investigator site. When we examined individual neurocognitive factors, the pattern remained the same. Patients with TD had higher levels of psychopathology (Positive and Negative Syndrome Scale [PANSS] total score) [56] even after the covariates and investigator site were included in the analysis.

The severities of parkinsonism and akathisia were significantly related to TD in unadjusted models and after covariate adjustment.

In conclusion, our results confirm previously suggested relationships between age, duration of treatment with an antipsychotic, treatment with FGAs, treatment with an anticholinergic agent, presence of acute EPS, increased psychopathology, current substance abuse, and the presence of TD. Of note, the correlation between TD and FGAs at baseline contrasts with the lack of differences between perphenazine and SGAs observed in the prospective outcome data of the study. This could be explained by the long-term effect of past exposure to high doses of more potent D2 receptor antagonists, like haloperidol, in patients prior to entry in the study, whereas the mid-potency antipsychotic perphenazine was less likely to induce dyskinesias during the shorter trial period itself. Moreover, data on TD from the randomized, controlled prospective phases of CATIE provide a more rigorous test of the causal nature of the association between TD and drug class compared with the cross-sectional analysis of the correlation at a single point in time. Finally, we found no support for the hypothesis that diabetes or hypertension increase the risk for TD, or that TD is associated with cognitive impairment. This suggests that older patients with schizophrenia who have a long duration of treatment with potent FGAs, who experience EPS, are treated with anticholinergic agents, have higher ratings of psychopathology, and who are current substance abusers are at higher risk for developing TD.

Methodological limitations of the CATIE trial in relation to EPS

The strengths of the CATIE study include its large sample size, diverse representation of clinical settings, independence from industry sponsorship, and the head-to-head comparison of four SGAs and a representative FGA. Based on the sample size and event rates for EPS, the study had 80% power to detect with a p value < 0.05, a 15% difference between any two treatment groups for parkinsonism events, a 14% difference for akathisia, and a 7% difference in TD.

Nevertheless, there are a number of design features to consider in interpreting the findings on EPS and generalizability of the study data to other patient populations. First, the use of perphenazine, an intermediate potency FGA given at modest doses, was likely at least partially responsible for the lack of difference in the incidence of treatment-emergent EPS seen between the FGA and SGA groups in the study that might have been expected if haloperidol had been used as the FGA. The daily mean modal dose for the perphenazine group was 20.8 mg/day. Using the dose equivalency of 4:1 (perphenazine to haloperidol) proposed by Kane *et al.* [57], this would be equivalent to a dose of 5.2 mg/day of haloperidol, which is lower than was used in the initial trials for the SGA agents. At this dose, perphenazine was no less effective than olanzapine, quetiapine, risperidone, and ziprasidone measured as time to discontinuation of treatment for any cause [34]. Similarly, there were no differences between perphenazine and SGAs on measures of symptoms or quality of life, or on neurocognitive functioning [25,58,59].

Second, since most subjects in the trial had received antipsychotic medications for many years, the patients may be less likely to develop EPS than the general population of persons with schizophrenia, especially those with first-episode psychosis. In addition, it is possible that, for subjects who developed TD during the trial, the onset of TD could have been related to prior antipsychotic exposure. However, previous studies that showed advantages of SGAs over FGAs usually were conducted on patient samples of similar age and duration of illness, so these sample characteristics may not account for the differences in findings [60].

Like other studies comparing the incidence of TD in patients treated with FGAs and SGAs, some subjects may have been experiencing withdrawal dyskinesia or unmasking of TD related to switching from one antipsychotic to another. The majority of subjects in the CATIE schizophrenia trial switched antipsychotics at baseline. It is possible that the antipsychotic prior to entry into the study or the antipsychotic that they were randomized to may have had an influence on the rates of withdrawal dyskinesia although investigators were allowed to cross-titrate the previous and new antipsychotics for up to a month. In fact, we saw very few cases of TD within the first month of the trial, and our findings did not change substantially whether we included the data from the 1-month visit or not, suggesting that withdrawal dyskinesia did not significantly affect our findings.

Another potential limitation of the study was the relatively short duration of exposure to each drug due to high switch rates. Nonetheless, the duration of exposure was similar to or longer than those in prior studies with SGAs [19,60]. Our findings were corrected for duration of exposure, and it is unlikely that the results for parkinsonism and akathisia were affected by the duration of exposure as they tend to occur early in treatment.

Another substantial difference between the CATIE data and previously reported trials was that patients with a history of TD at baseline were excluded from analyses that compared SGAs and perphenazine. The CATIE design is more consistent than previous studies with the basic principle of risk assessment research which states that patients who already have the outcome being studied should be excluded from the study cohort [61]. Such patients already *are* "cases" and thus cannot be at any risk of *becoming* "cases" and add uninformative variance that biases results toward the null. The exclusion of TD patients from our statistical analysis allowed *more* precise comparison of treatment-emergent TD incidence than in studies that included mixed samples. It has previously been reported that there is a relationship between the development of parkinsonism, akathisia, and TD. Various investigators have shown that antipsychotic-induced parkinsonism and/or akathisia are associated with a higher risk of developing TD [52–55], and the baseline analysis of the CATIE data showed a significant correlation of parkinsonism and akathisia with TD [22,55,62–65] However, inclusion of acute EPS as a covariate in adjusted analyses of the incidence of TD did not alter the lack of significance between treatment groups.

We also excluded subjects who were experiencing parkinsonism and akathisia at baseline from the corresponding analysis comparing the incidence of treatment-emergent parkinsonism and akathisia to avoid potential biases. Although we feel that this was the best method for comparing rates of EPS, our findings may not directly relate to patients who are already experiencing an EPS on their current antipsychotic agent. It is also possible that patients with TD at baseline who were only randomized to an SGA may have been at a greater risk for developing parkinsonism and akathisia, which could potentially bias these results. However, in analyses between perphenazine and SGAs in the incidence of acute EPS, patients receiving perphenazine were compared only with patients receiving SGAs who were not in Phase 1A, i.e., patients with TD were excluded from these analyses. Moreover, there were no significant differences between antipsychotics in the incidence of acute EPS in the initial CATIE trial analyses regardless of whether patients with TD were included or not [34].

Another limitation of the study was that, as with most randomized trials of antipsychotic medications, training for the scales used to rate EPS and TD was not as rigorous as training for ratings of psychopathology. Given that the trial was double-blind, this fact should have influenced all treatment groups equally. Another issue related to scale scores concerns criteria used in the study to define EPS events. The S-K criteria for TD based on the AIMS scale have been standardized and widely used in antipsychotic trials, and the rate of TD events found in the CATIE study based on S-K criteria are comparable to previous results ranging from 1.1% to 4.5% [41]. Use of modified S-K data or use of an AIMS global score of 2 or more in the initial CATIE analysis yielded substantially higher rates of dyskinesia (8.3% to 11.8% and 13% to 17%, respectively) [34,40]. In any case, the criteria were applied uniformly to all treatment groups in double-blind fashion, and we found no significant differences regardless of the criteria used.

With respect to acute EPS, there is a lack of standardization among trials in diagnostic criteria. Most previous studies report data either on comparative analysis of continuous measures of rating scale scores between treatments or spontaneous adverse reports without specified symptom criteria. In contrast, we applied pre-defined criteria for identifying EPS events similar to the method used by Schooler and Kane for TD [41]. In the initial analysis, parkinsonism was defined by an SAS mean score of 1 or more post-baseline (4% to 8%), whereas in the second analysis, parkinsonism was defined by more sensitive criteria of 1 or more on two items or 2 on one item of the SAS (28.1% to 32.5%). Similarly, akathisia was defined initially by a BAS global score of 3 or more post-baseline (5% to 9%), whereas in the second analysis akathisia was defined by a lower threshold of 2 or more on the BAS (15% to 23%). For both parkinsonism and akathisia, treatments were also compared by discontinuations, concomitant medications, and continuous measures of scale scores. Regardless of the criteria used, there were no significant differences between treatments. However, results may be difficult to compare to other trials if different methods for case ascertainment were used.

There is a need for standardization of the definition of "caseness" for acute EPS similar to the current consensus on TD. For example, the need for further study of the sensitivity and specificity of EPS criteria is underscored by the findings in Phase 1B, during which the patients seemed to be affected by the shared neurological properties of perphenazine and risperidone, even though no differences were found using the less sensitive criteria for EPS employed in the initial CATIE study analysis [34,52].

Conclusions

Using a variety of measures of dystonia, parkinsonism, akathisia, and TD, the analysis of incidence rates and continuous measures from CATIE shows no substantial or statistically significant differences between modest doses of the intermediate potency FGA perphenazine and four SGAs in patients with chronic schizophrenia requiring maintenance antipsychotic treatment.

However, there was evidence from secondary measures scattered through phases of the trial suggesting that subtle differences in extrapyramidal effects between the drugs, which correlate with D2 dopamine receptor affinity, were noted by patients and their doctors, although these findings could be explained by chance due to multiple comparisons. For example, in the initial analysis, perphenazine was associated with more discontinuations for all EPS effects combined, and perphenazine-treated patients received the most concomitant anticholinergic drugs and quetiapine-treated patients the least. In the second analysis, the overall rate of parkinsonian events was not different between drugs, but there was a lower rate of discontinuations due to parkinsonism for quetiapine and ziprasidone, and addition of anticholinergic drugs was most likely for risperidone and least likely for quetiapine. Finally, in Phase 1B, among patients who discontinued perphenazine, quetiapine was significantly more effective and less likely to be discontinued because of intolerability than risperidone, and this was especially true for patients who discontinued perphenazine because of EPS and intolerability in general.

Nevertheless, the conclusion that must be drawn from the CATIE study is that there were no significant differences in primary outcome measures of acute EPS and TD overall, while at the same time perphenazine was shown to be not significantly different in overall effectiveness compared with olanzapine, risperidone, quetiapine, and ziprasidone. Therefore, one could surmise that the advantages of SGAs over haloperidol used without anticholinergics in the incidence and significance of acute EPS and TD shown in previous trials are diminished when modest doses of a low or mid-potency antipsychotic like perphenazine are used as the representative FGA. This is entirely consistent with data emerging from other recent studies [21,26–32]. Furthermore, this implies that haloperidol cannot be considered paradigmatic of all FGAs in comparison with SGAs, and therefore, the dichotomy between first- and second-generation drugs and the concept of SGA "atypicality" based on EPS liability may be misleading. It can be compellingly argued that antipsychotic drugs should be conceptualized as a single drug class with a spectrum of risk for treatment-emergent EPS dependent upon dopamine D2 receptor affinity and patient susceptibility.

References

1. Rifkin A. Extrapyramidal side effects: A historical perspective. *Journal of Clinical Psychiatry* 1987;**48**(Suppl):3–6.

2. Delay J, Deniker P, Harl JM. [Therapeutic use in psychiatry of phenothiazine of central elective action (4560 RP).] *Annales Médcio-Psychologiques* 1952;**110**:112–7.

3. Sigwald J, Bouttier D, Raymondeau C and Piot C. Quatre cas de dyskinesie facio-bucco-linguo-masticatrice a evolution prolongee secondaire a un traitment pas les neuroleptiques. *Revue Neurologique* 1959;**100**:751–5.

4. Druckman R, Seelinger D and Thulin B. Chronic involuntary movements induced by phenothiazines. *The Journal of Nervous and Mental Disorders* 1962;**135**:69–76.

5. Van Putten T. Why do schizophrenic patients refuse to take their drugs?. *Archives of General Psychiatry* 1975;**31**:67–72.

6. Caroff S. The Neuroleptic malignant syndrome. *Journal of Clinical Psychiatry* 1980;**41**:79–83.

7. Kane J, Honigfeld G, Singer J and Meltzer H. Clozapine for the treatment-resistant schizophrenic. A double-blind comparison with chlorpromazine. *Archives of General Psychiatry* 1988;**45**:789–96.

8. Arvanitis LA and Miller BG. Multiple fixed doses of "Seroquel" (quetiapine) in patients with acute exacerbation of schizophrenia:

A comparison with haloperidol and placebo. The Seroquel Trial 13 Study Group. *Biological Psychiatry* 1997;**42**:233–46.

9. Potkin SG, Saha AR, Kujawa MJ, *et al.* Aripiprazole, an antipsychotic with a novel mechanism of action, and risperidone vs placebo in patients with schizophrenia and schizoaffective disorder. *Archives of General Psychiatry* 2003;**60**:681–90.

10. Tollefson GD, Beasley CM Jr, Tran PV, *et al.* Olanzapine versus haloperidol in the treatment of schizophrenia and schizoaffective and schizophreniform disorders: Results of an international collaborative trial. *American Journal of Psychiatry* 1997;**154**:457–65.

11. Marder SR and Meibach RC. Risperidone in the treatment of schizophrenia. *American Journal of Psychiatry* 1994;**151**:825–35.

12. Caroff SN, Mann SC, Campbell EC and Sullivan KA. Movement disorders associated with atypical antipsychotic drugs. *Journal of Clinical Psychiatry* 2002;**63**(Suppl. 4):12–9.

13. Daniel DG, Zimbroff DL, Potkin SG, Reeves KR, Harrigan EP and Lakshminarayanan M. Ziprasidone 80 mg/day and 160 mg/day in the acute exacerbation of schizophrenia and schizoaffective disorder: A 6-week placebo-controlled trial. Ziprasidone Study Group. *Neuropsychopharmacology* 1999;**20**:491–505.

14. Tarsy D, Baldessarini RJ and Tarazi FI. Effects of newer antipsychotics on extrapyramidal function. *CNS Drugs* 2002;**16**:23–45.

15. Dossenbach M, Arango-Davila C, Silva Ibarra H, *et al.* Response and relapse in patients with schizophrenia treated with olanzapine, risperidone, quetiapine, or haloperidol: 12-month follow-up of the Intercontinental Schizophrenia Outpatient Health Outcomes (IC-SOHO) study. *Journal of Clinical Psychiatry* 2005;**66**:1021–30.

16. Kane JM, Woerner M and Lieberman J. Tardive dyskinesia: Prevalence, incidence, and risk factors. *Journal of Clinical Psychopharmacology* 1988;**8**(Suppl):52S–6S.

17. Jeste DV, Lacro JP, Bailey A, Rockwell E, Harris MJ and Caligiuri MP. Lower incidence of tardive dyskinesia with risperidone compared with haloperidol in older patients. *Journal of the American Geriatrics Society* 1999;**47**:716–9.

18. Glazer WM. Expected incidence of tardive dyskinesia associated with atypical antipsychotics. *Journal of Clinical Psychiatry* 2000;**61**(Suppl. 4):21–6.

19. Correll CU, Leucht S and Kane JM. Lower risk for tardive dyskinesia associated with second-generation antipsychotics: A systematic review of 1-year studies. *American Journal of Psychiatry* 2004;**161**:414–25.

20. Tenback DE, van Harten PN, Slooff CJ, Belger MA and van Os J. Effects of antipsychotic treatment on tardive dyskinesia: A 6-month evaluation of patients from the European Schizophrenia Outpatient Health Outcomes (SOHO) Study. *Journal of Clinical Psychiatry* 2005;**66**:1130–3.

21. Leucht S, Pitschel-Walz G, Abraham D and Kissling W. Efficacy and extrapyramidal side-effects of the new antipsychotics olanzapine, quetiapine, risperidone, and sertindole compared to conventional antipsychotics and placebo. A meta-analysis of randomized controlled trials. *Schizophrenia Research* 1999;**35**:51–68.

22. Glazer WM. Extrapyramidal side effects, tardive dyskinesia, and the concept of atypicality. *Journal of Clinical Psychiatry.* 2000;**61**(Suppl. 3):16–21.

23. Meltzer HY. The mechanism of action of novel antipsychotic drugs. *Schizophrenia Bulletin* 1991;**17**:263–87.

24. Davis JM, Chen N and Glick ID. A meta-analysis of the efficacy of second-generation antipsychotics. *Archives of General Psychiatry* 2003;**60**:553–64.

25. Rosenheck RA, Leslie DL, Sindelar J, *et al.* Cost-effectiveness of second-generation antipsychotics and perphenazine in a randomized trial of treatment for chronic

schizophrenia. *American Journal of Psychiatry* 2006;**163**:2080–9.

26. Geddes J, Freemantle N, Harrison P and Bebbington P. Atypical antipsychotics in the treatment of schizophrenia: Systematic overview and meta-regression analysis. *British Medical Journal* 2000;**321**:1371–6.

27. Leucht S, Wahlbeck K, Hamann J and Kissling W. New generation antipsychotics versus low-potency conventional antipsychotics: A systematic review and meta-analysis. *Lancet* 2003;**361**:1581–9.

28. Leucht S, Barnes TR, Kissling W, Engel RR, Correll C and Kane JM. Relapse prevention in schizophrenia with new-generation antipsychotics: A systematic review and exploratory meta-analysis of randomized, controlled trials. *American Journal of Psychiatry* 2003;**160**:1209–22.

29. Rosenheck R, Perlick D, Bingham S, *et al.* Effectiveness and cost of clanzapine and haloperidol in the treatment of schizophrenia: A randomized controlled trial. *Journal of the American Medical Association* 2003;**290**:2693–702.

30. Hugenholtz GW, Heerdink ER, Stolker JJ, Meijer WE, Egberts AC and Nolen WA. Haloperidol dose when used as active comparator in randomized controlled trials with atypical antipsychotics in schizophrenia: Comparison with officially recommended doses. *Journal of Clinical Psychiatry* 2006;**67**:897–903.

31. Rosenheck R, Stroup S, Keefe RS, *et al.* Measuring outcome priorities and preferences in people with schizophrenia. *British Journal of Psychiatry* 2005;**187**:529–36.

32. Jones PB, Barnes TR, Davies L, *et al.* Randomized controlled trial of the effect on quality of life of second- vs first-generation antipsychotic drugs in schizophrenia: Cost Utility of the Latest Antipsychotic Drugs in Schizophrenia Study (CUtLASS 1). *Archives of General Psychiatry* 2006;**63**:1079–87.

33. Correll CU and Schenk EM. Tardive dyskinesia and new antipsychotics. *Current Opinion in Psychiatry* 2008;**21**:151–6.

34. Lieberman JA, Stroup TS, McEvoy JP, *et al.* Effectiveness of antipsychotic drugs in patients with chronic schizophrenia. *New England Journal of Medicine* 2005;**353**:1209–23.

35. Stroup TS, McEvoy JP, Swartz MS, *et al.* The National Institute of Mental Health Clinical Antipsychotic Trials of Intervention Effectiveness (CATIE) project: Schizophrenia trial design and protocol development. *Schizophrenia Bulletin* 2003;**29**:15–31.

36. Davis SM, Koch GG, Davis CE and LaVange LM. Statistical approaches to effectiveness measurement and outcome-driven re-randomizations in the Clinical Antipsychotic Trials of Intervention Effectiveness (CATIE) studies. *Schizophrenia Bulletin* 2003;**29**:73–80.

37. Simpson GM and Angus JW. A rating scale for extrapyramidal side effects. *Acta Psychiatrica Scandinavica. Supplementum* 1970;**212**:11–9.

38. Barnes TR. A rating scale for drug-induced akathisia. *British Journal of Psychiatry* 1989;**154**:672–6.

39. Guy W. *ECDEU Assessment Manual for Psychopharmacology-Revised*. Rockville, MD: Department of Health; 1976.

40. Miller DD, Caroff SN, Davis SM, *et al.* Extrapyramidal side effects of antipsychotics in a randomized trial. *British Journal of Psychiatry* 2008;**193**:279–88.

41. Schooler NR and Kane JM. Research diagnoses for tardive dyskinesia. *Archives of General Psychiatry* 1982;**39**:486–7.

42. Tarsy D. Neuroleptic-induced extrapyramidal reactions: Classification, description, and diagnosis. *Clinical Neuropharmacology* 1983;**6**(Suppl. 1):S9–26.

43. Gelenberg AJ. General principles of treatment of extrapyramidal syndromes. *Clinical Neuropharmacology* 1983;**6** (Suppl. 1):S52–6.

44. Simpson GM and Lindenmayer JP. Extrapyramidal symptoms in patients treated with risperidone. *Journal of Clinical Psychopharmacology* 1997;**17**:194–201.

45. Hirsch SR, Kissling W, Bauml J, Power A and O'Connor R. A 28-week comparison of ziprasidone and haloperidol in outpatients with stable schizophrenia. *Journal of Clinical Psychiatry* 2002;**63**:516–23.

46. Barnes TR and McPhillips MA. Critical analysis and comparison of the side-effect and safety profiles of the new antipsychotics. *British Journal of Psychiatry. Supplement* 1999;(38):34–43.

47. Kane JM. Tardive dyskinesia. In: Bloom FE, Kupfer DJ, eds. *Psychopharmacology: The Fourth Generation of Progress.* Nashville, TN: American College of Neuropsychopharmacology; 1995. pp 1485–95.

48. Tarsy D. History and definition of tardive dyskinesia. *Clinical Neuropharmacology* 1983;6:91–9.

49. Chakos MH, Alvir JM, Woerner MG, *et al.* Incidence and correlates of tardive dyskinesia in first episode of schizophrenia. *Archives of General Psychiatry* 1996;53:313–9.

50. Beasley CM, Dellva MA, Tamura RN, *et al.* Randomised double-blind comparison of the incidence of tardive dyskinesia in patients with schizophrenia during long-term treatment with olanzapine or haloperidol. *British Journal of Psychiatry* 1999;174:23–30.

51. Kane JM. Tardive dyskinesia circa 2006. *American Journal of Psychiatry* 2006;163:1316–8.

52. Stroup TS, Lieberman JA, McEvoy JP, *et al.* Effectiveness of olanzapine, quetiapine, and risperidone in patients with chronic schizophrenia after discontinuing perphenazine: A CATIE study. *American Journal of Psychiatry* 2007;164:415–27.

53. McEvoy JP, Lieberman JA, Stroup TS, *et al.* Effectiveness of clozapine versus olanzapine, quetiapine, and risperidone in patients with chronic schizophrenia who did not respond to prior atypical antipsychotic treatment. *American Journal of Psychiatry* 2006;163:600–10.

54. Stroup TS, Lieberman JA, *et al.* Effectiveness of olanzapine, quetiapine, risperidone, and ziprasidone in patients with chronic schizophrenia following discontinuation of a previous atypical antipsychotic. *American Journal of Psychiatry* 2006;163:611–22.

55. Miller DD, McEvoy JP, Davis SM, *et al.* Clinical correlates of tardive dyskinesia in schizophrenia: Baseline data from the CATIE schizophrenia trial. *Schizophrenia Research* 2005;80:33–43.

56. Kay SR, Fiszbein A and Opler LA. The positive and negative syndrome scale (PANSS) for schizophrenia. *Schizophrenia Bulletin* 1987;13:261–76.

57. Kane JM, Leucht S, Carpenter D and Docherty JP. The expert consensus guideline series. Optimizing pharmacologic treatment of psychotic disorders. Introduction: Methods, commentary, and summary. *Journal of Clinical Psychiatry* 2003;64(Suppl. 12):5–19.

58. Keefe RS, Bilder RM, Davis SM, *et al.* Neurocognitive effects of antipsychotic medications in patients with chronic schizophrenia in the CATIE Trial. *Archives of General Psychiatry* 2007;64:633–47.

59. Swartz MS, Perkins DO, Stroup TS, *et al.* Effects of antipsychotic medications on psychosocial functioning in patients with chronic schizophrenia: Findings from the NIMH CATIE study. *American Journal of Psychiatry* 2007;164:428–36.

60. Rosenheck R, Stroup S, Swartz M, *et al.* Dr. Rosenheck and colleagues reply. *American Journal of Psychiatry* 2007;164:678–80.

61. Kelsey JL, Whittemore AS, Evans AS and Thompson DS. *Methods in Observational Epidemiology.* New York: Oxford University Press; 1996.

62. Crane GE. Prevention and management of tardive dyskinesia. *American Journal of Psychiatry* 1972;129:466–7.

63. Kane JM, Woerner M, Borenstein M, Wegner J and Lieberman J. Integrating incidence and prevalence of tardive dyskinesia. *Psychopharmacology Bulletin* 1986;22:254–8.

64. Saltz BL, Woerner MG, Kane JM, *et al.* Prospective study of tardive dyskinesia incidence in the elderly. *Journal of the American Medical Association* 1991;266:2402–6.

65. Umbricht D and Kane JM. Medical complications of new antipsychotic drugs. *Schizophrenia Bulletin* 1996;22:475–83.

Chapter 1

Metabolic side effects and risk of cardiovascular disease

Jonathan M. Meyer, Donald C. Goff, and Joseph P. McEvoy

Introduction

The understanding of cardiovascular (CV) risk continues to evolve, as does the ongoing search for novel biomarkers to improve risk prediction [1]. The use of new markers for lipid metabolism [2] and systemic inflammation [3] has yet to be fully integrated into CV risk assessment algorithms, but emerging data document the potential utility of novel biomarkers in refining CV risk estimates. For now, clinical CV assessment continues to be based on well-established cardiac risk factors derived from cohort studies, such as the community-based Framingham Heart Study (FHS) [4], the longitudinal nature of which have provided robust means to assess the relative impact of clinical factors on cardiac morbidity and mortality. The additive CV effects of cigarette smoking, hypertension, total cholesterol, and high density lipoprotein (HDL) cholesterol have been found to predict the risk of major cardiac events (angina, myocardial infarction [MI], and sudden cardiac death) over a 10 year period, and can be calculated with empirically derived CV risk algorithms [4,5]. The FHS derived formula may overestimate CV risk in Hispanic men and Native Americans compared to Whites and African-Americans [6], but is considered a standard and important method for clinical CV risk calculations [5].

Although the standard FHS algorithm and the gender-specific charts from the National Cholesterol Education Program (NCEP) [5] are based on extensive clinical data, there are limitations to these predictive models. Particularly problematic is the fact that a substantial fraction (20%) of subjects in the FHS experienced major CV events without evidence of one of the major CV risk factors [4]. Another issue for CV risk assessment rests in the use of serum low density lipoprotein (LDL) as the primary target for lipid lowering therapy [5]. Although numerous trials have demonstrated the benefits of LDL reduction, there is often a poor correlation between baseline LDL and future MI risk during statin treatment [7]; moreover, 46% of CV events in the longitudinal Women's Health Study occurred in those with serum LDL below 130 mg/dL [8].

These limitations with CV risk algorithms and the standard conceptualization of treatment goals has impelled the search for new physiological CV risk predictors including novel lipid fractions such as apolipoprotein B (apo-B), and measures of inflammation and endothelial injury such as interleukin-6 (IL-6), intracellular adhesion molecule (ICAM), and C-reactive protein (CRP). Among these newer measures, quantification of CRP using high sensitivity assays (hS-CRP) has shown superior predictive power by itself compared to other biomarkers, including LDL, HDL, total cholesterol:HDL ratio, IL-6, ICAM, and apo-B [9].

Antipsychotic Trials in Schizophrenia, ed. T. Scott Stroup and Jeffrey A. Lieberman. Published by Cambridge University Press. © Cambridge University Press 2010.

Moreover, the use of CRP provides added CV risk information after controlling for traditional CV risk factors [8], and, in global risk models, is second to systolic blood pressure and ahead of smoking as a predictor of CV risk [10,11]. The use of hS-CRP assays during large statin trials has also raised the question of whether the CV effects from treatment are driven by changes in LDL or changes in CRP. Patients in a large randomized pravastatin vs. atorvastatin trial with lower post-treatment CRP experienced fewer CV events than those with higher CRP, regardless of LDL levels [12]; moreover, agents that reduce LDL but increase CRP (e.g. hormone replacement therapy) are associated with increased CV risk.

Another source of CV risk often not captured by the NCEP algorithm is that related to insulin resistance. Type 2 diabetes mellitus (DM) has long been recognized as a strong predictor of future CV events [13,14], and the original FHS derived algorithms accounted for glycemic status [4]. As long-term follow-up studies indicated equal risk for major CV events and CV-related mortality between type 2 DM patients and non-diabetic patients with a history of MI [15], the latest NCEP algorithm removed type 2 DM as a CV risk factor, and deemed it a coronary heart disease (CHD) risk-equivalent condition [5]. For DM patients, the 10-year MI risk is so great (>20%) that the clinical approach to risk reduction must be as aggressive as for those who have already suffered an MI.

Type 2 DM represents the endpoint of a 10- to 20-year process in which increased adiposity leads to insulin resistance, and, in some individuals, to β-cell failure and hyperglycemia. Type 2 DM itself is associated with markedly elevated CV risk, but within the group of non-diabetic insulin resistant individuals, there is a cohort that is particularly predisposed to adverse CV outcomes. The metabolic syndrome concept was first elaborated over two decades ago [16], and describes the fact that, in certain susceptible individuals, central adiposity results not only in compensatory hyperinsulinemia, but co-occurring hypertension, atherogenic dyslipidemia (decreased high density lipoprotein cholesterol, elevated triglycerides), and increased levels of prothrombotic proteins and inflammatory markers. These metabolic parameters define a continuum of risk, such that those individuals who have more features of this syndrome appear more greatly predisposed to type 2 DM [17] and CV disease [18]. There has been an ongoing debate in recent literature over the value of the metabolic syndrome concept [19,20], since the metabolic syndrome diagnosis itself confers no greater predictive value for CV events than traditional estimating algorithms [21]. Nonetheless, there is a strong association between the number of metabolic syndrome criteria met and increased risk of CHD [22]; moreover, the concept is of value by highlighting clinical findings that, by themselves, may not generate significant attention, and are associated with future risk for DM and CHD [23]. The commonly used definitions of the metabolic syndrome [24] noted in Table 10.1 provide clinicians with a useful means for conceptualizing the association between central adiposity, serum triglycerides (TG), insulin resistance, and DM risk. Serum TG was not included in FHS and other CV risk algorithms since, by itself, TG was not superior to either total cholesterol or HDL; however, there is convincing data to indicate that, for any level of HDL, elevated TG confers additional risk [25]. Importantly, fasting TG levels highly correlate with insulin resistance among non-diabetics [26]. Elevations in fasting TG are a direct result of adipocyte insulin resistance to the inhibitory effects on insulin-dependent lipase. As insulin resistance worsens, inappropriately high levels of lipolysis release excess free fatty acids into circulation that are hepatically transformed into TG [27]. Among laboratory markers of CV risk in schizophrenia patients, hypertriglyceridemia assumes particular importance for two reasons: the association with metabolic syndrome, a highly prevalent problem in this population, and the fact that elevated TG may be frequently seen during treatment with certain atypical antipsychotics [28].

Table 10.1. Metabolic syndrome criteria syndrome criteria

Criterion	NCEP ATP III [5] (≥3 criteria)	IDF [24] (abdominal obesity plus ≥2 other criteria)
Abdominal obesity (waist circumference)		Europid South Asian/Chinese
Men	>40 cm	≥37 cm ≥ 35.4 cm
Women	>35 cm	≥31.5 cm ≥ 31.5 cm
Fasting triglycerides	≥150 mg/dL	≥150 mg/dL
HDL		
Men	<40 mg/dL	<40 mg/dL
Women	<50 mg/dL	<50 mg/dL
Blood pressure	≥130/85 mm Hg or use of antihypertensive medication	≥130/85 mm Hg
Fasting glucose	≥110 mg/dL* or use of insulin or hypoglycemic medication	≥100 mg/dL or use of insulin or hypoglycemic medication

Note: *Now decreased to 100 mg/dL [73].

Schizophrenia has long been associated with early mortality from natural causes [29,30], but literature published in the past decade has convincingly demonstrated that CV disease is the leading natural cause of excess mortality [31–34]. Importantly, the standardized mortality ratio from CV causes is twofold greater among schizophrenia patients than the general population [31–33], with evidence suggesting that the mortality gap may be widening [34]. In the past decade, the increased concern over CV disease risk factors and metabolic disorders has assumed a prominent place in the schizophrenia literature [35], with expert recommendations for the comprehensive care of schizophrenia patients now including monitoring for CV risk factors, and other common medical co-morbidities [36–38], as a means to mitigate the high mortality rates from natural causes seen in this patient population [31,33,34].

Multiple factors contribute to high levels of CV risk in schizophrenia patients [35], including lifestyle habits, particularly the high rates of cigarette smoking [39], undertreatment of common conditions [40,41], and possibly the biology of schizophrenia itself [42–47], yet it is the metabolic effects of antipsychotic treatment that have emerged as one of the most important elements in the risk equation. Early articles documented adverse effects of low potency phenothiazines on weight, glucose, and lipid parameters [48–51]; however, there has been an exponential increase in the literature on antipsychotic metabolic effects since 2001, along with litigation and regulatory action in this area [52]. Consensus panels recognize that certain newer antipsychotics such as clozapine and olanzapine are associated with higher metabolic risk, while others are more neutral [38], but much of the literature emanates from industry-sponsored clinical trials whose study population often excludes the common medical co-morbidities and risks seen among the general population of schizophrenia patients. With its broad enrollment criteria and large sample size [53], the CATIE schizophrenia trial offered a unique opportunity to examine the CV and metabolic health status of a representative sample of schizophrenia patients, and assess comparative antipsychotic effects in the context of a double-blind randomized trial.

The cardiovascular and metabolic risk profile of subjects entering the CATIE schizophrenia trial

By the time the initial CATIE analysis of metabolic syndrome prevalence was performed in 2005, there was already a signal that schizophrenia patients had 2–4 times higher prevalence than that expected from general population estimates [54,55]. The largest published study at that time was from a Canadian sample of 240 subjects with schizophrenia or schizoaffective disorder (65% male, mean age 43.3 years), which found a prevalence of 42.6% for males and 48.5% for females using the NCEP criteria [55]. Cohn also reported similar prevalence between those under age 45 (43.8%) and those age 45 and over (45.8%), a finding in stark contrast to the age-related increase in metabolic syndrome prevalence noted in the general population.

The CATIE schizophrenia trial yielded baseline information on 1,460 subjects with chronic schizophrenia to perform metabolic and CV risk analyses. In addition to descriptive statistics, comparisons were performed between the CATIE baseline sample and individuals in the general population, using a 1:1 matching on the basis of age, gender, race, and ethnicity with subjects randomly drawn from the 3rd National Health and Nutrition Examination Survey (NHANES III). Among the 689 CATIE subjects with fasting laboratory measures at study baseline, the metabolic syndrome prevalence was 40.9% using NCEP criteria [56]. Broken down by gender, the metabolic syndrome prevalence in CATIE females was 51.6%, compared to 36.0% for CATIE males ($p = 0.0002$). A logistic regression model was performed in the CATIE and matched NHANES cohorts, with metabolic syndrome status as the outcome variable, and age, race, and ethnicity as covariates. CATIE male subjects were more than twice as likely to have metabolic syndrome than the NHANES males (odds ratio [OR] 2.38; 95% confidence interval [CI] 1.78–3.18), and CATIE females had three times greater odds for metabolic syndrome (odds ratio [OR] 3.51; 95% confidence interval [CI], 2.19–5.62). Even when controlling for differences in body mass index, CATIE males were still 85% more likely to have metabolic syndrome than the NHANES male cohort, and CATIE females 137% more likely than females in NHANES. When compared to the matched NHANES sample (Table 10.2), the CATIE subjects also had greater prevalence of every metabolic syndrome criterion, with fasting glucose among males the sole exception. This finding illustrates the concept that elevated fasting glucose is a late manifestation of insulin resistance, and, as such, may be a relatively insensitive marker of changes in insulin sensitivity.

Previously an association has been observed between medical co-morbidity and lower self-rated physical and mental health among schizophrenia patients [57], so the CATIE baseline population was examined for correlations between the metabolic syndrome diagnosis, and both symptom severity and neurocognitive measures. Of 1,460 subjects enrolled at baseline, metabolic syndrome status could be assigned for 1,231 subjects, primarily using criteria which did not depend on fasting laboratory values (e.g. serum HDL, blood pressure, waist circumference) [58]. The glucose criterion could only be met by documented use of hypoglycemic medications or insulin, or by having a value in the diabetic range as defined for random glucose measurements (≥ 200 mg/dL). In this larger group of CATIE subjects, the metabolic syndrome prevalence was 35.8% using NCEP derived criteria. After

Table 10.2. Comparison of metabolic syndrome prevalence and measurements by gender between fasting CATIE subjects and randomly selected age-, gender-, and race/ethnicity-matched NHANES III subjects [56]

	Males (N = 509)			Females (N = 180)		
	CATIE	NHANES	p	CATIE	NHANES	p
Metabolic syndrome prevalence	36.0%	19.7%	0.0001	51.59%	25.1%	0.0001
Mean waist circumference (inches)	39.0	37.0	0.0001	40.0	36.2	0.0001
Met. waist circumference criterion	35.5%	24.8%	0.0001	76.3%	57.0%	0.0001
Mean triglyceride (mg/dL)	194.7	143.6	0.0001	173.8	118.9	0.0001
Met. triglyceride criterion	50.7%	32.1%	0.0001	42.3%	19.6%	0.0001
Mean HDL (mg/dL)	42.3	47.2	0.0001	47.7	55.2	0.0001
Met. HDL criterion	48.9%	31.9%	0.0001	63.3%	36.3%	0.0001
Systolic BP (mm Hg)	124.4	123.4	0.2948	122.3	119.0	0.0626
Diastolic BP (mm Hg)	79.3	77.4	0.0046	80.0	73.3	0.0001
Met. BP criterion	47.2%	31.1%	0.0001	46.9%	26.8%	0.0001
Glucose (mg/dL)	97.7	102.4	0.0340	100.9	99.9	0.7925
Met. glucose criterion ($\geq$110 mg/dL)	14.1%	14.2%	0.9635	21.7%	11.2%	0.0075

Reprinted from Schizophrenia Research, Copyright 2005, with permission from Elsevier.

adjustment for age, gender, race, ethnicity, and site variance, those with metabolic syndrome rated significantly lower on physical health by SF-12 ($p < 0.001$) [59] and scored higher on somatic preoccupation (Positive and Negative Syndrome Scale [PANSS] item G1 [60]) ($p = 0.03$). There were no significant differences between those patients with and without metabolic syndrome on measures of symptom severity, depression, quality of life, neurocognition, or self-rated mental health.

The FHS analysis found that 10-year CHD risk was significantly elevated in male (9.4% vs. 7.0%) and female (6.3% vs. 4.2%) schizophrenia patients in the CATIE baseline sample compared to matched NHANES controls ($p = 0.0001$) [61]. Schizophrenia patients also had significantly higher rates of smoking (68% vs. 35%), diabetes (13% vs. 3%), and hypertension (27% vs. 17%) compared to controls ($p < 0.001$). Ten-year CHD risk remained elevated among CATIE patients compared to controls after controlling for body mass index ($p = 0.0001$), as did diabetes ($p = 0.0001$), HDL cholesterol ($p = 0.0001$) and hypertension ($p = 0.002$).

The impact of antipsychotic treatment on cardiovascular and metabolic outcomes in the CATIE schizophrenia trial

Metabolic outcomes

The initial CATIE publications [53,62] provided summary information on a core group of metabolic parameters, including weight, serum cholesterol, hemoglobin A1C, glucose, and TG (including fasting and non-fasting values for both) (Table 10.3). These data provide

Table 10.3. CATIE metabolic outcomes: change from baseline for basic laboratory results in Phase I [53] and Phase II tolerability arm [62]

	Olanzapine	Quetiapine	Risperidone	Perphenazine	Ziprasidone
Weight (lb/mo)					
Phase I mean ± SE	2.0 ± 0.3	0.5 ± 0.2	0.4 ± 0.3	−0.2 ± 0.2	−0.3 ± 0.3
Phase II mean ± SE	1.3 ± 0.6	0.1 ± 0.6	−0.2 ± 0.4	XXX	−1.7 ± 0.5
Glucose (mg/dL)					
Phase I mean ± SE	13.7 ± 2.5	7.5 ± 2.5	6.6 ± 2.5	5.4 ± 2.8	2.9 ± 3.4
Phase II mean ± SE	13.8 ± 5.9	1.2 ± 6.0	6.9 ± 5.8	XXX	0.8 ± 5.6
Hemoglobin A1C (%)					
Phase I mean ± SE	0.40 ± 0.07	0.04 ± 0.08	0.07 ± 0.04	0.09 ± 0.09	0.11 ± 0.09
Phase II mean ± SE	0.97 ± 0.30	0.61 ± 0.30	0.49 ± 0.30	XXX	0.46 ± 0.30
Cholesterol (mg/dL)					
Phase I mean ± SE	9.4 ± 2.4	6.6 ± 2.4	−1.3 ± 2.4	1.5 ± 2.7	−8.2 ± 3.2
Phase II mean ± SE	17.5 ± 5.2	6.5 ± 5.3	−3.1 ± 5.2	XXX	−10.7 ± 5.1
Triglycerides (mg/dL)					
Phase I mean ± SE	40.5 ± 8.9	21.2 ± 9.6	−2.4 ± 9.1	9.2 ± 10.1	−16.5 ± 12.2
Phase II mean ± SE	94.1 ± 21.8	39.3 ± 22.1	−5.2 ± 21.6	XXX	−3.5 ± 20.9

sound confirmation of olanzapine's metabolic liabilities, particularly the effects on weight, TG, and glycemic control by A1C (but not serum glucose), while ziprasidone was associated with metabolic improvement in a manner seen in previously published switch studies [63,64]. Risperidone and quetiapine were previously believed to have equivalent metabolic profiles [38], but there was a clear signal for quetiapine having a significant adverse impact on TG not seen with risperidone.

Detailed analysis of the CATIE Phase 1 data for all metabolic syndrome components [65] noted that, after 3 months, there were significant between-drug differences for the change in the group meeting metabolic syndrome status among all subjects whose metabolic status could be determined (n = 660) (Table 10.4). The metabolic syndrome prevalence increased for olanzapine from 34.8% to 43.9%, but decreased for ziprasidone (from 37.7% to 29.9%) (p = 0.001). Although effect sizes varied across the treatments in Phase 1, at 3 months, both olanzapine and quetiapine had the largest mean increase in waist circumference (0.7 inches for both) followed by risperidone (0.4 inches), compared to no change for ziprasidone (0.0 inches) and a decrease in waist circumference for perphenazine (−0.4 inches). Olanzapine also demonstrated significantly different changes in fasting TG at 3 months (+21.5 mg/dL) compared to ziprasidone (−32.1 mg/dL). To examine the impact of longer exposure duration on metabolic parameters, an analysis was performed using the last Phase 1 data available for each subject (hereafter referred to as "end of phase"). As shown in Table 10.5, these data were obtained, on average, 9 months from baseline, and the findings were consistent with those at 3 months for mean changes in waist circumference and fasting TG, although between-group differences now emerged for HDL and systolic

Table 10.4. Proportion of subjects at baseline and 3 months meeting the criteria for metabolic syndrome – all classifiable subjects [65]

| | Metabolic syndrome prevalence | |
	Baseline	3 Mo
Olanzapine	34.8%	43.9%[†] (N = 164)
Risperidone	30.6%	30.6% (N = 147)
Quetiapine	37.8%	37.1% (N = 143)
Ziprasidone	37.7%	29.9%[†] (N = 77)
Perphenazine	37.2%	38.0% (N = 129)
Overall treatment difference		.015

Note: [†]Change from baseline to 3 months in proportion of subjects meeting criteria for metabolic syndrome is greater for olanzapine than for ziprasidone ($p = 0.001$) among all classifiable subjects. Reprinted from Schizophrenia Research, Copyright 2008, with permission of Elsevier.

blood pressure. A repeated measures mixed model analysis of waist circumference was also performed, since this outcome had the most usable data over the 18 months. The repeated measures analysis found a significant impact of baseline value on changes in waist circumference, with patients who were more centrally obese becoming thinner. For subjects with baseline values below the median (<39 inches), olanzapine caused greater increases in central adiposity (+1.92 inches) against all other medications (range + 0.35 inches [ziprasidone] to +0.97 inches [quetiapine]). Among subjects with baselines ≥39 inches, only the olanzapine-exposed cohort did not experience an adjusted mean decrease in waist circumference; moreover, perphenazine (−0.97 inches) was found to be significantly superior to both olanzapine (+0.17 inches; $p < 0.0001$) and quetiapine (−0.01 inches; $p = 0.0007$).

Fasting TG levels are important for their association with insulin resistance, but there has been recent interest in non-fasting TG for several reasons: 1) emerging evidence which indicates that atherosclerosis may be a postprandial phenomenon, during which small triglyceride-rich particles are at their highest concentrations and penetrate arterial intimal cells [66]; 2) the fact that individuals are in a non-fasting state most of the day, as TG levels peak 4 hours after an oral fat load, and return to baseline only after 8–10 hours [67]; and, 3) clinical data from long-term studies indicating a strong association between non-fasting TG and CV risk [68], and the superiority of non-fasting TG over fasting TG in predicting CV events [69]. Echoing findings from fasting TG samples, the analysis of CATIE Phase 1 non-fasting TG (Table 10.6) noted greater increases in median and adjusted mean non-fasting TG levels among those randomized to quetiapine (mean + 54.7 mg/dL, median + 26 mg/dL) and olanzapine (mean + 23.4 mg/dL, median + 26.5 mg/dL), with a significant between-group difference for perphenazine vs. olanzapine ($p = 0.002$) [69].

Framingham cardiovascular risk

Since the greatest metabolic impact of atypical antipsychotics is on weight [52] and serum TG, but much less on cholesterol measures [28], an important question for the FHS analysis is whether there would be between-treatment differences, given the fact that neither weight nor TG are part of FHS risk calculations [70]. The other question is, over a relatively short

Table 10.5. Mean changes in individual metabolic criteria at end of CATIE Phase 1 visit [65]

	Waist circumference[†] (inches)		Systolic BP[†] (mm Hg)		Diastolic BP (mm Hg)	HDL[@‡] (mg/dL) (Whites)	HDL[@] (mg/dL) (non-Whites)	Fasting glucose (mg/dL)	Fasting triglycerides[†] (mg/dL)	
	Below Median	Above Median	Below Median	Above Median					Below Median	Above Median
Mean exposure (months)	8.9	8.7	8.7	9.1	8.9	9.2	9.9	9.9	9.9	9.8
OLANZ	1.9 (SE=0.2) (N=146)	0.4 (SE=0.3) (N=147)	6.0 (SE=1.0) (N=159)	−3.6 (SE=1.2) (N=146)	0. (SE=0.6) (N=305)	−1.7 (SE=0.6) (N=171)	−0.9 (SE=0.9) (N=115)	4.5 (SE=2.3) (N=94)	49.0 (SE=10.8) (N=42)	5.2 (SE=17.4) (N=51)
RISP	0.9 (SE=0.2) (N=145)	−0.7 (SE=0.3) (N=143)	5.6 (SE=1.1) (N=136)	−9.0 (SE=1.1) (N=162)	−1.3 (SE=0.6) (N=298)	0.1 (SE=0.6) (N=162)	0.9 (SE=0.9) (N=109)	−0.4 (SE=2.6) (N=74)	19.7 (SE=11.2) (N=39)	−67.1 (SE=21.2) (N=35)
QUET	0.7 (SE=0.2) (N=142)	0.0 (SE=0.2) (N=157)	8.6 (SE=1.0) (N=158)	−8.0 (SE=1.2) (N=145)	−0.1 (SE=0.6) (N=303)	−0.2 (SE=0.6) (N=186)	0.1 (SE=1.1) (N=85)	−1.8 (SE=2.4) (N=88)	29.8 (SE=10.8) (N=42)	−13.0 (SE=18.4) (N=46)
ZIP	0.0 (SE=0.3) (N=77)	−0.4 (SE=0.3) (N=78)	8.8 (SE=1.5) (N=78)	−7.6 (SE=1.6) (N=80)	−0.4 (SE=0.8) (N=158)	0.6 (SE=0.9) (N=90)	4.3 (SE=1.4) (N=51)	0.0 (SE=3.5) (N=39)	26.0 (SE=15.6) (N=20)	−96.4 (SE=28.5) (N=19)

PER	0.6 (SE=0.2) (N=126)	−1.1 (SE=0.3) (N=110)	6.0 (SE=1.2) (N=107)	−6.4 (SE=1.2) (N=137)	0.0 (SE=0.6) (N=243)	2.7 (SE=0.7) (N=130)	−1.3 (SE=1.0) (N=88)	−1.0 (SE=2.7) (N=68)	28.7 (SE=11.6) (N=36)	−27.5 (SE=22.3) (N=31)
Overall treatment difference	<0.001[1]	0.001[2]	NS	0.017[3]	NS	<0.001[4]	0.012[5]	NS	NS	0.011[6]

Notes: Table entries are ANCOVA least squares-adjusted means. All models include time to treatment discontinuation as a covariate, as well as baseline value of outcome. Demographic variables were analyzed, but only age and race entered the models for HDL, SBP, and DBP, and gender for HDL and SBP.

Note: NS = not significant ($p \geq 0.05$).

[†] Data presented in separate columns due to significant baseline by treatment effect. Median WC = 39 in, median SBP = 122 mm Hg, median TG = 148 mg/dL.

[@] Data presented in separate columns due to significant race by treatment effect.

[‡] There was a significant ziprasidone cohort effect, but the between-group results were not different for cohorts enrolled prior to, or after, the introduction of ziprasidone.

[1] Between-group comparison significant for olanzapine vs. risperidone ($p = 0.001$), quetiapine ($p < 0.001$), ziprasidone ($p < 0.001$), perphenazine ($p < 0.001$).

[2] Between-group comparison significant for perphenazine vs. olanzapine ($p < .001$), perphenazine vs. quetiapine ($p = 0.003$), and olanzapine vs. risperidone ($p = 0.003$).

[3] Between-group comparison significant for olanzapine vs. risperidone ($p = 0.001$).

[4] Between-group comparison significant for perphenazine vs. olanzapine ($p < 0.001$), and perphenazine vs. quetiapine ($p = 0.002$).

[5] Between-group comparisons significant for ziprasidone vs. olanzapine ($p = 0.002$), and ziprasidone vs. perphenazine ($p = 0.001$).

[6] Between-group comparisons significant for olanzapine vs. ziprasidone ($p = 0.003$).

Reprinted from Schizophrenia Research, Copyright 2008, with permission from Elsevier.

Table 10.6. 3-Month changes from baseline in non-fasting triglycerides (mg/dL) by treatment group [69]

	N	Observed		Adjusted[†]
		Median (interquartile range)	Mean ± SD	Least squares Mean ± SE
Olanzapine	62	26.5 (−20–80)	33.1 ± 159.1	23.4 ± 22.8
Perphenazine	39	−22 (−81–24)	−3.7 ± 243.8	−1.3 ± 28.6
Quetiapine	59	26 (−34–96)	36.0 ± 264.0	54.7 ± 23.5
Risperidone	56	−6.5 (−52–38)	−7.9 ± 85.3	−18.4 ± 24.0
Ziprasidone	30	8 (−48–58)	0.4 ± 145.0	0.0 ± 32.7
Overall treatment difference		0.016*		0.009**

Notes: [†]Model adjusted for baseline triglycerides. Age, gender, race, ethnicity, baseline antipsychotic medication, and smoking were allowed to enter the model but were not significant. The interaction between baseline triglycerides and treatment was also explored and was not significant.
*Unadjusted comparisons using the Kruskal-Wallis rank test revealed overall significant treatment differences ($p = 0.016$). Individual pairwise comparisons revealed a significant difference for olanzapine vs. perphenazine ($p = 0.002$).
**Rank ANCOVA adjusting for baseline triglycerides revealed overall significant treatment differences ($p = 0.009$). Individual pairwise comparisons revealed a significant difference for perphenazine vs. olanzapine ($p = 0.002$). The change in non-fasting TG was also numerically different for perphenazine vs. quetiapine, although not statistically significant with the Bonferroni correction ($p = 0.006$).
Reprinted from Schizophrenia Research, Copyright 2008, with permission from Elsevier.

time frame, the magnitude of any changes in CHD risk will be significant in those with higher baseline levels of risk (range 8.1%–9.1% across antipsychotic treatments). Using the 3-month outcomes, the covariate-adjusted mean change in 10-year FHS calculations of CHD risk did indeed find significant differences between treatments [70]. Olanzapine was associated with an absolute increase in risk of 0.5% (SE = 0.3) and quetiapine, a 0.3% (SE 0.3) increase; whereas risk decreased in patients treated with perphenazine, −0.5% (SE = 0.3), risperidone, −0.6% (SE = 0.3), and ziprasidone −0.6% (SE = 0.4). The difference in 10-year CHD risk between olanzapine and risperidone was statistically significant ($p = 0.004$). As seen with waist circumference, there was an impact of baseline risk. In this case, differences in estimated 10-year CHD risk changes between drugs were most marked in the tertile of subjects with higher baseline CHD risk ($\geq 10\%$).

Analysis of individual FHS cardiac risk factors revealed no difference between treatment groups for change in smoking status, new-onset DM, or hypertension during Phase 1. There was also no difference between treatment groups for change in HDL at 3 months, but in the end of phase analysis, covariate-adjusted HDL cholesterol levels decreased in olanzapine (−1.4 mg/dL SE = 0.5) compared to an increase in perphenazine (1.1 mg/dL, SE = 0.6, $p = 0.001$) and ziprasidone (1.9 mg/dL, SE = 0.7, $p < 0.001$). As noted in the analysis for Table 10.5, an effect of race was also seen in the FHS end of phase HDL outcomes. The end of phase analysis of change in total cholesterol found significant differences between risperidone (−11.2 mg/dL, SE = 2.0) compared to olanzapine (0.8 mg/dL, SE = 2.0, $p < 0.001$) and quetiapine (−2.2 mg/dL, SE = 2.0, $p = 0.002$), and for ziprasidone (−9.3, SE = 2.8) vs. olanzapine ($p = 0.003$). Results of mixed model analyses for total and HDL cholesterol were consistent with findings from the end of phase analyses.

Outcomes with novel biomarkers

The enormity of the data collected in the CATIE schizophrenia trial means that new findings will continue to emerge for years to come. As of this writing, samples are being analyzed to examine various markers associated with cardiometabolic risk, but the first of these to yield important results is the examination of CRP changes during Phase 1. As mentioned in the introduction, clinical data on CRP have greatly influenced our understanding of CV risk, and of possible targets for risk modification. As with waist circumference and HDL, baseline CRP was a significant predictor of 3-month change ($p < 0.001$), yet the 3-month analysis still found significant treatment differences in change from baseline after adjustment for baseline CRP ($p = 0.011$) [71]. At 3 months, olanzapine and quetiapine had the greatest increases. There were no significant treatment differences in those with higher baseline levels of systemic inflammation (CRP $\geq$ 1 mg/L), but for those with lower baseline CV risk (CRP < 1 mg/L), pairwise comparisons were significantly different for olanzapine vs. perphenazine ($p < 0.001$) and vs. risperidone ($p = 0.001$). The 12-month repeated measures analysis confirmed the association between baseline CRP and outcomes, and the deleterious impact of olanzapine compared to perphenazine ($p < 0.001$) and ziprasidone ($p = 0.003$) in those with baseline CRP < 1 mg/L.

Discussion

The CATIE data confirm the fact that metabolic differences exist between various antipsychotics, and pinpoint the metabolic outcomes (adiposity, TG) most greatly influenced by certain medications. Among patients with clinical and laboratory findings suggestive of insulin resistance, use of olanzapine is associated with further worsening in metabolic status in a manner previously documented with long-term clozapine exposure [72], risperidone and quetiapine have intermediate effects, and ziprasidone appears to be metabolically neutral. The 2004 APA/ADA Consensus paper placed quetiapine and risperidone in the central tier of metabolic risk [38], but the CATIE data suggest that quetiapine, when used at doses >400 mg for schizophrenia treatment, has significant adverse effects on non-fasting TG, HDL (in White subjects), and central adiposity in a manner not seen with risperidone, despite not having a greater impact on serum glucose than risperidone.

Prior literature noted minimal effects of atypical antipsychotic treatment on blood pressure compared to other metabolic parameters, and this is confirmed by CATIE. Weight gain is associated with hypertension, but the time frame of this study may be inadequate to manifest this effect. The absence of a significant signal for HDL changes in prior antipsychotic studies may have been the result of limited duration of exposure and smaller sample sizes [28], since the end of phase results here reveal a deleterious impact of olanzapine and quetiapine on serum HDL in Whites, and significant improvement in HDL with ziprasidone in non-Whites. CATIE also provided the first controlled data on the metabolic effects of a medium potency typical antipsychotic published in the past 40 years, with evidence that perphenazine is generally metabolically neutral. The lack of significant between-group differences for glucose should not reassure clinicians that there are no differences in future DM risk between antipsychotics. As previously described, DM develops over 10–20 years, so short-term changes in serum glucose may not be seen, despite worsening in other parameters associated with insulin resistance, especially waist circumference and TG.

183

The net result, as shown by change in traditional FHS risk or by CRP, is that choice of antipsychotic treatment may significantly influence CV risk, even over short time frames. While the absolute 3-month increase in FHS risk with olanzapine exposure seems small (+0.5%), this would translate to a 2% increase in CV risk over 12 months, assuming a linear change in CV risk over the course of the year. For an individual with a baseline CV risk of 9.0%, well within the range seen among CATIE subjects, this amounts to a 22% proportional change in CV risk. After several years, the net result would be a marked increase in CV events and mortality, a finding already documented during 10-year outcomes with clozapine treated patients [72].

Clinicians face significant challenges in modifying certain lifestyle risks in schizophrenia patients such as smoking, dietary habits, and activity levels. The CATIE schizophrenia trial data illustrate the possibility for improving metabolic health by switching patients from more offending medications, and for avoiding long-term CV consequences by preferential use of agents with metabolically benign profiles, such as ziprasidone and perphenazine. Although not studied in randomized phases of CATIE, aripiprazole has also been demonstrated to possess a benign cardiac risk profile [52]. Regardless of medication choice, the onus remains on clinicians to monitor all metabolic parameters associated with increased CV risk in schizophrenia patients, bearing in mind that medications are but one source of risk, and that many patients receive few or no primary care services. Future research may identify genetic markers associated with antipsychotic response and metabolic adverse effects, arming clinicians with the means to make more informed risk:benefit treatment decisions. Until such time, the health assessment of schizophrenia patients must continue to evaluate traditional elements of DM risk (age, family history, race/ethnicity, obesity, etc.), and track metabolic syndrome parameters and those attributable to FHS risk elements (age, gender, smoking status, lipids, blood pressure). While novel biomarkers such as CRP show promise for refining CV risk prediction, many schizophrenia patients continue to receive inadequate assessment of common medical conditions associated with increased CV risk such as hypertension, DM, and dyslipidemia [41]. The scale, the blood pressure cuff, and a tape measure (for waist circumference) are basic necessities for anyone prescribing antipsychotics for schizophrenia patients. The detailed data on relative antipsychotic metabolic liabilities provided by the CATIE schizophrenia trial provides clinicians with the basis for creating a nuanced approach to metabolic monitoring, by highlighting those parameters impacted by antipsychotic treatment, and those agents with the greatest adverse effects. Management of schizophrenia requires acknowledgment that CV disease remains a primary cause of excess mortality in this patient population. Psychiatrists and others who prescribe antipsychotic medications, and all those who care for the severely mentally ill, should use the emerging information from prospective, randomized trials such as CATIE to minimize the iatrogenic contributions to CV risk.

References

1. Gerszten RE and Wang TJ. The search for new cardiovascular biomarkers. *Nature* 2008;**451**:949–52.

2. Ingelsson E, Schaefer EJ, Contois JH, *et al.* Clinical utility of different lipid measures for prediction of coronary heart disease in men and women [see comment]. *Journal of the American Medical Association* 2007;**298**:776–85.

3. Dhingra R, Gona P, Nam BH, *et al.* C-reactive protein, inflammatory conditions, and cardiovascular disease risk. *The American Journal of Medicine* 2007;**120**:1054–62.

4. Wilson PW, D'Agostino RB, Levy D, *et al.* Prediction of coronary heart disease using risk factor categories [see comment]. *Circulation* 1998;**97**:1837–47.

5. Expert Panel on Detection, Evaluation, and Treatment of High Blood Cholesterol in Adults. Executive summary of the third report of The National Cholesterol Education Program (NCEP) Expert Panel on detection, evaluation, and treatment of high blood cholesterol in adults (Adult Treatment Panel III). *JAMA* 2001;**285**:2486–97.

6. D'Agostino RB Sr, Grundy S, Sullivan LM, *et al.* Validation of the Framingham coronary heart disease prediction scores: Results of a multiple ethnic groups investigation [see comment]. *Journal of the American Medical Association* 2001;**286**:180–7.

7. Heart Protection Study Collaborative Group. MRC/BHF Heart Protection Study of cholesterol lowering with simvastatin in 20,536 high-risk individuals: A randomised placebo-controlled trial.[see comment] [summary for patients in *Current Cardiology Reports* 2002;**4**:486–7; PMID: 12379169]. *Lancet* 2002;**360**:7–22.

8. Ridker PM, Rifai N, Rose L, *et al.* Comparison of C-reactive protein and low-density lipoprotein cholesterol levels in the prediction of first cardiovascular events [see comment]. *New England Journal of Medicine* 2002;**347**:1557–65.

9. Ridker PM, Hennekens CH, Buring JE, *et al.* C-reactive protein and other markers of inflammation in the prediction of cardiovascular disease in women. *New England Journal of Medicine* 2000;**342**:836–43.

10. Boekholdt SM, Hack CE, Sandhu MS, *et al.* C-reactive protein levels and coronary artery disease incidence and mortality in apparently healthy men and women: The EPIC-Norfolk prospective population study 1993–2003. *Atherosclerosis* 2006;**187**:415–22.

11. Cook NR, Buring JE and Ridker PM. The effect of including C-reactive protein in cardiovascular risk prediction models for women. *Annals of Internal Medicine* 2006;**145**:21–9.

12. Ridker PM, Cannon CP, Morrow D, *et al.* C-reactive protein levels and outcomes after statin therapy [see comment]. *New England Journal of Medicine* 2005;**352**:20–8.

13. Epstein FH. Hyperglycemia: A risk factor in coronary heart disease. *Circulation* 1967;**36**:609–19.

14. Kannel WB and McGee DL. Diabetes and cardiovascular risk factors: The Framingham study. *Circulation* 1979;**59**:8–13.

15. Haffner SM, Lehto S, Ronnemaa T, *et al.* Mortality from coronary heart disease in subjects with type 2 diabetes and in nondiabetic subjects with and without prior myocardial infarction [see comment]. *New England Journal of Medicine* 1998;**339**:229–34.

16. Reaven GM. Banting lecture 1988: Role of insulin resistance in human disease. *Diabetes* 1988;**37**:1595–607.

17. de Vegt F, Dekker JM, Jager A, *et al.* Relation of impaired fasting and postload glucose with incident type 2 diabetes in a Dutch population: The Hoorn Study. *Journal of the American Medical Association* 2001;**285**:2109–13.

18. Ford ES. The metabolic syndrome and mortality from cardiovascular disease and all-causes: Findings from the National Health and Nutrition Examination Survey II Mortality Study. *Atherosclerosis* 2004;**173**:309–14.

19. Kahn R, Buse J, Ferrannini E, *et al.* The Metabolic Syndrome: Time for a critical appraisal. *Diabetes Care* 2005;**28**:2289–304.

20. American Heart Association, National Heart Lung and Blood Institute; Grundy SM, Cleeman JI, Daniels SR, *et al.* Diagnosis and management of the metabolic syndrome. An American Heart Association/National Heart, Lung, and Blood Institute Scientific Statement. Executive summary. *Cardiology in Review* 2005;**13**:322–7.

21. Wannamethee SG, Shaper AG, Lennon L, *et al.* Metabolic syndrome vs Framingham risk score for prediction of coronary heart disease, stroke, and type 2 diabetes

mellitus. *Archives of Internal Medicine* 2005;**165**:2644–50.

22. Girman CJ, Dekker JM, Rhodes T, *et al.* An exploratory analysis of criteria for the metabolic syndrome and its prediction of long-term cardiovascular outcomes: The Hoorn study. *American Journal of Epidemiology* 2005;**162**:438–47.

23. Lorenzo C, Williams K, Hunt KJ, *et al.* The National Cholesterol Education Program – Adult Treatment Panel III, International Diabetes Federation, and World Health Organization definitions of the metabolic syndrome as predictors of incident cardiovascular disease and diabetes. *Diabetes Care* 2007;**30**:8–13.

24. Assmann G, Guerra R, Fox G, *et al.* Harmonizing the definition of the metabolic syndrome: Comparison of the criteria of the Adult Treatment Panel III and the International Diabetes Federation in United States American and European populations. *American Journal of Cardiology* 2007;**99**:541–8.

25. Jeppesen J, Hein HO, Suadicani P, *et al.* Triglyceride concentration and ischemic heart disease: An eight-year follow-up in the Copenhagen Male Study. *Circulation* 1998;**97**:1029–36.

26. McLaughlin T, Abbasi F, Cheal K, *et al.* Use of metabolic markers to identify overweight individuals who are insulin resistant [see comment][summary for patients in *Annals of Internal Medicine* 2003;**139**:I16; PMID: 14623638]. *Annals of Internal Medicine* 2003;**139**:802–9.

27. Smith DA. Treatment of the dyslipidemia of insulin resistance. *Medical Clinics of North America* 2007;**91**:1185–210.

28. Meyer JM and Koro CE. The effects of antipsychotic therapy on serum lipids: A comprehensive review. *Schizophrenia Research* 2004;**70**:1–17.

29. Allebeck P. Schizophrenia: A life-shortening disease. *Schizophrenia Bulletin* 1989;**15**:81–9.

30. Brown S. Excess mortality of schizophrenia. A meta-analysis. *British Journal of Psychiatry* 1997;**171**:502–8.

31. Osby U, Correia N, Brandt L, *et al.* Mortality and causes of death in schizophrenia in Stockholm county, Sweden. *Schizophrenia Research* 2000;**45**:21–8.

32. Osby U, Correia N, Brandt L, *et al.* Time trends in schizophrenia mortality in Stockholm county, Sweden: Cohort study. *British Medical Journal* 2000;**321**:483–4.

33. Colton CW and Manderscheid RW. Congruencies in increased mortality rates, years of potential life lost, and causes of death among public mental health clients in eight states. *Preventing Chronic Diseases* 2006;**3**:1–14.

34. Saha S, Chant D and McGrath J. A systematic review of mortality in schizophrenia: Is the differential mortality gap worsening over time? *Archives of General Psychiatry* 2007;**64**:1123–31.

35. Newcomer JW and Hennekens CH. Severe mental illness and risk of cardiovascular disease. *Journal of the American Medical Association* 2007;**298**:1794–6.

36. Meyer JM and Nasrallah HA, eds. *Medical Illness and Schizophrenia*. Washington, DC: American Psychiatric Press, Inc; 2003.

37. Marder SR, Essock SM, Miller AL, *et al.* Physical health monitoring of patients with schizophrenia. *American Journal of Psychiatry* 2004;**161**:1334–49.

38. American Diabetes Association, American Psychiatric Association, American Association of Clinical Endocrinologists, North American Association for the Study of Obesity. Consensus development conference on antipsychotic drugs and obesity and diabetes. *Journal of Clinical Psychiatry* 2004;**65**:267–72.

39. Brown S, Birtwistle J, Roe L, *et al.* The unhealthy lifestyle of people with schizophrenia. *Psychological Medicine* 1999;**29**:697–701.

40. Druss BG, Bradford DW, Rosenheck RA, *et al.* Mental disorders and use of cardiovascular procedures after myocardial infarction [see comments]. *Journal of the American Medical Association* 2000;**283**:506–11.

41. Nasrallah HA, Meyer JM, Goff DC, *et al.* Low rates of treatment for hypertension, dyslipidemia and diabetes in schizophrenia: Data from the CATIE Schizophrenia Trial sample at baseline. *Schizophrenia Research* 2006;**86**:15–22.

42. Braceland FJ, Meduna LJ and Vaichulis JA. Delayed action of insulin in schizophrenia. *Am J Psychiatry* 1945;**102**:108–10.

43. Lorenz WF. Sugar tolerance in dementia praecox and other mental disorders. *Archives of Neurology and Psychiatry* 1922;**8**:184–96.

44. Meduna LJ, Gerty FJ and Urse VG. Biochemical disturbances in mental disorders: Anti-insulin effect of blood in cases of schizophrenia. *Archives of Neurology and Psychiatry* 1941;**47**:38–52 (correction, v. **47**:1057).

45. Winkelmayer R. Diabetes mellitus in chronic mental patients. *The Psychiatic Quarterly* 1962;**36**:530–6.

46. Cohn TA, Remington G, Zipursky RB, *et al.* Insulin resistance and adiponectin levels in drug-free patients with schizophrenia: A preliminary report [erratum appears in *Canadian Journal of Psychiatry* 2006;**51**:552]. *Canadian Journal of Psychiatry – Revue Canadienne de Psychiatrie* 2006;**51**:382–6.

47. van Nimwegen LJM, Storosum JG, Blumer RME, *et al.* Hepatic insulin resistance in antipsychotic naive patients with schizophrenia, a detailed study of glucose metabolism with stable isotopes. *Journal of Clinical Endocrinology and Metabolism* 2008;**93**:572–7.

48. Mefferd RB, Labrosse EH, Gawienowski AM, *et al.* Influence of chlorpromazine on certain biochemical variables of chronic male schizophrenics. *Journal of Nervous and Mental Disease* 1958;**127**:167–79.

49. Efron HY and Balter AM. Relationship of phenothiazine intake and psychiatric diagnosis to glucose level and tolerance. *Journal of Nervous and Mental Disease* 1966;**142**:555–61.

50. Schwarz L and Munoz R. Blood sugar levels in patients treated with chlorpromazine. *American Journal of Psychiatry* 1968;**125**:253–5.

51. Clark ML, Ray TS, Paredes A, *et al.* Chlorpromazine in women with chronic schizophrenia: The effect on cholesterol levels and cholesterol-behavior relationships. *Psychosomatic Medicine* 1967;**29**:634–42.

52. Newcomer JW. Second-generation (atypical) antipsychotics and metabolic effects: A comprehensive literature review. *CNS Drugs* 2005;**19**(Suppl. 1):1–93.

53. Lieberman JA, Stroup TS, McEvoy JP, *et al.* Effectiveness of antipsychotic drugs in patients with chronic schizophrenia. *New England Journal of Medicine* 2005;**353**:1209–23.

54. Heiskanen T, Niskanen L, Lyytikainen R, *et al.* Metabolic syndrome in patients with schizophrenia. *Journal of Clinical Psychiatry* 2003;**64**:575–9.

55. Cohn T, Prud'homme D, Streiner D, *et al.* Characterizing coronary heart disease risk in chronic schizophrenia: High prevalence of the metabolic syndrome. *Canadian Journal of Psychiatry – Revue Canadienne de Psychiatrie* 2004;**49**:753–60.

56. McEvoy JP, Meyer JM, Goff DC, *et al.* Prevalence of the metabolic syndrome in patients with schizophrenia: Baseline results from the Clinical Antipsychotic Trials of Intervention Effectiveness (CATIE) schizophrenia trial and comparison with national estimates from NHANES III. *Schizophrenia Research* 2005;**80**:19–32.

57. Dixon L, Postrado L, Delahanty J, *et al.* The association of medical comorbidity in schizophrenia with poor physical and mental health. *Journal of Nervous and Mental Disease* 1999;**187**:496–502.

58. Meyer JM, Nasrallah HA, McEvoy JP, *et al.* The Clinical Antipsychotic Trials Of Intervention Effectiveness (CATIE) Schizophrenia Trial: Clinical comparison of subgroups with and without the metabolic syndrome. *Schizophrenia Research* 2005;**80**:9–18.

59. Ware JE, Kosinski M and Keller SD. A 12-item Short-Form Health Survey

(SF-12): Construction of scales and preliminary tests of reliability and validity. *Medical Care* 1996;**32**:220–33.

60. Kay SR, Fiszbein A and Opler LA. The positive and negative syndrome scale (PANSS) for schizophrenia. *Schizophrenia Bulletin* 1987;**13**:261–76.

61. Goff DC, Sullivan L, McEvoy JP, *et al.* A comparison of ten-year cardiac risk estimates in schizophrenia patients from the CATIE Study and matched controls. *Schizophrenia Research* 2005;**80**:45–53.

62. Stroup TS, Lieberman JA, McEvoy JP, *et al.* Effectiveness of olanzapine, quetiapine, risperidone, and ziprasidone in patients with chronic schizophrenia following discontinuation of a previous atypical antipsychotic. *American Journal of Psychiatry* 2006;**163**:611–22.

63. Weiden PJ, Daniel DG, Simpson GM, *et al.* Improvement in indices of health status in outpatients with schizophrenia switched to ziprasidone. *Journal of Clinical Psychopharmacology* 2003;**23**:1–6.

64. Weiden PJ, Newcomer JW, Loebel A, *et al.* Long-term changes in weight and plasma lipids during maintenance treatment with ziprasidone. *Neuropsychopharmacology* 2008;**33**:985–95.

65. Meyer JM, Davis VG, Goff DC, *et al.* Change in metabolic syndrome parameters with antipsychotic treatment in the CATIE Schizophrenia Trial: Prospective data from phase 1. *Schizophrenia Research* 2008;**101**:273–86.

66. Eberly LE, Stamler J, Neaton JD, *et al.* Relation of triglyceride levels, fasting and nonfasting, to fatal and nonfatal coronary heart disease. *Archives of Internal Medicine* 2003;**163**:1077–83.

67. Nordestgaard BG, Benn M, Schnohr P, *et al.* Nonfasting triglycerides and risk of myocardial infarction, ischemic heart disease, and death in men and women. *Journal of the American Medical Association* 2007;**298**:299–308.

68. Bansal S, Buring JE, Rifai N, *et al.* Fasting compared with nonfasting triglycerides and risk of cardiovascular events in women. *Journal of the American Medical Association* 2007;**298**:309–16.

69. Meyer JM, Davis VG, Goff DC, *et al.* Impact of antipsychotic treatment on nonfasting triglycerides in the CATIE Schizophrenia Trial phase 1. *Schizophrenia Research* 2008;**103**:104–9.

70. Daumit GL, Goff DC, Meyer JM, *et al.* Antipsychotic effects on estimated 10 year coronary heart disease risk in the CATIE Schizophrenia Study. *Schizophrenia Research* 2008;**105**:175–87.

71. Meyer JM, McEvoy JP, Davis VG, *et al.* Inflammatory markers in schizophrenia: Comparing antipsychotic effects in phase 1 of the CATIE Schizophrenia Trial. *Biological Psychiatry* 2009 [Epub ahead of print].

72. Henderson DC, Nguyen DD, Copeland PM, *et al.* Clozapine, diabetes mellitus, hyperlipidemia, and cardiovascular risks and mortality: Results of a 10-year naturalistic study. *Journal of Clinical Psychiatry* 2005;**66**:1116–21.

73. Grundy SM, Brewer B, Cleeman JI, *et al.* Definition of metabolic syndrome: report of the National Heart, Lung, and Blood Institute/American Heart Association conference on scientific issues related to definition. *Circulation* 2004;**109**:433–38.

Chapter

11

Substance use in persons with schizophrenia: incidence, baseline correlates, and effects on outcome

Fred Reimherr, Marvin S. Swartz, and John L. Olsen

One unintended consequence of shifting care for patients with schizophrenia away from institutional settings to the community has been exposing them to a much greater risk of using substances of abuse. Estimates of substance use/abuse in schizophrenia range from a low of 10% up to 70%, depending on variations in diagnostic assessment methods, use of collateral informants, and laboratory assessment techniques [1–10]. Because self-report of illicit behaviors is frequently unreliable, inclusion of laboratory assessments and collateral informants tends to increase rates of detections of substance use. Substance abuse is a significant risk factor for a variety of poor outcomes in schizophrenia, including treatment non-adherence [11,12], relapse [13], rehospitalization [11], violence [12,14], victimization [15], HIV and hepatitis [16], and criminal justice involvement [17].

On the whole, rates of substance use and their sequelae are underestimated. In fact, some surveys and treatment outcome studies continue to rely solely on self-report measures of illicit drug use, despite problems with reliability and validity. In a recent study comparing methods of detection of illicit substances in schizophrenia, use of urine drug testing combined with radioimmunoassay of hair specimens (RIAH) increased rates of detection of illicit drug use from 16% based solely on self-report to 38% [18]. This is because urine drug testing generally detects substance use in the past 24 hours, while RIAH can detect 90 days or more of use, depending on the length of hair sampled.

The importance of substance use is underappreciated in schizophrenia research. First, obtaining a more precise estimate of the level of substance abuse in a population of schizophrenic patients is somewhat more labor intensive and costly than use of simple self-report or urine drug screening. Next, the FDA, in their review of any of the currently approved antipsychotic medications, has not required subgroup analyses of schizophrenic patients comparing substance abusing and non-abusing groups. Finally, it is not clear that many genetic or biological studies in schizophrenia have adequately evaluated the potential impact of co-morbid substance abuse within their subject populations.

The NIMH Clinical Antipsychotic Trials of Intervention Effectiveness (CATIE) [19] project has provided an important opportunity to comprehensively characterize patterns and consequences of substance abuse co-morbidity in moderately ill patients with chronic schizophrenia enrolled in the trial and to examine the effects of substance abuse on clinical outcomes in these patients. CATIE used comprehensive methods of assessment of substance use including self,

---

Antipsychotic Trials in Schizophrenia, ed. T. Scott Stroup and Jeffrey A. Lieberman. Published by Cambridge University Press. © Cambridge University Press 2010.

189

family, and clinician report of substance use, combined with urine drug testing and RIAH. Consequently, CATIE provided the most detailed data on substance abuse in a clinical trial in schizophrenia to date. In addition, by not systematically excluding schizophrenia patients with substance use or other co-morbid conditions, as is common in clinical trials, CATIE provided an opportunity to better study the effects of substance use on treatment outcomes. Three analyses of CATIE substance use data have now been published.

In an initial report [20], approximately 60% of the CATIE sample was documented to use at least one substance of abuse (including illicit substances and alcohol) and 37% of the total sample had evidence of a substance use disorder. Three substance use groups (users – Substance Use Without Impairment; abusers – Substance Abuse or Dependence; and these two groups combined – Any Substance Use) were compared to a "No Substance Use" category. In multivariable analyses, compared to non-users, individuals with "Any Substance Use" were significantly more likely to be male, less educated, have more childhood conduct problems, have higher positive and lower negative symptom scores on the Positive and Negative Syndrome Scale (PANSS), have had a recent illness exacerbation, and a history of major depression in the past 5 years. Similar variables differentiated abusers from users, including male gender, childhood conduct problems, positive PANNS scores, and recent illness exacerbation, all of which were more common among abusers.

A second report contrasted abusers, users, and non-users without including the combined group "any use" category. The paper presented a detailed examination of the effects of substance abuse on psychosocial functioning as evaluated on the Quality of Life Scale in schizophrenia [21]. Somewhat counterintuitively, substance users and substance abusers (those with abuse and dependence disorders) were rated by clinicians to have *higher* psychosocial functioning than non-users in several domains, possibly because some drug-seeking behaviors require higher functioning. However, if cocaine was one of the substances used then there was great disruption in several domains of psychosocial functioning. Contrary to speculation that schizophrenic patients might use substances to ameliorate negative symptoms or a deficit syndrome, this was not evident.

Because of the wealth of CATIE data on alcohol and illicit substance use, several comparisons of use patterns have been conducted. For example, while illicit substance and alcohol use and abuse disorders were grouped together in "any use" analyses, preliminary analyses suggested that the small group of patients who used alcohol alone and not with illicit drugs were not representative of most substance-using patients and would best be grouped with non-users of illicit drugs in terms of level of functioning. Additionally, our initial analyses differentiated illicit drug use into users and abusers; it is not known whether this distinction is clinically meaningful. In fact, one published report indicated that few individuals with mental illness maintain low levels of use without progressing to substance use disorders [8].

A third CATIE publication [22] followed this logic and combined illicit substance use and abuse into a single comparison group. This additional analysis sought to contrast treatment outcomes among illicit substance users and non-users on time to discontinuation. In this article, patients with schizophrenia who used or abused only alcohol and showed no evidence of illicit drug use or abuse were assigned to the non-user group. In addition, illicit substance users and abusers were combined. Differences between non-users and users seen in the previous baseline CATIE substance use analyses were replicated in this alternative analysis, i.e., users were more likely to be male, less educated, have more childhood conduct problems, have higher positive and lower negative symptom scores on the PANSS, have had a recent illness exacerbation, and a history of major depression in the past 5 years. This suggests that many of the differences between users and non-users reported in the first two reports were attributable to the use of illicit substances and not alcohol when used alone.

Among non-users of illicit substances, time to treatment discontinuation was significantly longer for patients treated with olanzapine (median 13.0 months) than perphenazine (5.9 months), risperidone (5.6 months), or quetiapine (5.0 months). In contrast, there were no significant differences between treatment groups in time to treatment discontinuation among patients who use illicit drugs (median 3.3 to 6.8 months).

This chapter further addresses three critical questions using published and unpublished data:

1. What was the pattern of substance abuse found in a carefully evaluated sample of patients with schizophrenia?
2. What were the differences between patients with schizophrenia who did not use illicit drugs and those who used or abused illicit substances of abuse?
3. Were there differences in treatment outcome related to the use or abuse of illicit substances?

Methods
Study design and sample characteristics
The data for this study were collected as part of the NIMH CATIE project. Study details have been presented elsewhere [19] and in Chapters 1 and 2. The study was approved by an institutional review board at each site. Each patient provided written informed consent. The data on demographic variables and substance use were collected at the time of enrollment, i.e., before randomization and the initiation of experimental treatments.

In these analyses, subjects were categorized as illicit drug users (either users or abusers) or non-users of illicit drugs. Patients with evidence of alcohol use or abuse but no evidence of illicit drug use were included in the illicit drug non-user group. Second, group comparisons were made between patients on each of the five study antipsychotic medications (olanzapine, perphenazine, quetiapine, risperidone, and ziprasidone).

Measures
The diagnosis of schizophrenia was made using DSM-IV criteria as confirmed by the SCID [23]. The following sources of information were utilized to more accurately ascertain substance use in each patient: positive hair assay or urine screen for illicit drug use, self-reported drug use, clinician ratings on the initial screening inventory, clinician rating from the Alcohol or Drug Use Scale [24], clinician diagnostic assessment using the SCID [23], and family report of a problem with alcohol or illicit drugs. At study entry, few subjects endorsed enough substance use symptoms to make a current SCID abuse or dependence diagnosis but many more endorsed symptoms consistent with a past or 5 year diagnosis of substance use or dependence. Patients with such a *past* diagnosis of abuse or dependence on the SCID were re-categorized as *current* users or abusers based on other concurrent sources of information such as a positive collateral report of use or a positive urine drug screen. Thus, those with a past, but not current SCID substance abuse and dependence diagnosis were re-diagnosed using the positive SCID 5-year assessment of abuse/dependence *plus* any concurrent validation from one of the other indicators. Using these sources of information,

patients were divided into three categories: Abusers: current substance use disorders (alcohol and/or illicit drug abuse or dependence); Users: current alcohol and/or illicit drug use without impairment; and Non-users. A compete presentation of these data is provided in Table 11.1 and Figure 11.1. For later additional analyses below, patients who only used alcohol were re-categorized into the illicit substance non-use group.

The following demographic variables were collected: age; gender; racial status in three categories: White, African-American, or several other categories (Hispanic or non-Hispanic [reported separately from race]); marital status (married or cohabiting versus single); education (9-point scale from 0 = did not complete high school to 8 = advance degree completed); homelessness (homeless in the past 30 days); restrictive housing (restrictive housing in past 30 days); employment activity (employed, prevocational, or no vocational activity in the past 30 days).

The following items regarding clinical history were collected: history of physical or sexual abuse prior to age 15; childhood conduct problems prior to age 15 (skips school a lot, ran away from home more than once, ever deliberately destroyed someone else's property, often started physical fights, ever arrested or sent to juvenile court, ever suspended from school); years in treatment; years since onset; history of major depression in the past 5 years.

The clinical status of each patient was assessed using the following scales and assessments: Clinical Global Impressions – Severity Scale (CGI-S); Calgary Depression Scale for Schizophrenia [25]; PANSS [26]; recent illness exacerbation (defined as hospitalization or treatment in a crisis center in the previous 3 months; recent victimization as defined as being the victim of 1) any violent crime, such as assault, rape, mugging, or robbery; and 2) any non-violent crime, such as burglary, property theft, or being cheated; and Quality of Life Scale [27].

Measures of treatment outcome include the following: compliance rating as assessed by a count of pills taken; Kaplan-Meier survival in months for all-cause treatment discontinuation; Kaplan-Meier survival in months for treatment discontinuation due to all causes, lack of efficacy, intolerable side effects, or patient decision; change in PANSS total; percentage of patients completing 18 months in Phase 1; percentage of responders based on a 20-point PANSS drop; percentage of responders based on Scores of ≤ 2 on CGI-I; and Calgary Depression Scale.

Results

Nearly 1,500 subjects from 57 clinics completed the baseline evaluation and entered the study. Information on patterns of substance use, abuse, and dependence is presented in Figure 11.1 and Table 11.1.

Figure 11.1 demonstrates the yield of different methods of detection of illicit substances (excluding alcohol) in this population comparing self-report, urine drug testing, and RIAH among subjects with these sources of information available. In these methods, roughly one-third of subjects were classified as users. By self-report, only 21.4% would be classified as users, by urine drug testing, 15.9% and by RIAH, 22.4%. Urine drug testing yielded the fewest unique positive results (2.0%) when other methods are negative, compared to 6.4% for self-report and 7.4% for RIAH. Thus, the combined use of detection methods yields the highest sensitivity for detection of illicit substance use.

Table 11.1 excludes the 40% of the patients who showed no evidence of use/abuse dependence of either alcohol or illicit substances. In addition, 22% of the entire study population only used or abused alcohol. Overall, 38% of the sample used or abused illicit drugs.

Table 11.1. Patterns of substance use and abuse/dependence

	Use by type (N = 334)*		Abuse by type (N = 532)**	
	Frequency	Percentage	Frequency	Percentage
Any alcohol	221	66.2	465	91.9
Any THC	87	26.1	240	47.4
Any cocaine	78	23.4	187	37.0
Any opiates	26	7.8	34	6.7
Any stimulants	7	2.1	33	6.5
Any other	34	10.2	77	15.2
	Use by number*		**Abuse by number****	
	Frequency	Percentage	Frequency	Percentage
One drug	216	64.7	198	37.2
Two drugs	74	22.2	161	30.3
Three drugs	23	6.9	106	19.9
Four drugs	5	1.5	26	4.9
Five drugs	0	0.0	15	2.8
Six drugs	0	0.0	3	0.6
Other/missing	16	4.7	23	4.3
	Use by pattern*		**Abuse by pattern****	
	Frequency	Percentage	Frequency	Percentage
Alcohol (only)	151	45.2	172	32.3
THC (only)	33	9.9	15	2.8
Cocaine (only)	33	9.9	9	1.7
Stimulants (only)	0	0.0	0	0.0
Opiates (only)	0	0.0	0	0.0
Other drug (only)	1	0.3	2	0.2
Alcohol/THC	27	8.1	94	17.6
Alcohol/cocaine	20	6.0	53	9.9
Alcohol/other	0	0.0	5	0.9
THC/cocaine	10	3.0	8	1.5
Opiates/other	15	4.5	1	0.2
Stimulants/other	2	0.6	0	0.0
Alcohol/THC/cocaine	12	3.6	81	15.2
Others/missing	30	8.9	92	17.3

Notes: Table does not include those who were abstinent.
*Substance use without dependence or abuse.
**Includes patients with abuse or dependence.

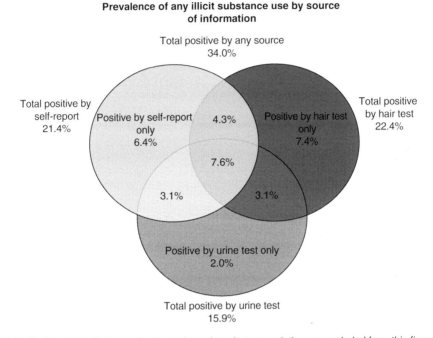

Prevalence of any illicit substance use by source of information

Total positive by any source
34.0%

Total positive by self-report 21.4%

Positive by self-report only 6.4%

4.3%

Positive by hair test only 7.4%

Total positive by hair test 22.4%

7.6%

3.1%

3.1%

Positive by urine test only 2.0%

Total positive by urine test 15.9%

Note: Positive lab tests for medications where there is a prescription are excluded from this figure.

Figure 11.1. Prevalence of any illicit substance use by source of information.

As can be seen in Table 11.1, the most common substance used or abused, in descending order, were alcohol, marijuana, cocaine, and to a lesser extent, opiates. Among patients with abuse/dependence, nearly one-half used marijuana and one-third used cocaine, while among users, marijuana and cocaine were used by roughly one-quarter each. These patterns of use of substances mirror rates of use in comparable US populations [25] and suggest substance use patterns are similar to the general population rather than somehow being specific to schizophrenia. Among users, nearly two-thirds used only one drug, while among those with abuse/dependence, only about one-third used only one substance. Roughly another third used two drugs, and nearly 20% used three drugs. Hence, those with abuse/dependence evidenced more complex patterns of polydrug use. The most common pattern of multiple drug use among users and those with abuse/dependence was alcohol and marijuana followed by alcohol and cocaine. Further, use of alcohol, marijuana, and cocaine was a relatively prevalent pattern of use among users (3.6%) but especially those with abuse/dependence (15.2%).

Tables 11.2 and 11.3 compare the baseline characteristics of CATIE subjects, contrasting those who used illicit substances to non-users (including users of alcohol). (For purposes of these analyses, the sample includes subjects at baseline for whom key follow-up data were available.) As can be seen in Table 11.2, in contrast to non-users, illicit substance users were younger, more likely to be male, non-White, and less educated. Users were also more likely to have a history of physical or sexual abuse prior to age 15, have a greater number of childhood conduct disorder symptoms, and a history of major depression in the past 5 years.

As can be seen in Table 11.3, illicit substance users were more likely to have been recently homeless, more likely to live in restrictive housing, such as a group home, and had

Table 11.2. Demographic and past clinical characteristics for patients with and without illicit substance use [22]

	Statistic	No illicit substance use (N = 789)	Illicit substance use (N = 643)	Probability
Demographics				
Age (years)	Mean ± SD	42.6 ± 10.9	38.1 ± 10.8	<0.0001
Sex: male	N (%)	541 (69%)	521 (81%)	<0.0001
Race				<0.0001
White	N (%)	540 (63%)	323 (37%)	
Black	N (%)	208 (42%)	290 (58%)	
Other	N (%)	39 (57%)	30 (43%)	
Hispanic	N (%)	103 (13%)	62 (10%)	0.0443
Marital status – married or cohabiting	N (%)	156 (20%)	118 (18%)	
Education (years)	Mean ± SD	12.3 ± 2.4	11.8 ± 2.0	0.0001
Prior clinical history				
Physical or sexual abuse prior to age 15	N (%)	231 (29%)	234 (36%)	.0049
Childhood conduct disorder symptoms	Median (25%–75%)	0 (0–1)	1 (0–3)	<0.0001
Major depression (past 5 years)	N (%)	191 (24%)	206 (32%)	0.001

Reprinted from Schizophrenia Research, Copyright 2008, with permission from Elsevier.

suffered recent victimization at twice the rate of non-users. They were also more likely to have had an exacerbation of their illness in the past 3 months, including hospitalization of crisis stabilization, had fewer years of treatment, and a more recent illness onset. At baseline, the illicit users' clinical status was notable for higher levels of clinical severity, depressive symptoms as measured on the Calgary Depression Scale, and higher severity ratings on the total, general psychopathology, and positive symptom scales of the PANSS, but lower negative symptom severity.

Figure 11.2 compares Kaplan-Meier plots of time to discontinuation for study anti-psychotic treatment groups for non-illicit substance users and users. As can be seen for all-cause treatment discontinuation among non-users, olanzapine appears to be superior to other antipsychotics, but this advantage appears to be attenuated among illicit substance users. Time to discontinuation due to intolerability appears to be comparable between all treatment groups. For efficacy, olanzapine appears to have modest advantage compared to other antipsychotic treatment groups and parallels the all-cause treatment discontinuation pattern. For discontinuation due to patient decision, illicit substance users assigned to olanzapine appear to discontinue comparably to other antipsychotic treatment groups. Thus, although illicit users appear to find olanzapine more efficacious compared to other

Table 11.3. Sample characteristics for patients with and without illicit substance use [22]

	Statistic	No illicit substance use (N=789)	Illicit substance use (N=643)	Probability
Current social history				
Recent homeless – yes	N (%)	16 (2%)	35 (5%)	0.0005
Restrictive housing	N (%)	84 (11%)	94 (15%)	0.0223
Employment activity (employed, prevocational or no vocational activity in the past 30 days)	N (%)	61 (8%)	36 (6%)	0.1123
Recent victimization	N (%)	105 (13%)	166 (26%)	<0.0001
Current clinical assessments				
Recent exacerbation past 3 months:	N (%)	181 (23%)	208 (32%)	<0.0001
Years treatment	Median (25%–75%)	17 (8–26)	14 (5–23)	<0.0001
Years since onset	Median (25%–75%)	14 (6–24)	11 (4–22)	0.0003
Alcohol abuse or dependence	N (%)	82 (10%)	268 (42%)	<0.0001
Drug abuse or dependence	N (%)	0 (0%)	409 (64%)	<0.0001
Alcohol/drug abuse or dependence	N (%)	83 (10%)	447 (70%)	<0.0001
Clinical status:				
CGI-S	Mean ± SD	3.9 ± 1.0	4.0 ± 1.0	0.0297
Calgary Depression Scale	Median (25%–75%)	3 (1–7)	4 (1–8)	0.0011
Calgary Depression Scale > 4	N (%)	304 (39%)	291 (45%)	0.0112
PANSS:				
Total	Mean ± SD	75.0 ± 17.6	76.4 ± 17.6	0.0002
Positive symptoms	Mean ± SD	18.0 ± 5.6	19.1 ± 5.6	
Negative symptoms	Mean ± SD	20.4 ± 6.4	19.9 ± 6.5	
General psychopathology	Mean ± SD	36.7 ± 9.2	37.4 ± 9.4	

Reprinted from Schizophrenia Research, Copyright 2008, with permission from Elsevier.

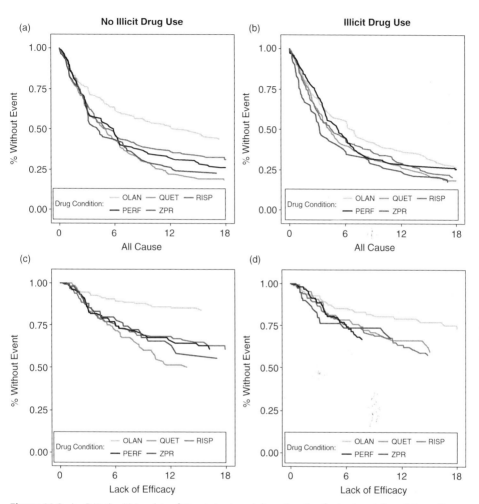

Figure 11.2. (a–d) Kaplan-Meier plots of time to treatment discontinuation for treatment. See plate section for color version [22]. Reprinted from Schizophrenia Research, Copyright 2008, with permission from Elsevier.

antipsychotic treatment groups, they had a somewhat greater tendency than non-illicit olanzapine users to discontinue treatment due to patient decision.

Table 11.4A and 11.4B stratifies users and non-users of illicit substances to compare discontinuation rates. Among non-users, the discontinuation rate was lower and time to all-cause discontinuation was significantly longer for olanzapine (discontinuation rate, 56%; median time, 13.02 months) compared to quetiapine (discontinuation rate, 81%; median time, 5.02 months), risperidone (discontinuation rate, 69%, median time, 5.57 months), perphenazine (discontinuation rate, 74%, median time, 5.89 months), but not ziprasidone (discontinuation rate, 77%, median time, 4.34 months). Among non-users there were significant differences in odds of discontinuation between olanzapine and quetiapine (hazard ratio (HR = 0.52; confidence interval [CI] 0.40, 0.67; $p < 0.001$), risperidone (HR = 0.70; CI 0.53, 0.92; $p = 0.01$) and perphenazine (HR = 0.59; CI 0.56, 1.08;

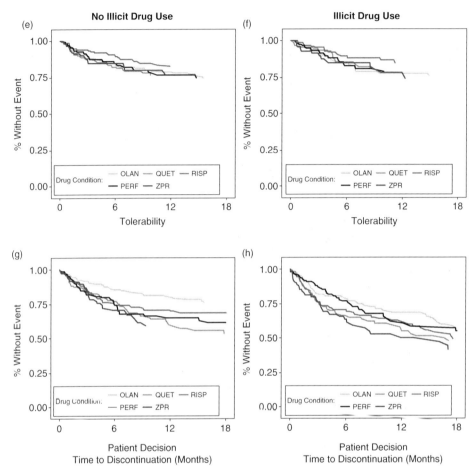

Figure 11.2. (*cont.*) (e–h)

$p = < 0.001$), but not ziprasidone (HR = 0.78; CI 0.56, 1.08; $p = 0.13$). Odds of discontinuation were also significantly higher for subjects randomized to quetiapine relative to risperidone (HR = 1.35; CI 1.05, 1.73; $p = 0.021$). Rates of medication compliance were higher for non-users, but were not different across treatment groups.

Among illicit substance users, there were no significant differences in discontinuation rates and time to all-cause discontinuation. Outcomes were similar among all treatment groups: olanzapine (discontinuation rate, 74%; median time, 6.75 months) compared to quetiapine (discontinuation rate, 82%; median time, 4.36 months), risperidone (discontinuation rate, 79%; median time, 4.61 months), perphenazine (discontinuation rate, 75%; median time, 5.25 months), and ziprasidone (discontinuation rate, 82%; median time, 3.29 months). Hazard rates for olanzapine relative to the other four antipsychotic drugs were as follows: quetiapine (HR = 0.90; CI 0.67, 1.20; $p = 0.47$), risperidone (HR = 0.93; CI 0.70, 1.24; $p = 0.63$), perphenazine (HR = 1.16; CI 0.84, 1.60; $p = 0.36$), and ziprasidone (HR = 0.75; CI 0.53, 1.07; $p = 0.11$). The contrast between quetiapine and risperidone also was not significant (HR = 1.04; CI 0.78, 1.37; $p = 0.79$).

Table 11.4A. Time to all-cause treatment discontinuation [22]

Condition: no illicit substance use

Assessment	Statistic	OLAN (N = 188)	QUET (N = 192)	RISP (N = 176)	PERF (N = 133)	ZPR (N = 100)
Modal dose (mg)/ no. patients	Mean	20.2/183	562.8/183	4.0/165	21.2/128	112.4/90
Number discontinuing	N (%)	105 (56)	156 (81)	121 (69)	99 (74)	77 (77)
Kaplan-Meier	Median	13.02	5.02	5.57	5.89	4.34
Time to discontinuation — mo.	[95%CI]	[8.14][1]	[3.79,6.21]	[3.93,7.57]	[3.32,6.50]	[3.11,7.04]
Compliance % (SE)		87.3 (21.0)	82.0 (27.5)	81.1 (28.1)	83.0 (26.7)	79.1 (29.9)

Condition: illicit substance use

Assessment	Statistic	OLAN (N = 142)	QUET (N = 137)	RISP (N = 157)	PERF (N = 124)	ZPR (N = 83)
Modal dose (mg)	Mean	20.0/129	515.1/126	3.8/140	20.4/117	113.3/75
Number discontinuing	n (%)	105 (74)	113 (82)	124 (79)	93 (75)	68 (82)
Kaplan-Meier	Median	6.75	4.36	4.61	5.25	3.29
Time to discontinuation — mo.	[95%CI]	[4.57,9.1]	[3.54,5.54]	[3.36,6.3]	[4.00,6.50]	[2.75,5.36]
Compliance % (SE)		78.7 (28.7)	71.9 (33.3)	75.9 (29.2)	78.1 (28.0)	75.7 (31.4)

Note: [1]Upper bound confidence interval not estimable.
Reprinted from Schizophrenia Research, Copyright 2008, with permission from Elsevier.

Table 11.5 presents estimated changes in PANSS (and its subscales) and CGI ratings from baseline to the end of Phase 1, adjusted to duration of Phase 1 treatment, in an effort to examine whether differences in discontinuation were mirrored in these efficacy measures. The total PANSS score decreased more from baseline to the end of Phase 1 for subjects randomized to olanzapine (approximately seven units, or roughly 10%) relative to the other treatment groups (generally a 0–3 unit decrease). Overall, there were no differences between olanzapine substance users and non-users or between other treatment groups comparing substance users and non-user subgroups for duration-adjusted change from baseline. Olanzapine illicit use and non-use treatment groups made greater improvements relative to other user and non-user treatment groups on PANSS subscales, but there were no significant differences between olanzapine illicit users and non-users. CGI severity measurements decreased significantly more from baseline to the end of Phase 1 among subjects randomized to olanzapine relative to other treatment groups, but as above, the decrease was not affected by illicit substance use (see Table 11.5).

Table 11.4B. Time to all-cause treatment discontinuation: Cox models [22]

Condition: no illicit substance use

Assessment	Statistic	OLAN (N = 188)	QUET (N = 192)	RISP (N = 176)	PERF (N = 133)	ZPR (N = 100)	p value[2]
	HR[1]		0.52	0.7	0.59	0.78	<0.001
OLANZAPINE	[95%CI]		[0.40,0.67]	[0.53,0.92]	[0.43,0.81]	[0.56,1.08]	
	p value		<0.001	0.010	0.001	0.134	
	HR			1.35	1.16	1.12	
QUETIAPINE	[95%CI]			[1.05,1.73]	[0.88,1.54]	[0.82,1.53]	
	p value			0.021	0.288	0.464	
	HR				0.87	1.02	
RISPERIDONE	[95%CI]				[0.64,1.17]	[0.75,1.40]	
	p value				0.354	0.877	
	HR					1.05	
PERPHENAZINE	[95%CI]					[0.74,1.49]	
	p value					0.79	

Condition: illicit substance use

Assessment	Statistic	OLAN (N = 142)	QUET (N = 137)	RISP (N = 157)	PERF (N = 124)	ZPR (N = 83)	p value[2]
OLANZAPINE	HR		0.9	0.93	1.16	0.75	0.827
	[95%CI]		[0.67,0.1.20]	[0.70,1.24]	[0.75,1.60]	[0.53,1.07]	
	p value		0.471	0.627	0.357	0.11	
QUETIAPINE	HR			1.04	1.1	0.89	
	[95%CI]			[0.79,1.37]	[0.80,1.51]	[0.63,1.24]	
	p value			0.793	0.55	0.486	
RISPERIDONE	HR				1.11	0.76	
	[95%CI]				[0.81,1.52]	[0.0.53,1.09]	
	p value				0.513	0.132	
PERPHENAZINE	HR					0.76	
	[95%CI]					[0.53,1.10]	
	p value					0.15	

Notes: [1]Hazard ratios are obtained from analysis of four cohorts defined by the stratified randomization for TD patients and the addition of ziprasidone. [2]The p value column is the overall 3 degree of freedom test comparing olanzapine, quetiapine, risperidone, and perphenazine for patients without TD. Reprinted from Schizophrenia Research, Copyright 2008, with permission from Elsevier.

Table 11.5. Efficacy measures at end of Phase 1–LS mean estimates of last observation carried forward differences from baseline, adjusted for average treatment duration [22]

	OLAN	QUET	RISP	PERF	ZIP
Positive and Negative Syndrome Scale (PANSS) Total Scale[1]:					
	Units (SE)	Units (SE)	Units (SE)	Units (SE)	Units (SE)
No use	−7.44 (1.19)	0.12 (1.32)	−2.46 (1.57)	−3.32 (1.62)	0.34 (1.85)
Illicit substance use	−7.56 (1.53)	−3.14 (1.49)	−3.03 (1.51)	−2.45 (1.50)	−1.07 (1.95)
PANSS Negative Symptom Scale:					
No use	−1.57 (0.45)	−0.41 (0.44)	−0.51 (0.49)	−2.27 (0.49)	−0.46 (0.62)
Illicit substance use	−1.76 (0.59)	−0.67 (0.53)	−0.17 (0.54)	−0.09 (0.49)	0.01 (0.57)
PANSS Positive Symptom Scale:					
No use	−2.28 (0.38)	0.34 (0.43)	−0.96 (0.44)	−1.16 (0.55)	−0.06 (0.65)
Illicit substance use	−2.79 (0.43)	−0.70 (0.53)	−0.98 (0.51)	−0.88 (0.53)	−0.31 (0.72)
PANSS General Psychopathology Scale:					
No use	−3.58 (0.63)	0.19 (0.70)	−0.99 (0.86)	−0.89 (0.88)	0.74 (0.91)
Illicit substance use	−3.02 (0.79)	−1.78 (0.79)	−1.88 (0.76)	−1.47 (0.81)	−0.77 (1.04)
Clinical Global Impression–Severity Scale:					
No use	−0.26 (0.08)	0.16(0.08)	−0.11 (0.09)	−0.16 (0.10)	0.01 (0.12)
Illicit substance use	−0.53 (0.09)	−0.12 (0.09)	−0.03 (0.09)	−0.10 (0.10)	−0.04 (0.13)

Note: [1]Final Phase 1 measurement less baseline measurement.
SE indicates standard error.
Reprinted from Schizophrenia Research, Copyright 2008, with permission from Elsevier.

Olanzapine stood out in analyses of efficacy in that the olanzapine treatment group improved more compared to other treatment groups. Interestingly, although olanzapine had an advantage over other drugs in time to discontinuation for non-users but not users of illicit substances, efficacy measures improved comparably for illicit substance users and non-users taking olanzapine. This suggests that patients were doing equally well on olanzapine whether or not they were using illicit substances, but were more likely to discontinue treatment for other reasons, probably related to poor treatment adherence.

Discussion

The CATIE study incorporated arguably the most exhaustive substance use assessment methods ever conducted in patients with schizophrenia in a clinical trial setting, combining reports from multiple informants, clinical assessment, drug urine testing, and RIAH. In contrast to most clinical trials, patients with co-morbid substance disorders and other co-morbidities were actively recruited into the trial and, in fact, 38% of the subject population met criteria for an illicit substance abuse diagnosis or used illicit drugs, while 40% of the sample showed no evidence of use of illicit drugs or alcohol. Approximately 22% used or abused only alcohol and were very distinct from patients with illicit substance involvement in terms of clinical characteristics. As a result, users of alcohol alone were grouped as non-illicit drug users for analyses of treatment outcomes.

The careful substance abuse screening conducted in the CATIE trial provides important information for the planning of future research. Most studies rely on a combination of self-report and urine drug testing to assess patients for the presence of substance abuse. Of the 38% of the sample that used illicit drugs, only 16% had positive urine tests. Consequently, reliance on urine drug testing alone might mean that, in many patients, the substance abuse problems could go undetected.

Illicit drug abusers or users were more likely to be younger, male, Black, had recent major depression, had a recent period of homelessness, and had a more recent exacerbation of symptoms. Most notable was the history of childhood conduct symptoms among illicit substance users. Illicit drug users and abusers were less compliant with study medications and were more likely to discontinue their initial study medication.

Earlier CATIE Phase 1 reports demonstrated that olanzapine had a significantly longer time to all-cause treatment discontinuation than quetiapine or risperidone, but not per-phenazine or ziprasidone [28]. In those analyses, illicit drug use was not a specific focus of analyses and it was unclear whether illicit substance use might affect discontinuation rates.

As we review here, among illicit substance users, there were no differences in time to all-cause discontinuation across treatment groups—hence no advantage for olanzapine. Compared to other antipsychotic groups, olanzapine had a marginally longer time to discontinuation (median of 6.7 vs. between 3.29–5.25 months across the other treatment groups) among illicit substance users. Among non-users, olanzapine's superiority in time-to-discontinuation was strengthened substantially and significantly (olanzapine median 13.0 versus 4.34–5.89 months for other antipsychotic treatment groups). The difference in median time to discontinuation between non-users and illicit drug users in the olanza-pine group is 6.3 months, while for other antipsychotic treatment groups the difference among users and non-users was a month or less, suggesting perhaps that better treatment compliance, or other unknown factor, in the non-users accentuated olanzapine's advantage in time to discontinuation.

As expected, substance users and non-users experienced more weight gain on olanza-pine than other treatment [22,29], suggesting that increased time to discontinuation with olanzapine still came at the cost of weight gain.

It appears that the primary cause of earlier discontinuation among olanzapine illicit substance users, compared to non-users, was patient decision to discontinue treatment, which was likely compounded by poorer treatment adherence overall in the illicit substance use. Patient decision discontinuations were those which were idiosyncratic to the patient and in the judgment of the study physician not clearly related to inefficacy or side effects, and these decisions may have also been related to the lower medication compliance seen in this group.

It remains somewhat puzzling why olanzapine's time to discontinuation was affected more by illicit substance use than other treatment groups, or conversely, why in the absence of illicit use, the other antipsychotic treatment groups did not demonstrate longer times to discontinuation comparable to olanzapine. Our analyses suggest that illicit drug users differ from non-users in ways that might affect treatment discontinuation: users had higher psychopathology severity scores at baseline, were clinically less stable, and during the course of the study were less treatment adherent. Treatment non-adherence may have been a key pathway to discontinuation, but these other characteristics no doubt contribute to shorter time to discontinuation and may have disproportionately affected olanzapine's superiority in time to discontinuation in the illicit user group.

Taken as a whole, these results underscore the need for concurrent substance abuse treatment and efforts to improve treatment adherence in order for patients to benefit from antipsychotic treatment. These results also suggest that the many clinical trials that exclude substance users may offer an incomplete picture of clinical effectiveness in real-world populations.

There are several limitations to these findings. While we carefully characterized patterns of use, we did not *quantify* illicit substance use and cannot assess the potential impact of quantities of use. Furthermore, these analyses do not assess the potential benefit of substance abuse treatment, although preliminary analyses showed that too few patients were actively engaged in substance abuse treatment for this to have affected the results. It is also possible that these differential outcomes were not a direct function of illicit substance use because individuals with illicit substance use were different in many ways and substance use could merely have served as a proxy for a host of negative predictors of clinical status, course, and outcome. Finally, only a well-powered randomized trial of antipsychotic treatment among illicit substance users and non-users could definitively shed light on which antipsychotics fare better or worse in these populations.

Conclusions

CATIE included perhaps the most complete evaluation of substance abuse ever conducted in a clinical trial of schizophrenia. As opposed to almost all clinical trials, patients with co-morbid substance disorders were included and almost 4 out of 10 subjects qualified for an illicit substance abuse diagnosis or used illicit drugs. A small minority used or abused only alcohol. Illicit drug abusers or users were younger, more often male, more often black, more often had a recent major depression, more often had a recent period of homelessness, and a more recent exacerbation of symptoms. One striking difference was the history of childhood conduct symptoms in illicit drug users. Illicit drug users and abusers were less compliant with medication and were more likely to discontinue their assigned medication. While non-drug abusers did better in treatment, much of this difference was due to non-drug using subjects doing particularly well on olanzapine and in remaining in treatment for almost twice as long as the other groups.

References

1. Blanchard JJ, Brown SA, Horan WP and Sherwood AR. Substance use disorders in schizophrenia: Review, integration, and a proposed model. *Clinical Psychology Review* 2000;**20**:207–34.

2. Cantor-Graae E, Nordstrom LG and McNeil TF. Substance abuse in schizophrenia: A review of the literature and a study of correlates in Sweden. *Schizophrenia Research* 2001;**48**:69–82.

3. Dixon L. Dual diagnosis of substance abuse in schizophrenia: Prevalence and impact on outcomes. *Schizophrenia Research* 1999;**35**: S93–S100.

4. Goswami S, Mattoo SJ, Basu D and Singh G. Substance-abusing schizophrenics: Do they self-medicate? *The American Journal on Addictions* 2004;**13**:139–50.

5. Kavanagh DJ, McGrath J, Saunders JB, Dore G and Clark D. Substance misuse in patients with schizophrenia: Epidemiology and management. *Drugs* 2002;**62**:743–55.

6. Kessler RC, Crum RM, Warner LA, Nelson CB, Schulenberg J and Anthony JC. Lifetime co-occurrence of DSM-III-R alcohol abuse and dependence with other psychiatric disorders in the National

Comorbidity Survey. *Archives of General Psychiatry* 1997;**54**:313–21.

7. McCreadie RG. Use of drugs, alcohol and tobacco by people with schizophrenia: Case-control study. *British Journal of Psychiatry* 2002;**181**:321–5.

8. Mueser KT, Drake RE and Wallace MA. Dual diagnosis: A review of etiological theories. *Addictive Behaviors* 1998; **23**:717–34.

9. Regier DA, Farmer ME, Rae DS, *et al.* Comorbidity of mental disorders with alcohol and other drug abuse. Results from the Epidemiologic Catchment Area (ECA) Study. *Journal of the American Medical Association* 1990;**264**:2511–8.

10. Salyers MP and Mueser KT. Social functioning, psychopathology, and medication side effects in relation to substance use and abuse in schizophrenia. *Schizophrenia Research* 2001;**48**:109–23.

11. Haywood TW, Kravita HM, Grossman LS, Cavanaugh JL Jr, Davis JM and Lewis DA. Predicting the "revolving door" phenomenon among patient with schizophrenic, schizoaffective, and affective disorders. *American Journal of Psychiatry* 1995;**151**:856–61.

12. Swartz MS, Swanson JW, Hiday VA, Borum R, Wagner HR and Burns BJ. Violence and severe mental illness: The effects of substance abuse and nonadherence to medication. *American Journal of Psychiatry* 1998;**155**:226–31.

13. Swofford CD, Kasckow JW, Scheller-Gilkey G and Inderbitzin LB. Substance use: A powerful predictor of relapse in schizophrenia. *Schizophrenia Research* 1996;**20**:145–51.

14. Swanson J, Estroff S, Swartz M, *et al.* Violence and severe mental disorder in clinical and community populations: The effects of psychotic symptoms, comorbidity, and lack of treatment. *Psychiatry* 1997;**60**:1–22.

15. Goodman LA, Salyers MP, Mueser KT, *et al.* Recent victimization in women and men with severe mental illness: Prevalence and correlates. *Journal of Traumatic Stress* 2001;**14**:615–32.

16. Rosenberg SD, Goodman LA, Osher FC, *et al.* Prevalence of HIV, Hepatitis B and Hepatitis C in people with severe mental illness. *American Journal of Public Health* 2001;**91**:31–7.

17. Abram K and Teplin L. Co-occurring disorders among mentally ill jail detainees: Implications for public policy. *The American Psychologist* 1991;**46**:1036–44.

18. Swartz MS, Swanson JW and Hannon MJ. Detection of illicit substance use in persons with schizophrenia. *Psychiatric Services* 2003;**54**:891–5.

19. Stroup TS, McEvoy JP, Swartz MS, *et al.* The National Institute of Mental Health Clinical Antipsychotic Trials of Intervention Effectiveness (CATIE) project: Schizophrenia trial design and protocol development. *Schizophrenia Bulletin* 2003;**29**:15–31.

20. Swartz MS, Wagner HR, Swanson JW, *et al.* Substance use in persons with schizophrenia: Baseline prevalence and correlates from the NIMH CATIE study. *The Journal of Nervous and Mental Disease* 2006;**194**:164–72.

21. Swartz MS, Wagner HR, Swanson JW, *et al.* Substance use and psychosocial functioning in schizophrenia among new enrollees in the NIMH CATIE study. *Psychiatric Services* 2006; **57**:1110–6.

22. Swartz MS, Wagner HR, Swanson JW, *et al.* The effectiveness of antipsychotic medications in patients who use or avoid illicit substances: Results from the CATIE study. *Schizophrenia Research* 2008;**100**:39–52.

23. First MB, Spitzer RL, Gibbon M, *et al. Structured Clinical Interview for Axes I and II DSM-IV Disorders-Patient Edition (SCID-I/P).* New York: Biometrics Research Department, New York State Psychiatric Institute; 1996.

24. Drake R, Osher FC, Noordsy DL, Hurlbut SC, Teague GB and Beaudett MS. Diagnosis of alcohol use disorders in schizophrenia. *Schizophrenia Bulletin* 1990;**16**:57–67.

25. Addington D, Addington J and Schissel B. A depression rating scale for schizophrenics. *Schizophrenia Research* 1990;**3**:247–51.

26. Kay SR, Fiszbein A and Opler, LA. The positive and negative syndrome scale (PANSS) for schizophrenia. *Schizophrenia Bulletin* 1987;**13**:261–76.

27. Heinrichs DW, Hanlon TE and Carpenter WT Jr. The Quality of Life Scale: An instrument for rating the schizophrenic deficit syndrome. *Schizophrenia Bulletin* 1984;**10**:388–98.

28. US Department of Health and Human Services, Substance Abuse and Mental Health Services Administration, Office of Applied Studies. *National Survey on Drug Use and Health*. Washington, DC: HHS; 2006.

29. Lieberman JA, Stroup TS, McEvoy JP, *et al.* Effectiveness of antipsychotic drugs in patients with chronic schizophrenia. *New England Journal of Medicine* 2005;**353**:1209–23.

Chapter 2

Violence in schizophrenia: prevalence, correlates, and treatment effectiveness

Jeffrey Swanson and Richard Van Dorn

Among the possible complications and adverse outcomes of schizophrenia, perhaps none is more troubling and tragic—albeit infrequent—than violence. Aside from causing physical harm to its victims, violent behavior is ruinous to its perpetrators and costly to the public. It precipitates the loss of personal liberty, necessitates expensive interventions, perpetuates stigma, and disrupts continuity of care.

Despite a substantial amount of research literature [1,2], key questions remain about the link between schizophrenia and violence. Questions include: How common is serious violence compared to minor violence among schizophrenia patients, and what causes these different behaviors? To what extent is violence associated with acute psychopathology, rather than other factors, including those that may precede the onset of schizophrenia? How effective are various antipsychotic medications in reducing violence, and for which types of patients?

Definitive answers to these questions remain elusive. However, the Clinical Antipsychotic Trials of Intervention Effectiveness (CATIE) study provides a wealth of new evidence about violence and schizophrenia.

Research questions

In this chapter, we present three sets of analyses, adapted from published primary reports [3–5]. First, we examine baseline data to estimate the prevalence of serious and minor violence, and to identify significant correlates of each. We also develop an overarching explanatory model of any violence. With this first set of analyses we focus most specifically on clinical factors, particularly the link between violence and psychotic symptoms.

Second, we consider whether there might be a subgroup of patients whose risk of violence is distinct in its etiology, and is perhaps unexplained by the acute psychopathology of schizophrenia. To address this question, we divide the baseline sample into two strata— those with a history of childhood conduct problems and those without. We model the correlates of violence in each of these groups.

Third, we utilize the longitudinal CATIE data to examine the impact of treatment on violence, specifically comparing the effectiveness of five medications, that is, olanzapine, risperidone, quetiapine, ziprasidone, and perphenazine, in reducing violence. We also present the results of a subgroup analysis of the effects of medication compliance on violence within the two strata identified above—those with and without childhood conduct problems.

Antipsychotic Trials in Schizophrenia, ed. T. Scott Stroup and Jeffrey A. Lieberman. Published by Cambridge University Press. © Cambridge University Press 2010.

Prior research

In this section, we review research as it pertains to our three research questions and briefly indicate how the CATIE data are able to address limitations associated with prior research. First, the nature and importance of the link between violence and psychotic symptoms remains unresolved [6,7]. Despite lack of scientific consensus, clinicians continue to believe that psychotic symptoms play a key role in violent behavior for some persons with schizophrenia [8]. The CATIE project offers several advantages relevant to this debate: a large sample, a specific measure of community-based violence, and comprehensive clinical assessments, including those related to psychotic symptoms.

Second, prior to the CATIE study, researchers had begun to characterize two distinct patterns of criminality and violence among persons with schizophrenia [9]. In the first pattern, violent behavior seems to result directly from psychopathology, including disorders of perception, cognition, or mood. In contrast, in the second pattern, antisocial behavior begins in childhood, typically before the onset of psychosis in late adolescence or adult life.

That there is a strong link between childhood conduct problems and adult crime (and violent behavior in particular) has been well established in general population studies [10]; perhaps not surprisingly, the same association can be found among schizophrenia patients [11]. Still, the precise extent to which violence differs in the conduct problem subgroup compared to a larger population of schizophrenia patients was poorly understood. The CATIE data go a long way toward clarifying this matter.

Third, and finally, while the primary means of treating persons with schizophrenia are based on pharmacological interventions, information regarding the effectiveness of particular medications in reducing violence was lacking. Whether second-generation antipsychotics (SGAs) were more effective at preventing community violence than first-generation antipsychotics (FGAs) had not been established in a double-blind randomized controlled trial. Moreover, no trial had examined whether medication compliance reduces community violence differentially when violence is related to psychosis or other causes. The CATIE study thus fills an important scientific gap in this area as well.

Study design and methods

The CATIE project provides new evidence in all three of the areas described above, overcoming some key shortcomings of previous studies and offering several advantages. Full details of the study design, randomized intervention, medication dosing, and assessments are described elsewhere in this volume (see Chapters 1 and 2).

For the first two sets of analyses, we report findings from the baseline sample; for these analyses, assessments were conducted before randomization and experimental treatments began. For the third set of analyses, we use data from a 6-month intention-to-treat analysis, with last-observation-carried-forward for missing data, and from a subset of patients who completed 6 months on their initially assigned study medication. (Sample sizes for all analyses are included in the Tables throughout the chapter.)

Measures

Clinical assessment instruments are described elsewhere in this volume. Specific to the analyses in this chapter, the MacArthur Community Violence Interview [12] was used to measure violent behavior at two levels during the past 6 months: *minor violence*, corresponding to simple assault without injury or weapon use; and *serious violence*, corresponding to any assault using a lethal weapon or resulting in injury, any threat with a lethal weapon in hand, or any sexual assault. A composite measure of any violence was also analyzed.

Self-report information was supplemented with family collateral reports on parallel questions for minor violence and any violence. A positive report from either party was treated as a positive indicator of any violence. Family collateral information was available for 617 participants at baseline.

Childhood conduct problems prior to the age of 15 were assessed using six questions from the Structured Clinical Interview for Axes I and II DSM-IV Disorders-Patient Edition. Respondents scoring *above* the median (i.e., those reporting two or more of the six items; see Figure 12.5 for a listing of the questions) were compared to those at or below the median (i.e., those reporting none or one of the behaviors). (Note: Throughout the chapter the comparison group is referred to as the "no-conduct-problems sample"; however, persons in this group could have actually endorsed zero or one conduct problems.) It was this variable on which the sample was stratified for the second analysis and the medication compliance–violence relationship for the third analysis.

Analysis

The assumption that guides our empirical examination of schizophrenia and violence is that that no single variable explains this relationship. Rather, we conceptualize violent behavior as a multi-determined phenomenon. It involves persons with particular characteristics and life histories as well as states of health or disease, interacting with others in a social environment [13]. Thus, we assess violence risk in five domains: *dispositional* (demographic characteristics and socioeconomic position); *social-contextual* (household composition, social contact, and social support); *life-historical* (childhood victimization and childhood conduct problems); *clinical* (current symptomatology, impairment, and functioning); and *treatment* (hospitalization and institutional contact).

For the first series of analyses, multivariable models were estimated using mixed-model logistic regression [14] with three dichotomous measures of violence: 1) minor violence vs. no violence, 2) serious violence vs. no serious violence, and 3) any violence vs. no violence. Site was entered as a random effect.

For each outcome, bivariate associations with individual risk factors were first estimated, then followed by multivariable models for each of the five domains. Covariates were retained in the domain models at $p < 0.15$. Finally, all covariates that were selected in the domain models were entered together into a final model, with selection at $p < 0.15$.

For the second set of analyses, the sample was stratified by history of childhood conduct problems. The two strata were compared on demographic and clinical variables using Chi-square tests confirming that the two groups were sufficiently different to warrant a stratified analysis. Next, logistic regression analysis was used to examine violence risk within each stratum, using the domain-modeling approach described above.

For the final series of analyses, we utilized longitudinal data to examine the unadjusted rates of violence from baseline to follow-up. We then compared the unadjusted rates in the intention-to-treat group to rates from the retained group. Next, we tested treatment effects controlling for baseline violence, site, design effects, and compliance. Then we conducted multivariable analysis of predictors of violence. Finally, we performed subgroup analysis in the two strata described above, that is, patients with and without childhood antisocial conduct history.

Regarding statistical methods for the third set of analyses, the treatment effects on violence at 6 months for the retained sample were examined using mixed-model logistic regression analysis [14] with a dummy variable for each SGA compared to perphenazine, controlling for baseline violence and compliance with medication. Trends in the rate of violence across medication groups were tested using repeated-measures logistic regression analysis, comparing violence at baseline and 6 months, with controls for design and site effects and within-subject observations. The statistical models also included controls for whether the participant was recruited before or after the introduction of ziprasidone, and whether the participant had tardive dyskinesia at baseline. Site was entered as a random effect for all multivariable models. The violence prediction analyses followed a similar approach and were conducted in three stages, as described above.

Results

Prevalence and correlates of minor, serious, and any violence

At baseline, we found that the large majority of patients—about 8 out of 10—had *not* engaged in any violence in the past 6 months. Of the small subgroup who had behaved violently, only a fraction of those—about 1 in 5—had committed serious acts involving weapons or causing physical injury to others. The rest of the violent behaviors reported would qualify as simple battery: pushing, shoving, slapping, etc., without a weapon in hand and without causing injury. Figure 12.1 displays these results graphically for the participants at baseline.

The data also help explain why only some patients become violent, while most do not—and why some engage in minor violence while only a few commit serious violent acts. The study suggests that violence can have many different causes, or may result from a number of factors operating together. Schizophrenia is only one potential contributing factor, but is neither a necessary nor a sufficient cause of violence. Sometimes people with schizophrenia behave violently for the same reasons that other people do—reasons that have little directly to do with their illness or with acute psychotic symptoms. Moreover, the correlates for engaging in minor violence differ from those associated with serious violence—although they overlap. Along these lines, Table 12.1 presents bivariate odds ratios for the three measures of violence compared to no violence.

Table 12.2 presents adjusted odds ratios for the three measures of violence. The first column shows minor violent behavior was significantly more likely among participants with several non-clinical characteristics: younger age, female gender, limited or no vocational activity, residing in restrictive housing, residing with family or relatives, not feeling "listened to" by family members, and recent history of police contact. In the clinical/functional

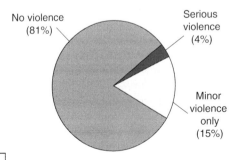

No violence (81%)

Serious violence (4%)

Minor violence only (15%)

Figure 12.1. Baseline prevalence of violence: past 6 months [3].

Table 12.1. Unadjusted odds ratios for minor, serious, and any violence [3]

	Unadjusted odds ratios								
	Minor violence			**Serious violence**			**Any violence**		
	OR	(95% CI)		OR	(95% CI)		OR	(95% CI)	
Model 1: Demographic characteristics, social stratification, and housing									
Age	0.95	(0.94 to 0.96)	***	0.95	(0.93 to 0.98)	***	0.95	(0.94 to 0.96)	***
Male	0.77	(0.56–1.05)		1.32	(0.72–2.42)		0.86	(0.64–1.16)	
Non-white	1.13	(0.83–1.54)		1.37	(0.81–2.33)		1.13	(0.85–1.51)	
Cohabitation	1.38	(0.98–1.94)		1.05	(0.56–1.97)		1.31	(0.95–1.80)	
High income	0.54	(0.40–0.73)	***	0.52	(0.30–0.89)	*	0.53	(0.40–0.70)	***
College	0.78	(0.58–1.05)		0.96	(0.58–1.60)		0.79	(0.60–1.04)	
Substantial vocational activity	0.20	(0.07–0.53)	***	0.84	(0.29–2.40)		0.29	(0.14–0.62)	**
Housing during the past 30 days. . .									
Extremely restrictive	3.04	(2.04–4.53)	***	1.85	(0.95–3.59)		2.96	(2.03–4.32)	***
Homeless	1.08	(0.52–2.23)		2.06	(0.79–5.35)		1.25	(0.66–2.38)	
Economic deprivation	1.93	(1.32–2.86)	***	1.12	(0.52–2.42)		1.75	(1.20–2.50)	**
Model 2: Household composition and social contact									
Currently live with. . .									
Alone [reference]									
Family/other relatives	2.64	(1.79–3.90)	***	1.21	(0.72–2.02)		2.41	(1.69–3.45)	***
Other people not related	1.77	(1.13–2.80)	**	1.27	(0.72–2.24)		1.77	(1.17–2.68)	**

Table 12.1. (cont.)

	Unadjusted odds ratios							
	Minor violence			Serious violence			Any violence	
	OR	(95% CI)		OR	(95% CI)		OR	(95% CI)
Frequent contact w/family and friends	1.29	(0.82–2.01)		0.79	(0.41–1.53)		1.13	(0.76–1.67)
Feel "listened to" most of the time by family	0.56	(0.41–0.77)	***	0.75	(0.43–1.29)		0.59	(0.44–0.78)	***
Model 3: Childhood risk factors								
Childhood physical abuse	1.52	(1.09–2.12)	**	2.28	(1.35–3.86)	**	1.67	(1.23–2.26)	***
Childhood sexual abuse	1.82	(1.31–2.52)	***	1.83	(1.06–3.16)	*	1.84	(1.36–2.48)	***
Childhood conduct problems (2+)	1.90	(1.42–2.55)	***	4.81	(2.69–8.62)	***	2.30	(1.75–3.01)	***
Model 4: Current clinical characteristics, impairment, and functioning								
Clinical Global Impression	1.18	(1.01–1.37)	*	1.22	(0.93–1.60)		1.19	(1.03–1.38)	*
PANSS Negative (above median)	1.06	(0.79–1.41)		0.31	(0.17–0.56)	***	0.87	(0.67–1.15)	
PANSS Positive (above median)	1.81	(1.35–2.43)	***	3.00	(1.69–5.31)	***	2.02	(1.53–2.67)	***
Calgary	1.05	(1.02–1.08)	**	1.09	(1.04–1.15)	**	1.06	(1.03–1.09)	***
Insight (above median)	0.89	(0.66–1.19)		1.16	(0.70–1.91)		0.94	(0.72–1.23)	
Years in treatment	0.97	(0.96–0.99)	***	0.98	(0.95–1.00)		0.97	(0.96–0.99)	***
Substance use								
Abstinent [reference]								
Use	1.54	(1.03–1.94)	*	2.46	(1.09–5.60)	*	1.60	(1.10–1.98)	**
Abuse/dependence	2.77	(1.96–3.93)	***	4.11	(1.99–8.52)	***	3.01	(2.17–4.18)	***

Recent victimization

Violently victimized (past 6 months)	3.53	(1.68–7.40)	***	4.88	(1.99–11.93)	***	4.00	(2.03–7.89)	***
Non-violently victimized (Past 6 months)	2.04	(1.27–3.27)	**	3.84	(2.08–7.09)	***	2.43	(1.60–3.69)	***
Heinrichs-Carpenter QOL									
Common Objects and Activities subscale	1.08	(0.88–1.34)		1.08	(0.88–1.34)		0.81	(0.73–0.91)	***
Instrumental Role subscale	0.97	(0.83–1.12)		0.97	(0.83–1.12)		0.94	(0.87–1.03)	
Intrapsychic Foundations subscale	1.11	(0.90–1.37)		1.11	(0.90–1.37)		0.89	(0.79–0.99)	*
Interpersonal Relations subscale	1.11	(0.92–1.34)		1.11	(0.92–1.34)		1.00	(0.91–1.11)	
Leisure activities (past week)	0.61	(0.44–0.86)	**	1.19	(0.60–2.36)		0.67	(0.48–0.92)	**
Instrumental ADLs (past week)	0.85	(0.28–2.54)					1.13	(0.38–3.38)	
Satisfaction with life	0.86	(0.78–0.95)	**	0.83	(0.46–1.51)		0.87	(0.80–0.96)	**
Model 5: Institutional contact									
Total prior hospitalizations (lifetime 4+)	0.96	(0.72–1.27)		0.93	(0.57–1.53)		0.95	(0.73–1.23)	
Total prior hospitalizations (past year 2+)	2.16	(1.60–2.91)	***	1.44	(0.86–2.40)		2.02	(1.53–2.67)	***
Arrested or picked up for crime (past 6 months)	4.28	(2.67–6.84)	***	5.85	(3.18–10.76)	***	4.93	(3.20–7.60)	***

Notes: *$p < 0.05$; **$p < 0.01$; ***$p < 0.001$.
Reprinted with permission of Archives of General Psychiatry.

Table 12.2. Adjusted odds ratios for minor, serious, and any violence [3]

	Adjusted odds ratios					
	Minor violence		Serious violence		Any violence	
	OR	(95% CI)	OR	(95% CI)	OR	(95% CI)
Model 1: Demographic characteristics, social stratification, and housing						
Age	0.94	(0.92–0.96) ***	0.96	(0.94–0.99) **	0.94	(0.92–0.96) ***
Male	0.52	(0.35–0.78) **			0.51	(0.35–0.74) ***
Non-white						
Cohabitation						
High income						
College						
Substantial vocational activity	0.17	(0.06–0.50) ***			0.21	(0.09–0.51) ***
Housing during the past 30 days...						
Extremely restrictive	1.70	(1.01–2.84) *			1.93	(1.23–3.03) **
Homeless			2.34	(0.80–6.82)		
Economic deprivation						
Model 2: Household composition and social contact						
Currently live with...						
Alone [reference]						
Family/other relatives	2.62	(1.47–4.57) ***			2.64	(1.56–4.47) ***
Other people not related	1.61	(0.81–3.21)			1.55	(0.83–2.89)

	OR	(95% CI)		OR	(95% CI)	
Frequent contact w/family and friends						
Feel "listened to" most of the time by family	0.63	(0.44–0.91)	**	0.61	(0.44–0.85)	**
Model 3: Childhood risk factors						
Childhood physical abuse						
Childhood sexual abuse						
Childhood conduct problems (2+)	3.29	(1.79–6.07)	***	1.50	(1.06–2.11)	*
Model 4: Current clinical characteristics, impairment, and functioning						
Clinical Global Impression						
PANSS Negative (above median)	0.25	(0.13–0.47)	***	0.72	(0.51–1.02)	***
PANSS Positive (above median)	2.71	(1.46–5.06)	**	1.86	(1.32–2.62)	***
Calgary	1.08	(1.02–1.14)	**			
Insight (above median)						
Years in treatment	1.03	(1.00–1.05)	*	1.02	(1.00–1.05)	*
Substance use						
Abstinent [reference]						
Use	1.41	(0.87–2.28)		1.35	(0.86–2.12)	
Abuse/dependence	2.42	(1.59–3.69)	***	2.28	(1.53–3.41)	***
Recent victimization						
Violently victimized (past 6 months)						
Non-violently victimized (past 6 months)	2.10	(1.12–3.94)	*	2.36	(1.34–4.15)	**

Table 12.2. (cont.)

	Adjusted odds ratios					
	Minor violence		Serious violence		Any violence	
	OR	(95% CI)	OR	(95% CI)	OR	(95% CI)
Heinrichs-Carpenter QOL						
Common Objects and Activities subscale						
Instrumental Role subscale						
Intrapsychic Foundations subscale						
Interpersonal Relations subscale	1.15	(0.98–1.34)			1.13	(0.98–1.30)
Leisure activities (past week)	0.56	(0.36–0.87)**			0.57	(0.37–0.87)**
Instrumental ADLs (past week)						
General life satisfaction	0.89	(0.78–1.00)*				
Model 5: Institutional contact						
Total prior hospitalizations (lifetime 4+)						
Total prior hospitalizations (past year 2+)	1.35	(0.92–1.98)				
Arrested or picked up for crime (past 6 months)	3.16	(1.76–5.69)***	3.45	(1.74–6.85)***	3.26	(1.91–5.56)***
	N = 1,115		N = 1,401		N = 1,161	

Notes: *p < 0.05; **p < 0.01; ***p < 0.001.
Reprinted with permission of Archives of General Psychiatry.

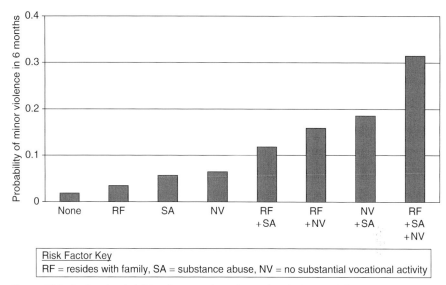

Figure 12.2. Predicted probabilities of minor violence by combined selected risk factors [3].

domain, minor violence was significantly associated with positive psychotic symptoms (higher Positive and Negative Syndromes Scale [PANSS] positive scores), more years in treatment, co-occurring substance abuse/dependence, recent non-violent victimization, and functional impairment in the area of leisure activities.

Additional analyses (not shown) revealed that the gender effect in the final model was influenced by a subgroup of younger females with substance abuse problems and history of arrest. Females in the sample were also more likely to live with family, thereby presumably having more opportunities for physical fights with social network members.

Figure 12.2 illustrates how these risk factors can operate in a cumulative fashion. Having any one of three risk factors—substance abuse, lacking vocational activity, or residing with family rather than alone—resulted in a predicted probability of minor violence that is slightly higher than having none of these characteristics, but not greater than 10%. Having any two of these risk factors together increased minor violence prevalence to the range of 10–20%. Finally, having all three risk factors simultaneously resulted in a predicted probability of over 30%. These results suggest that the combination of impairment, poor social functioning, and opportunity result in a high cumulative risk of minor violence.

What factors are associated with serious violence? The second column in Table 12.2 presents adjusted odds ratios (ORs) for serious violence compared to no violence. This model shows that three non-clinical covariates—younger age, childhood conduct problems, and arrest history—were significantly associated with serious violence.

Among the clinical or functional variables, higher scores on the Calgary depression scale and PANSS positive symptoms were correlated with greater likelihood of serious violence. However, above-median PANSS *negative* scores significantly lowered risk. Figure 12.3 depicts the pattern of opposite-directional effects of PANSS positive vs. PANSS negative symptoms on serious violence risk.

Is the association of violence with positive schizophrenia symptoms conditioned on the relative absence of negative symptoms? To answer this question, we tested the categorical

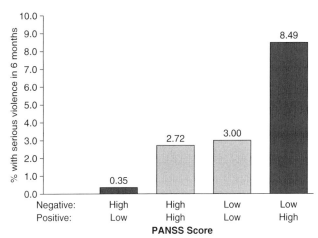

Figure 12.3. Percentage of CATIE study participants with serious violence in 6 months, by PANSS score combination.

Source: Swanson JW, Swartz MS, Van Dorn RA, Elbogen EB, Wagner HR, Rosenheck RA, Stroup TS, McEvoy JP, Lieberman JA (2006). A national study of violent behavior in persons with schizophrenia. *Archives of General Psychiatry* **63**:490–499. Used with permission.

interaction effect of positive and negative symptoms. Participants with a combination of above-median positive and below-median negative symptoms were at significantly elevated risk for serious violence (OR = 3.05, $p < 0.001$), compared to those with below-median scores on both types of symptoms. However, those with a combination of above-median positive and above-median negative symptoms were not more violent (OR = 0.95, not significant); those with below-median positive and above-median negative symptoms were less violent (OR = 0.12, $p < 0.05$).

In bivariate analysis, substance abuse/dependence was associated with a fourfold increase in the odds of serious violence (Table 12.1, second column). However, in the final model, covariates including psychotic symptoms and childhood conduct disorder rendered the effect of substance abuse non-significant. Thus, the effect of substance abuse on serious violence in this population may be mediated by psychopathology, pre-morbid conditions, and other factors.

We estimate that these models account for approximately 18% of the variance in both minor and serious violence. Significant site differences (which would incorporate urban population density, neighborhood crime rate, and other social-environmental characteristics) may explain an additional 7% of the variance in minor violence and an additional 16% of the variance in serious violence. These estimates suggest that, even taking into account significant demographic, clinical, and site effects, the majority of the variability in violence in this population remains unexplained by these statistical models.

We conducted additional item-level analyses to elucidate the association between serious violence and positive vs. negative psychotic symptoms. Among the seven symptom ratings that comprise the PANSS positive subscale, five specific symptoms—hostility, suspiciousness/persecution, hallucinatory behavior, grandiosity, and excitement—were significantly associated with increased risk of serious violence. The rating of hostility assessed "verbal and non-verbal expressions of anger and resentment." For each unit increase on the 7-point rating of hostility, the odds of serious violence increased by a factor of 1.65 ($p < 0.001$).

Suspiciousness and persecutory symptoms also showed a strong association with serious violence (OR = 1.46, $p < 0.001$). This symptom is characterized by "unrealistic or exaggerated ideas of persecution, as reflected in guardedness, a distrustful attitude, suspicious hypervigilance, or frank delusions that others mean one harm." The highest score was given when the patient manifested a "network of systematized persecutory delusions [which] dominates the patient's thinking, social relations, and behavior."

Serious violence was also strongly associated with hallucinatory behavior (OR = 1.43, $p < 0.001$). This symptom is characterized by auditory, visual, or other perceptions that are not generated by external stimuli; the highest score was assigned when the patient reported these false perceptions and also gave the perceptions "a rigid delusional interpretation," and when the perceptions "provoke[d] verbal and behavior responses, including obedience to command hallucinations."

Finally, serious violence was significantly associated with grandiosity (OR = 1.31, $p < 0.001$), characterized as "exaggerated self-opinion and unrealistic conviction of superiority, including delusion of extraordinary abilities," and excitement symptoms (OR = 1.30, $p < 0.05$), characterized as "hyperactivity as reflected in accelerated motor behavior, heightened responsivity to stimuli, hypervigilance, or excessive mood lability."

Two other PANSS positive symptoms were not, by themselves, associated with serious violence: conceptual disorganization, characterized by incoherent thinking, and a general rating of delusions, denoting "beliefs which are unfounded, and idiosyncratic." However, an interaction analysis showed that the combination of delusional thinking with suspiciousness/persecutory ideation was highly associated with serious violence: patients scoring above the median on both the general delusions scale and the suspiciousness/persecution scale were 2.9 times ($p < 0.001$) more likely to be seriously violent than those scoring below the median on both of these symptom ratings. Patients with above-median scores on general delusions combined with below-median scores on suspiciousness/persecution did not display a higher risk of serious violence (OR = 0.77, not significant). These patterns are shown in Figure 12.4. In contrast, participants with above-median scores on suspiciousness/persecution and below-median scores on general delusions were significantly more likely to be seriously violent (OR = 2.6, $p < 0.05$). However, it should be noted this last symptom combination was rare. Because suspiciousness and delusions were highly correlated ($\chi^2 = 248$, 1 DF, $p < 0.0001$), the combination of high suspiciousness with low delusions affected a relatively small subgroup (12% of the total sample), of which nine individuals reported serious violent behavior.

Among the seven symptoms that comprise the PANSS negative subscale, five specific symptom ratings were significantly associated with decreased risk of serious violence: lack of spontaneity and flow of conversation (OR = 0.66, $p < 0.001$), passive/apathetic social withdrawal (OR = 0.67; $p < 0.001$), blunted affect (OR = 0.75, $p < 0.001$), poor rapport (OR = 0.79, $p < 0.05$), and difficulty in abstract thinking (OR = 0.84, $p < 0.001$).

A final model at baseline predicted any (minor or serious) violence. The third column in Table 12.2 displays these results. The overall picture of correlates of any violence is similar to that for minor violence, except that history of childhood conduct problems is significant in the final model of any violence, but not in the final model of minor violence only.

Alternative pathways to violence: the role of early antisocial conduct

The overarching multivariable models of minor and serious violence are informative as far as they go; they are built on data from the baseline sample and thus have the advantage of being generalizable to schizophrenia patients resembling those enrolled in the CATIE trial. However, the foregoing analysis leaves open the question of whether there could be a

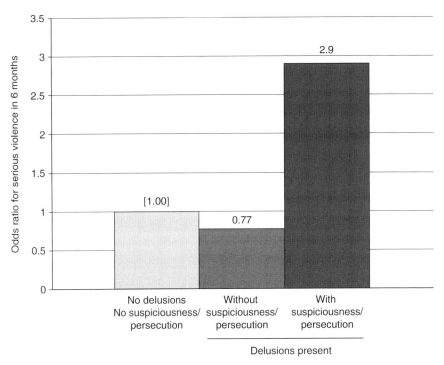

Figure 12.4. Delusions, suspiciousness/persecution, and risk of serious violence: odds ratios [3].

subgroup of individuals with schizophrenia with an increased risk of violence that is largely unexplained by psychotic illness. In particular, could there be a subgroup of schizophrenia patients characterized by a pattern of antisocial behavior dating back to childhood—preceding the typical age of onset of psychosis?

To address this question, we conducted a stratified analysis of the prevalence and correlates of violence in two groups: those with and without a self-reported history of childhood antisocial history. Figure 12.5 lists these items and shows that the number of conduct problems is associated with increased odds of violence, but the association is non-linear. No increase in risk occurs moving from one to two conduct problems. However, a substantial increase is seen at the level of three problems. Beyond three conduct problems, the odds ratios increase in magnitude with each increment. These findings remain significant when controlling for substance use and abuse/dependence.

Considering antisocial conduct history as a dichotomy, we found that adult violence was reported twice as frequently in the group of patients with two or more of these childhood conduct problems than in the group with less than two of the problems (28.3% vs. 14.4%, $p < 0.0001$). Table 12.3 shows that the two groups differed significantly in the proportions with minor violence as well as serious violence.

The social-demographic and clinical profiles of those in the conduct-problems group differed substantially from those without conduct problems. Specifically, those in the conduct-problem group were younger and had less education. They were more likely to have experienced physical or sexual victimization during childhood. They had more severe

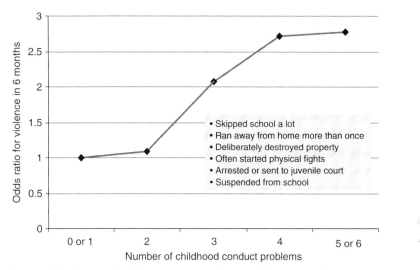

Figure 12.5. Number of childhood antisocial problems and risk of adult violence in schizophrenia patients [5].

clinical symptomatology and impairment: higher PANSS positive symptoms, Calgary depression symptoms, and substance abuse. They also had more recent violent victimization history, and exhibited lower functioning on the Heinrichs-Carpenter scale of working with common objects and activities.

Table 12.4 presents adjusted odds ratios for any violence within each of the two subgroups. For the conduct problems sample (first column in Table 12.4), the final model shows violent behavior was significantly more likely among participants residing in restrictive housing, residing with family or relatives, and those with a recent history of being arrested or picked up by police. In the clinical/functional domain, violence was significantly associated with co-occurring substance use and abuse/dependence, and recent non-violent victimization. Controlling for all other violence risk factors in the final model, being older, engaging in substantial vocational activity, and feeling listened to most of the time by family were significantly and negatively associated with violence in the conduct-problems group.

The second column in Table 12.4 presents parallel findings for the no-conduct-problems sample. The final model shows that violence was significantly more likely among participants with several non-clinical characteristics: residing with family or relatives, childhood sexual abuse, reporting one or more psychiatric hospitalization in the past year, and recent history of being arrested or picked up by police. Other non-clinical factors had a significant and negative association with violence for this subgroup: age and reporting substantial vocational activity. Among the clinical/functional variables, violence was significantly associated with positive psychotic symptomatology (higher PANSS positive scores), substance abuse/dependence, recent violent victimization, and functional impairment in the area of leisure activities.

Antipsychotic treatment effects on reducing violence

Incorporating the follow-up data from Phase I of the CATIE trial enables us to address several key questions of particular relevance to treatment and management of violence risk

Table 12.3. Prevalence of sample characterisitcs by conduct problems [5]

	Percentage with characteristic		
	Conduct problems (N = 488)	Non-conduct problems[1] (N = 956)	χ^2
Violence			
All violence	28.28	14.44	40.05***
Minor violence	22.22	13.16	18.51***
Serious violence	7.80	1.47	37.20***
Demographic characteristics, social stratification			
Age			
Below median (less than 42)	61.07	38.93	19.35***
Sex			
Male	79.30	71.44	10.4
Race			
Non-white	41.77	38.7	1.27
Marital status			
Married, co-habitating	19.67	18.93	0.11
Income			
Above median ($\geq$ $620/month)	52.32	44.97	6.95
Education			
College	26.43	45.61	49.86***
Substantial vocational activity			
Yes	8.25	6.09	2.35
Extremely restrictive housing (past 30 days)			
Yes	11.93	12.68	0.17
Homeless			
Yes	3.92	3.56	0.11
Enough money for necessities			
Yes	85.01	88.91	4.52
Household composition and social contact			
Currently live with . . .			
Alone	23.20	25.05	0.60
Family	52.25	55.65	1.50
Others not related	26.49	20.13	7.54

Table 12.3. (cont.)

	Percentage with characteristic		
	Conduct problems (N = 488)	Non-conduct problems[1] (N = 956)	χ^2
Frequent contact with family and friends			
Yes	83.57	85.43	0.86
Feel listened to most of the time by family			
Yes	48.17	51.80	1.45
Childhood history			
Childhood physical abuse			
Yes	34.43	12.57	96.62***
Childhood sexual abuse			
Yes	30.80	14.88	50.55***
Current clinical characteristics, impairment and functioning			
Clinical Global Impression			
Moderately to very severely ill	75.10	71.01	2.70
PANSS Negative			
Above median	45.88	47.43	0.31
PANSS Positive			
Above median	55.97	46.18	12.35***
Calgary			
Above median	43.74	28.38	34.13***
Insight			
Above median	47.13	44.13	1.17
Years in Treatment			
Above median (16 or more years)	47.35	46.78	0.04
Substance use			
Abstinent	24.80	46.97	66.47***
Use	23.57	22.70	0.14
Abuse/dependence	51.64	30.33	62.54***
Violently victimized (past 6 months)			
Yes	4.31	1.36	12.17***
Nonviolently victimized (past 6 months)			
Yes	10.29	6.29	7.30

Table 12.3. *(cont.)*

	Percentage with characteristic		
	Conduct problems (N = 488)	Non-conduct problems[1] (N = 956)	χ^2
Heinrichs-Carpenter QOL			
Common objects and activities subscale			
Above median	47.33	57.04	12.21***
Instrumental role subscale			
Above median	47.84	48.26	0.02
Intrapsychic foundations subscale			
Above median	55.07	53.20	0.45
Interpersonal relations subscale			
Above median	53.09	50.74	0.71
Leisure activities (past week)			
Yes	82.96	81.32	0.58
How do you feel about your life in general?			
Delighted to mixed	74.69	78.15	2.17
Service utilization, institutional contact, treatment engagement			
Total hospitalizations lifetime			
Above median (4+)	50.10	49.95	0.00
Total hospitalizations past year			
Above median (1+)	42.71	39.48	1.40
Arrested or picked up for crime (past 6 months)			
Yes	9.65	5.03	11.17***

Notes: [1]Throughout the paper the comparison group is referred to as the "no-conduct-problems sample"; however, persons in this group could have actually endorsed zero or one conduct problems.
***$p < 0.001$ (Bonferroni adjustment)

in schizophrenia. Does treatment with antipsychotic medications significantly reduce violence? If so, do the newer, more expensive medications work better, perhaps because they are more tolerable? And for which patients do the medications work, or not work as well, in reducing violence?

Table 12.5 displays rates of violence for the medication groups at baseline and 6 months for the retained sample. The observed rate of violence declined from 16% to 9% in the retained sample. Figure 12.6 displays the pattern of decline in violence across all treatment

Table 12.4. Adjusted odds ratios for any violence in the conduct problems and non-conduct problems samples [5]

	Any violence					
	Conduct problems sample			Non-conduct problems sample		
	OR	(95% CI)		OR	(95% CI)	
Model 1: Demographic characteristics, social stratification and housing						
Age	0.94	(0.92–0.97)	***	0.96	(0.94–0.97)	***
Male				0.66	(0.41–1.04)	†
Non-white						
Cohabitation						
High income						
College						
Substantial vocational activity	0.35	(0.13–0.98)	*	0.07	(0.01–0.47)	**
Housing during the past 30 days . . .						
Extremely restrictive	2.33	(1.21–4.48)	*			
Homeless						
Low on economic scarcity				0.63	(0.37–1.08)	†
Model 2: Household composition and social contact						
Currently live with . . .						
Alone [Reference]						
Family/other relatives	2.22	(1.23–4.00)	**	1.91	(1.13–3.21)	*
Other people not related	1.82	(0.96–3.43)	†	0.84	(0.44–1.61)	
Frequent contact w/family and friends						
Feel "listened to" most of the time by family	0.55	(0.34–0.89)	*			
Model 3: Childhood risk factors						
Childhood physical abuse						
Childhood sexual abuse				2.23	(1.36–3.65)	**
Model 4: Current clinical characteristics, impairment and functioning						
Clinical Global Impression (Mod. to very severely ill)						
PANSS Negative (above median)	0.71	(0.45–1.11)				
PANSS Positive (above median)				1.99	(1.33–2.98)	***
Calgary	1.05	(1.00–1.10)	†			

Table 12.4. (cont.)

	Any violence					
	Conduct problems sample			Non-conduct problems sample		
	OR	(95% CI)		OR	(95% CI)	
Insight (above median)						
Years in treatment	1.03	(1.00–1.06)	†			
Substance use						
Abstinent [reference]						
Use	2.12	(1.03–4.36)	*	1.23	(0.72–2.08)	
Abuse/dependence	2.59	(1.42–4.73)	**	2.00	(1.25–3.18)	**
Recent victimization						
Violently victimized (past 6 months)				3.59	(1.13–11.47)	*
Non-violently victimized (past 6 months)	2.74	(1.38–5.44)	**			
Heinrichs-Carpenter QOL						
Common objects and activities subscale						
Instrumental role subscale						
Intrapsychic foundations subscale						
Interpersonal relations subscale						
Leisure activities (past week)				0.58	(0.36–0.94)	*
General life satisfaction (delighted to mixed)						
Model 5: Institutional contact						
Total prior hospitalizations (Lifetime 4+)	0.73	(0.46–1.17)				
Total prior hospitalizations (Past Yr. 1+)				2.29	(1.53–3.42)	***
Arrested or picked up for crime (past 6 months)	2.89	(1.43–5.81)	**	3.04	(1.53–6.01)	**
	n = 466			n = 947		

Notes: $^{†}p < 0.10$; $^{*}p < 0.05$; $^{**}p < 0.01$; $^{***}p < 0.001$.

Table 12.5. Treatment groups and rate of violence for the retained sample (N = 653) [4]

Phase 1 treatment group	Retained sample (6 months) Percent with any violence			
	N	Baseline	6-month follow-up	% Change
Perphenazine	114	19.3	7.0	−63.6
Risperidone	153	15.1	11.8	−22.3
Olanzapine	185	16.8	7.6	−54.8
Ziprasidone	70	15.7	4.3	−72.7
Quetiapine	131	14.5	13.7	−5.2
Total	653	16.3	9.3	−42.6

	Odds ratios				
	Unadjusted			Adjusted	
	OR	(95% CI)		OR	(95% CI)
Baseline violence	6.05	(3.46–10.57)	***	6.28	(3.63–10.86) ***
Medication					
Perphenazine [reference]	[1.0]			[1.0]	
Risperidone	1.21	(0.91–1.60)		1.29	(0.96–1.72) †
Olanzapine	1.09	(0.46–2.60)		1.20	(0.49–2.95)
Ziprasidone	0.90	(0.69–1.17)		0.96	(0.73–1.27)
Quetiapine	1.47	(0.96–2.24)	†	1.65	(1.07–2.57) *
Non-compliant (Q1 v. Q2–Q4)	1.73	(1.01–3.01)	*	1.45	(0.82–2.57)

Notes: $^†p < 0.10$; $^*p < 0.05$; $^{**}p < 0.01$; $^{***}p < 0.001$.

Adjusted model is controlled for design and site effects.

Reprinted with permission from British Journal of Psychiatry 2008.

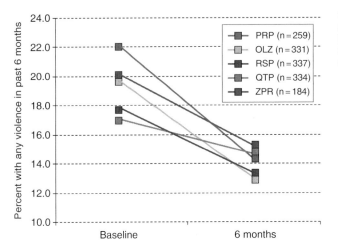

Figure 12.6. Violence by assigned CATIE treatment group: intention-to-treat sample (N = 1,445). See plate section for color version [4].

groups for the intention-to-treat sample. While the rates of violence were slightly more dispersed at baseline, the trend of reduced violence is quite consistent over 6 months in all the groups, with the rates converging around 14%. The proportional magnitude of decline in violence was substantially greater in the retained sample than in the intention-to-treat sample (43% vs. 27% decline).

We used repeated-measures logistic regression analysis to examine the significance of the decline in violence risk across the whole sample from baseline to 6 months. Among participants retained in the study, the adjusted odds of violence were approximately cut in half (OR = 0.52; 95% CI = 0.38 to 0.71; $p < 0.001$); among those who discontinued medication or dropped out, the finding was less dramatic (OR = 0.77; 95% CI = 0.60 to 0.99; $p < 0.05$) (results not shown).

The treatment groups did not differ significantly from each other on violence outcomes in the intention-to-treat sample. In the retained sample, patients assigned to perphenazine showed a greater reduction in violence risk—from 19% at baseline to 7% at follow-up—when compared to patients assigned to quetiapine, whose risk of violence declined from 15% to 14% over the same period. Perphenazine did not differ from olanzapine, risperidone, or ziprasidone. Table 12.5 (far right column) presents a test of these treatment effects using logistic regression. Baseline violence was also a strong predictor of violence at 6 months (OR = 6.28; 95% CI = 3.63 to 10.86; $p < 0.001$), and was included as a control in the model along with controls for site, design effects, and compliance with assigned medication.

Overall, medication compliance was not significantly associated with 6-month violence. However, when the sample was stratified into those with a history of childhood antisocial conduct problems, and those without a history of conduct problems, compliance with antipsychotic medications was found to significantly reduce violence only in the group *without* a history of conduct problems (OR = 0.47; 95% CI = 0.27 to 0.81; $p < 0.01$). In the conduct-problems group, the effect of medication compliance on violence reduction was in the same direction, but not statistically significant (OR = 0.59; 95% CI = 0.32 to 1.09; not significant) (results not shown).

Finally, Table 12.6 presents bivariate and adjusted odds ratios for baseline covariates *prospectively* predicting violence at 6 months for the retained sample. In multivariable

Table 12.6. Baseline risk factors predicting any violence at 6 months [4]

	Any violence					
	Bivariate associations		Domain models		Violence prediction Final model	
	OR	(95% CI)	OR	(95% CI)	OR	(95% CI)
Model 1: Demographic characteristics, social stratification, and housing						
Age	0.96	(0.93–0.98) ***	0.96	(0.94–0.99) **	0.97	(0.95–1.00) †
Male	1.05	(0.58–1.91)				
White	1.31	(0.75–2.28)				
Cohabitation	1.16	(0.61–2.23)				
High income	0.47	(0.27–0.81) **	0.47	(0.26–0.85) *	0.54	(0.28–1.03) †
Education (beyond high school)	0.87	(0.51–1.48)				
Substantial vocational activity	0.94	(0.33–2.63)				
Housing during the past 30 days . . .						
Extremely restrictive	0.76	(0.30–1.94)				
Homeless	1.02	(0.14–7.64)				
Economic deprivation	2.83	(0.91–8.73) †	3.31	(1.01–10.82) *	4.84	(1.29–18.09) *
			N = 646			
Model 2: Household composition and social contact						
Currently live with . . .						
Alone [reference]						
Family/other relatives	2.99	(1.41–6.37) **	2.96	(1.37–6.38) **	2.73	(1.14–6.56) *
Other people not related	3.14	(1.37–7.20) **	3.23	(1.40–7.42) **	3.29	(1.28–8.47) *

Table 12.6. (cont.)

	Any violence Bivariate associations			Domain models			Violence prediction Final model		
	OR	(95% CI)		OR	(95% CI)		OR	(95% CI)	
Frequent contact with family and friends	1.17	(0.52–2.59)							
Feel "listened to" most of the time by family	0.78	(0.46–1.31)							
Model 3: Childhood risk factors				N = 650					
Childhood physical abuse	1.74	(0.98–3.10)	†						
Childhood sexual abuse	1.92	(1.07–3.48)	*						
Childhood conduct problems (above median 2+)	2.80	(1.54–5.09)	***	2.77	(1.53–4.99)	***	2.07	(1.05–4.11)	*
Model 4: Baseline clinical characteristics, impairment and functioning				N = 653					
Clinical Global Impression	0.95	(0.54–1.68)							
PANSS Negative	0.96	(0.92–0.99)	*	0.96	(0.91–1.00)	†	0.94	(0.90–0.99)	*
PANSS Positive	1.03	(0.99–1.08)							
Calgary	1.07	(1.01–1.13)	*	1.07	(1.01–1.14)	*	1.07	(0.99–1.14)	†
Insight (median)	0.83	(0.49–1.40)							
Years in treatment	0.99	(0.96–1.01)							

	Model A			Model B			Model C		
Substance use									
Abstinent [reference]									
Use	3.73	(1.64–4.55)	**	3.38	(1.46–7.86)	**	3.31	(1.33–8.23)	*
Abuse/dependence	4.91	(2.29–10.53)	***	4.46	(2.04–9.75)	***	3.85	(1.65–9.02)	**
Victimization prior to study enrollment									
Violently victimized (12 months)	3.97	(1.24–12.73)	*	3.81	(1.09–13.38)	*	4.51	(1.06–19.20)	*
Non-violently victimized (12 months)	0.70	(0.22–2.23)							
Heinrichs-Carpenter QOL									
Common Objects and Activities subscale	0.84	(0.67–1.05)							
Instrumental Role subscale	0.82	(0.69–0.97)	*	0.79	(0.65–0.96)	*	0.83	(0.68–1.02)	†
Intrapsychic Foundations subscale	0.92	(0.74–1.15)							
Interpersonal Relations subscale	1.12	(0.93–1.35)		1.20	(0.95–1.52)				
Satisfaction with life	0.79	(0.44–1.43)							
				N = 645					

Model 5: Institutional contact prior to study enrollment

Total prior hospitalizations (lifetime 4+)	1.28	(0.76–2.14)	
Total prior hospitalizations (12 months 1+)	1.15	(0.67–1.97)	
Arrested or picked up for crime (6 months)	1.71	(0.71–4.13)	
		N = 642	

Notes: †$p < 0.10$; *$p < 0.05$; **$p < 0.01$; ***$p < 0.001$.
Reprinted with permission from The British Journal of Psychiatry.

analysis across domains, a final model identified several significant longitudinal predictors of violence: living with family or unrelated others vs. living alone, history of childhood conduct problems, substance use or abuse/dependence, and history of violent victimization. Negative psychotic symptoms and being low on economic scarcity were associated with lower risk of violence.

Discussion

While not designed as an epidemiological study, the CATIE project makes an important contribution to our understanding of the overall prevalence and correlates of violence among schizophrenia patients. The study also provides new evidence of alternative pathways to violence among patients with a history of childhood conduct problems. It suggests that compliance with antipsychotic medications may reduce violence irrespective of which specific medication is taken, but only for patients with no substantial history of childhood conduct problems. As a corollary, antipsychotic medications may not significantly reduce violence in the subgroup of schizophrenia patients who tend to be violent for reasons unrelated to psychosis.

The CATIE study offers several methodological advantages over previous studies, including a large and diverse sample of schizophrenia patients who were enrolled from both outpatient and inpatient settings in 57 cites throughout the US; thus, it is quite representative of the schizophrenia patient population encountered by clinicians. The study measured violent behavior in the community providing estimates for two levels of severity. Finally, the study also included valid and reliable measures of a wide range of both clinical and non-clinical covariates.

To summarize, we conducted three sets of analyses using CATIE data to examine violent behavior. In the first set of analyses, we focused on the baseline prevalence and correlates of minor and serious violence. We found that about 81% of patients had not been violent; about 15% had engaged in only minor acts of physical aggression toward others, while about 4% had committed serious violent acts involving the use of weapons and/or causing physical injury to others. We found distinct, but overlapping profiles of risk linked to minor vs. serious violent behavior. Based on these findings, we conclude that violence in schizophrenia patients is associated with multiple factors, with an important role attributable to psychotic symptoms, pre-morbid developmental events such as childhood conduct problems, and current social situation such as increased opportunity for violence presented by living with family members.

Specifically, we found that both minor and serious violence were significantly more prevalent among patients with a higher level of positive psychotic symptoms. However, high negative psychotic symptoms were significantly associated with reduced risk of serious violence, and they moderated the effect of the positive symptoms. This finding has intuitive clinical plausibility. A certain level of initiative, organization, psychomotor activation, and social contact may be necessary to carry out violent acts; those conditions tend to be absent in persons with high negative symptoms of schizophrenia.

We also found that patients living alone were less likely to engage in any violence than their counterparts who were living with family. Non-clinical variables—such as family co-residence—may affect violence risk in complex ways, either preventing or provoking violent behavior.

Consistent with prior research [15], our study presents a complex picture of the linkage between violence, social contact, and social support. Respondents living with family were more likely to report engaging in any violent behavior. Female participants, in particular, were more likely than males to live with family—thereby presumably having more opportunities for physical fights with social network members [16]—and indeed, females in this sample were significantly more likely to engage in minor violence than their male counterparts. A subgroup of younger females with substance abuse problems largely accounted for this (unusual) finding, and there was no gender association with serious violence.

This pattern in the data could have been due to a treatment selection effect; whereas males were more likely in general to be selected in this treated sample of schizophrenia patients, it is possible that some females with schizophrenia may not have been identified by the service system until, or unless, they engaged in socially problematic behavior such as minor violence. Moreover, as mentioned, since women with this disease are more likely to be living with family, it may be that family members who become targets of assaultive behavior are instrumental in bringing their mentally ill relative into treatment.

At the same time, family relationships that apparently provided a supportive "audience" were protective. We found that subjects who felt "listened to. . .most of the time" by their family members were only about half as likely to behave violently as subjects who did not report feeling listened to by family.

Our baseline findings regarding substance abuse also warrant comment. The significant bivariate effect of substance abuse on serious violence was rendered non-significant in the final model when controlling for age, PANSS positive symptoms, childhood conduct problems, and recent victimization. This suggests that the effect of substance abuse on serious violence may be mediated by these other covariates.

In the second set of analyses, we developed two separate models of any violence distinguished by the presence or absence of childhood conduct problems. Our evidence suggests that these early problems constitute a particularly salient life-historical variable, which conditions both the magnitude of risk and the specific precipitants of later violent behavior in these patients. We find that a history of childhood conduct problems is significantly associated with adult violence, and also potentiates the effects of alcohol and illicit drug use on violent behavior—even at levels below the diagnostic threshold of substance abuse and dependence disorder. In contrast, we find that positive psychotic symptoms have a stronger connection to violence in schizophrenia patients *without* early conduct problems. And in both groups alike, opportunity factors, such as living at close quarters with family members, may contribute to violence in individuals at risk.

In the third set of analyses, we found that violence was reduced across all treatment groups, declining from a prevalence of 16.3% to 9.3% in the retained sample; and from 19.1% to 14.0% in the intention-to-treat sample. No differences by medication were found, with the exception that perphenazine showed greater reduction in violence than quetiapine in the retained sample only. Medication compliance across all treatment groups was significantly associated with reduced violence, except in patients with a history of childhood conduct problems. Significant prospective predictors of violence included childhood conduct problems, substance use, victimization history, economic deprivation, and social living situation; living with others, rather than alone, increased violence risk. Negative psychotic symptoms predicted lower violence.

These findings provoke new questions about prior research on SGAs and violence, and about the role of medication in managing violence risk in some schizophrenia patients who may be violent for reasons unrelated to psychosis. On the surface, there appear to be inconsistencies between the current results and previous research suggesting an advantage for the SGAs [17]. However, in several ways the studies are not fully comparable. First, some of the previous studies that found an advantage for SGAs over FGAs in reducing violence have included clozapine among the SGAs and haloperidol among the FGAs. Clozapine has the most convincing body of evidence for an anti-aggressive effect, while very high doses of haloperidol have been associated with some poorer outcomes including aggression [18]. Neither of these drugs was included in CATIE Phase 1. Another difference is that naturalistic studies have tended to include more stable patients and have followed them over a longer period of time [17]. Finally, some previous studies have used continuous measures to describe violence [19], whereas we used a dichotomous indicator of the presence or absence of any violence. All of these methodological and design differences may help explain why there are discrepant findings, and may also temper the impulse to discount the older research.

The prospective analysis of violence predictors was generally consistent with the baseline analysis. However, some significant correlates that were identified in the baseline analysis were not found to be significant as prospective predictors. Such differences may be explained by the lack of temporal contiguity between the assessment of risk and the follow-up assessment; for example, patients with psychotic symptoms at baseline may not have had psychotic symptoms after treatment during the follow-up period, which was the period of observation for violence. Differences may also be explained by attrition associated with baseline violence, and the reduction in statistical power resulting from patients who discontinued medication or dropped out of the study by 6 months.

In considering possible anti-aggressive mechanisms for antipsychotic medications, it is important to bear in mind that aggressive behavior may have a number of different causes, and that schizophrenia patients often have heterogeneous symptoms and co-occurring disorders that may increase violence risk. In particular, persistently violent schizophrenia patients with co-occurring antisocial personality or psychopathic features may not become less violent with antipsychotic medication alone. In the current study, the very strong predictive effect of baseline violence on future violence indicates its long-term persistence in some of these patients irrespective of treatment [5]. The fact that compliance with antipsychotic medication did not significantly reduce violent behavior in patients with childhood antisocial history is consistent with the view that much of the violence in these patients is not caused by their psychosis and, thus, is not likely to be reduced by antipsychotic medications. Differences among pharmacological drug effects may be obscured under such conditions.

Understanding the multiple and interacting causes of violence, and the role of anti-psychotic medication in reducing community-based violence, have long challenged researchers and clinicians alike. Findings from this study help to clarify both the import-ance and the inherent limitations of identifying violence risk factors, and then utilizing pharmacotherapy for violence risk management.

As a study of violence, CATIE is important but also limited in several ways. First, participants in CATIE may not be representative of all persons with schizophrenia. The CATIE sample is not a random sample, but a diverse group of treated schizophrenia patients who were willing to enroll in a medication trial. The study excluded first-episode patients (who might have been less violent), and wholly treatment refractory patients (who might have been more violent), and thus the findings cannot generalize to such patients. However, it is worth noting that the study population was shown to resemble a "usual care," quasi-random, observational, non-interventional study sample [3].

The absence of a placebo condition in the design prevents us from examining the effectiveness of antipsychotics compared to no medication, although examining non-compliance provides an uncontrolled finding of an effect for not taking medication as prescribed. A large proportion of the originally enrolled cohort discontinued their prescribed antipsychotic medication, which limits the evidence regarding the potential effectiveness of these drugs. The CATIE study did not selectively recruit patients with a history of serious violence, but rather, violence was one of many outcomes evaluated over the course of the study. For this reason, and because the population base rate of serious violence is very low, we were unable to examine effects of medication for different levels of severity of violence. Finally, we were only able to focus on Phase 1 and the first 6 months of the 18-month CATIE trial as too few patients remained on their assigned Phase 1 medication to allow for a valid longer-term analysis of violence.

In conclusion, contrary to high expectations and some previous research, CATIE did not show an advantage for SGAs in violence risk reduction when compared to perphenazine, among patients remaining on their medication for 6 months. Our violence prediction model suggests that a number of social and environmental factors may relate to violence independently of psychopathology. Therefore, more intensive psychosocial or family-based supportive interventions may be needed to substantially reduce violent behavior. Indeed, for patients with many developmental, social, and environmental risk factors, pharmacotherapy alone cannot be expected to mitigate essentially non-clinical predictors of violence [5]. Still, psychosis can play a central role in violence in some patients with schizophrenia [3], and may become intertwined with additional predictors of violence in other patients [5]. Effective antipsychotic medications are needed, along with psychosocial and supportive interventions to improve treatment adherence and social functioning, in order to effectively reduce violence risk in persons with schizophrenia.

References

1. Mullen PE. Schizophrenia and violence: From correlations to preventive strategies. *Advances in Psychiatric Treatment* 2006;**12**:239–48.

2. Walsh E, Buchanan A and Fahy T. Violence and schizophrenia: Examining the evidence. *British Journal of Psychiatry* 2002;**180**:490–5.

3. Swanson JW, Swartz MS, Van Dorn RA, *et al.* A national study of violent behavior in persons with schizophrenia. *Archives of General Psychiatry* 2006;**63**:490–9.

4. Swanson JW, Swartz MS, Van Dorn RA, *et al.* Comparison of antipsychotic drugs for reducing violence in persons with schizophrenia. *British Journal of Psychiatry* 2008;**193**:37–43.

5. Swanson JW, Van Dorn RA, Swartz MS, Smith A, Elbogen EB and Monahan J. Alternative pathways to violence in persons with schizophrenia: The role of childhood antisocial behavior problems. *Law and Human Behavior* 2008;**32**:228–40.

6. Bjorkly S. Psychotic symptoms and violence toward others – a literature review of some preliminary findings: Part 2. Hallucinations. *Aggression and Violent Behavior* 2002;**7**:605–15.

7. Bjorkly S. Psychotic symptoms and violence toward others – a literature review of some preliminary findings Part 1. Delusions. *Aggression and Violent Behavior* 2002;**7**:617–31.

8. Elbogen EB, Tomkins AJ, Pothuloori A and Scalora MJ. Documentation of violence risk factors in psychiatric facilities: An empirical examination. *Journal of the American Academy of Psychiatry and the Law* 2003;**31**:58–64.

9. Rutter M, Giller H and Hagell A. *Antisocial Behavior by Young People*. New York: Cambridge University Press; 1998.

10. Loeber R and Hay D. Key issues in the development of aggression and violence from childhood to early adulthood. *Annual Review of Psychology* 1997;**48**:371–410.

11. Hodgins S, Tiihonen J and Ross D. The consequences of conduct disorder for males who develop schizophrenia: Associations with criminality, aggressive behavior, substance use, and psychiatric services. *Schizophrenia Research* 2005;**78**:323–35.

12. Steadman HJ, Mulvey EP, Monahan J, *et al.* Violence by people discharged from acute psychiatric inpatient facilities and by others in the same neighborhoods. *Archives of General Psychiatry* 1998;**55**:393–401.

13. Susser M. *Causal Thinking in the Health Sciences: Concepts and Strategies of Epidemiology.* New York: Oxford University Press; 1973.

14. Fleiss JL, Williams JB and Dubro AF. The logistic regression analysis of psychiatric data. *Journal of Psychiatric Research* 1986;**20**:145–209.

15. Estroff S, Zimmer C, Lachicotte W and Benoit J. The influence of social networks and social support on violence by persons with serious mental illness. *Hospital and Community Psychiatry* 1994;**45**:669–79.

16. Swanson J, Swartz M, Estroff S, Borum R, Wagner R and Hiday V. Psychiatric impairment, social contact, and violent behavior: Evidence from a study of outpatient-committed persons with severe mental disorder. *Social Psychiatry and Psychiatric Epidemiology* 1998;**33**: S86–S94.

17. Swanson JW, Swartz MS and Elbogen EB. Effectiveness of atypical antipsychotic medications in reducing violent behavior among persons with schizophrenia in community-based treatment. *Schizophrenia Bulletin* 2004;**30**:3–20.

18. Herrera JN, Sramek JJ, Costa JF, Roy S, Heh CW and Nguyen BN. High potency neuroleptics and violence in schizophrenics. *Journal of Nervous and Mental Disease* 1988;**176**:558–61.

19. Volavka J, Czobor P, Nolan K, *et al.* Overt aggression and psychotic symptoms in patients with schizophrenia treated with clozapine, olanzapine, risperidone, or haloperidol. *Journal of Clinical Psychopharmacology* 2004;**24**:225–8.

Genetic investigations in the CATIE sample

James J. Crowley and Patrick F. Sullivan

Introduction

Rationale for gene hunting in schizophrenia

The rationale for searching for genes for schizophrenia comes from genetic epidemiological studies (family, adoption, and twin studies) [1]. Table 13.1 summarizes this body of work [2,3]. Taken together, these data suggest that genetic effects are the predominant component explaining the tendency of schizophrenia to run in families and thus provide a solid foundation for searches for genetic contributors to schizophrenia. In context, the heritability of schizophrenia is quite high in comparison to many other biomedical disorders. Schizophrenia is known as a "complex trait" in that its inheritance does not conform to a simple mode of inheritance (e.g., autosomal dominant, sex-linked, or mitochondrial). It is critical to note that the results in Table 13.1 are not from experimental studies and do not constitute rigorous proof of the involvement of genetic variation in the etiology of schizophrenia. Moreover, these results do not direct us to the locations of the relevant genomic regions much less describe their function or the mechanism by which schizophrenia might result.

Progress to date in identifying schizophrenia susceptibility genes

Until quite recently, the two major strategies to localize genetic variation for schizophrenia were candidate gene association studies and genomewide linkage studies. The conceptual basis of a candidate gene study is straightforward and entails the comparison of the genotype frequencies for a particular genetic marker in cases with schizophrenia to appropriately matched controls. Candidate gene selection is usually based on hypotheses about etiology and, for schizophrenia, most association studies have focused on the genes encoding proteins involved in some way with the neurotransmitter dopamine.

There have been at least 1,334 studies of 716 candidate genes in schizophrenia (http://www.schizophreniaforum.org/res/sczgene/dbindex.asp [accessed 30 June 2008]) with *COMT* the most intensively studied (73 reports). Despite the tremendous amount of work that has gone into these studies, the candidate gene approach has not yielded replicable associations with schizophrenia that meet a high standard of proof. The performance of the candidate gene approach in schizophrenia research, with no replicable associations, is not dissimilar to results from other complex traits of biomedical importance [4,5].

The conceptual basis of genomewide linkage studies is more complex, and is based on the correlations between genotypes and schizophrenia in families. These studies are based

Antipsychotic Trials in Schizophrenia, ed. T. Scott Stroup and Jeffrey A. Lieberman. Published by Cambridge University Press. © Cambridge University Press 2010.

Table 13.1. Summary of studies of the genetic epidemiology of schizophrenia*

Study Type	Conceptual basis	Studies	Findings
Family	Risk of schizophrenia in 1st degree relatives of cases with schizophrenia vs. controls	11	10/11 studies show familiality of schizophrenia
			Significant familial aggregation of schizophrenia – odds ratio: 9.8 (95% CI 6.2 to 15.5)
Adoption	Risk of schizophrenia in adoption cluster (offspring of one set of parents raised from early in life by unrelated strangers)	5	Effect of post-natal environment negligible
			Adoptees with schizophrenia: increased risk in biological vs. adoptive parents (OR = 5.0; 95% CI 2.4 to 10.4)
			Parents with schizophrenia: increased risk in biological vs. control offspring 3.5 (95% CI = 1.9 to 6.4)
Twin	Risk of schizophrenia in monozygotic vs. dizygotic twins	12	Heritability in liability to schizophrenia: 81% (95% CI = 73 to 90%)
			Environmental effects shared by members of a twin pair: 11% (95% CI = 3 to 19%)

Note: *Table adapted from: Sullivan PF. Schizophrenia genetics: the search for a hard lead. *Curr Opin Psychiatry* 2008;**21**:157–60 [1].

on families usually containing multiple affected individuals. Genetic markers for genome-wide linkage studies (previously ∼500, currently ∼10,000) are selected to be relatively evenly spaced across the genome. These studies are unbiased in that they are not based on prior etiological knowledge but rather can discover new and previously unsuspected knowledge about the locations of genes that might predispose or protect against the development of schizophrenia.

There have been genomewide linkage studies of 31 schizophrenia samples including 6,769 affected individuals. The results of these studies can now be searched and investigated on the web (http://slep.unc.edu [accessed 30 June 2008]) (http://slep.unc.edu [accessed 30 June 2008]). As Table 13.2 shows, these results do not appear to converge—no genomic region was identified by more than a few studies. Moreover, a meta-analysis of schizophrenia genomewide linkage studies was recently updated and showed that genomic regions that previously met genomewide significance were considerably less impressive and no longer exceeded genomewide significance [6].

Comprehensive evaluation of the accumulated work to date is consistent with the following impressions. First, despite considerable effort, genetic variation that predisposes or protects against schizophrenia has not yet been identified with definitive replication.

Table 13.2. Summary of schizophrenia genomewide linkage studies*

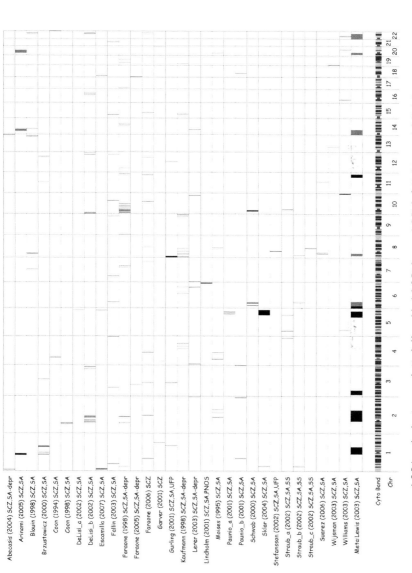

LOD/equivalents are plotted. Key: *black LOD≥3*, *gray LOD≥2*, & *light gray LOD≥1.5*

Note: *Table adapted from: http//slep.unc.edu

Second, evidence for several highly plausible candidate genes, e.g., *NRG1* [7,8], *DTNBP1* [9], or *DISC1* [10], is suggestive but inconclusive and is dissimilar to the pattern of highly consistent and compelling replications found for other complex traits. For example, associations of genetic markers in the *FTO* gene with body mass index were precisely replicated in 13 cohorts of over 38,000 individuals [11]. Finally, it is now clear that sample size requirements for adequate statistical power have almost always been underestimated in prior studies [12].

Genomewide association studies

Since about 2006, technical advances and reduced costs have made it possible to conduct genomewide association studies (GWAS) using large samples. These studies routinely genotype each individual for 300,000–1,000,000 genetic variants, and sample sizes usually exceed 1,000 cases and 1,000 controls. A typical GWAS might contain over a billion genotypes (in contrast, a large genomewide linkage study in the past might have had a million genotypes). Despite considerable skepticism prior to 2007, GWAS have identified strong evidence for ~100 new and previously unknown candidate genes for a variety of biomedical disorders. As an example, there were three candidate genes for type 2 diabetes mellitus (T2DM) identified prior to 2007 and there are now at least 10 with all of the new genes identified by GWAS [13].

There are at least seven ongoing GWAS for schizophrenia with results just beginning to come to light at the time of this writing. Our group used the CATIE sample to complete a GWAS [14] as described in the Results section. Three other small studies have been published [15–17], two of which used DNA pooling to reduce the cost of genotyping, and the remainder are in various stages of completion. Taken together, these studies total over 10,000 cases and 10,000 controls. The major studies include the International Schizophrenia Consortium coordinated by Dr. Pamela Sklar at the MIT/Harvard Broad Institute (~7,000 samples) and the Molecular Genetics of Schizophrenia group coordinated by Dr. Pablo Gejman of Northwestern University (~5,000 samples).

A welcome development that emerged in 2007 was the near-universal willingness of the investigators in the primary studies to participate in early data sharing. Nearly all investigators conducting GWAS of schizophrenia have agreed to participate in the Psychiatric GWAS Consortium (http://pgc.unc.edu), which will conduct integrated meta-analyses of schizophrenia along with ADHD, autism, bipolar disorder, and major depressive disorder. Results of these meta-analyses will be made available to the research community as soon as possible. The combined sample size across all these disorders should exceed 59,000 individuals with GWAS genotyping by early 2010.

It is now clear that GWAS can work in the sense of identifying highly replicable associations for human biomedical disorders of first-rank public health importance. Examples to date include T1DM, T2DM, Crohn's disease, cardiovascular disease, prostate cancer, breast cancer, body mass index, and height. Although the track record of GWAS in human genetics to date is exceptional and impressive, it is still unclear whether it will substantially increase our knowledge of schizophrenia genetics.

The CATIE clinical trial provided an excellent source of DNA samples from patients with schizophrenia for whom a great deal of clinical information was available. Because our group gained access to the CATIE samples shortly before GWAS was a possibility, we will first detail six candidate gene association studies that our group published prior to describing the results of our 2008 GWAS study below.

CATIE samples and reference controls
Cases

All cases were participants in the CATIE project, which was conducted between 1/2001–12/2004. CATIE was a multi-phase randomized controlled trial of antipsychotic medications involving 1,460 persons with schizophrenia followed for up to 18 months [18,19]. The philosophy of the trial was to assess controlled treatment with antipsychotic drugs in a broad range of patients with schizophrenia under "real-world" conditions. To maximize geographic representation, subjects were ascertained from an array of clinical settings across the United States. A total of 1,894 subjects were evaluated, and 1,460 (77.0%) were entered into CATIE. No subject was known to be related to any other subject. The optional genetic sub-study began about a year after the trial began, and 51% of CATIE participants donated a DNA sample.

Table 13.3 provides the descriptive data for the cases with schizophrenia and controls included in all of the genetic studies described in this chapter. Cases and controls were well-matched for age and ancestry but not for sex (due to insufficient numbers of African-American males in the control pool as described in the Methods section). There were large differences between cases and controls in education, marital status, and employment consistent with the adverse effects of a chronic mental illness with onset in early adulthood.

Table 13.3. Descriptive data for cases with schizophrenia and controls included in genetic studies*

Subject descriptor	Cases	Controls	Test
Number of subjects genotyped	738	733	–
Mean age in years (SD)	40.9 (11.1)	41.0 (11.6)	$F_{1,1469} = 0.09, p = 0.77$
Proportion male (N)	0.74 (544)	0.67 (493)	$\chi_1^2 = 7.37, p = 0.007$
Ancestry proportions (inferred from self-report)	0.29 (217)	0.30 (219)	$\chi_2^2 = 0.04, p = 0.98$
African only (N)	0.57 (417)	0.56 (411)	
European only (N)	0.14 (104)	0.14 (103)	
Other (N)			
Proportion with high school degree or more (N)	0.74 (543)	0.93 (684)	$\chi_1^2 = 100, p < 0.0001$
Proportion married (N)	0.11 (78)	0.57 (415)	$\chi_1^2 = 350, p < 0.0001$
Proportion employed (N)	0.06 (43)	0.75 (548)	$\chi_1^2 = 727, p < 0.0001$
Mean years since first antipsychotic prescribed	14.2 (10.8)	–	
Mean PANSS total score	74.0 (17.2)	–	
Mean PANSS positive symptom score	17.8 (5.5)	–	
Mean PANSS negative symptom score	19.9 (6.4)	–	

Note: *Table adapted from: Sullivan PF, Lin D, Tzeng JY, et al. Genomewide association for schizophrenia in the CATIE study: results of stage 1. Mol Psychiatry 2008;13:570–84 [14].

Cases had been ill for a mean of 14 years and the mean Positive and Negative Syndromes Scale (PANSS) scores [20] are consistent with a moderately ill sample. As described previously [21], CATIE subjects who provided DNA samples had lower symptom severity (PANSS total 74 vs. 77), less current drug/alcohol abuse/dependence (29% vs. 36%), and were less likely to describe themselves as African-American (29% vs. 40%) in comparison to CATIE subjects who did not provide a DNA sample.

Preliminary diagnoses were established by referring psychiatrists, and final study diagnoses of DSM-IV schizophrenia [22] were independently established by CATIE personnel using the Structured Clinical Interview for DSM-IV (SCID) [23] including review of all available information (including psychiatric and general medical records) along with one or more subject interviews. Interviewers were experienced Master's-level clinicians who were trained to criterion via a standard protocol [23]. Any diagnostic uncertainties were resolved via discussion with one of the CATIE senior clinicians. Study inclusion and exclusion criteria are described in detail in Chapter 1.

Controls

Controls were ascertained from a US national sampling frame as part of the NIMH Genetics repository (MH059571, PI Dr. Pablo Gejman, release v4.0, 6/2006). Controls were collected by Knowledge Networks (KN), a survey and market research company whose panel contains approximately 60,000 households (>120,000 unrelated adults). Households were selected via random digit dialing and proportionally from 25 major US population areas, and financial incentives were provided for participation. The KN panel is generally representative of the US population but with a slight bias toward higher income and education. To be eligible for matching to cases, we required that potential controls deny any history of schizophrenia, schizoaffective disorder, bipolar disorder, auditory hallucinations, and delusional beliefs. These controls are being used for multiple additional GWAS, and meta analysts need to use caution when combining results or data across studies that use these common controls.

There were 3,487 individuals in v4.0 of the control dataset and 2,645 controls were eligible for matching to CATIE cases; 842 individuals were removed from consideration due to at least one of the following: a self-reported possible history of a psychotic disorder (schizophrenia, schizoaffective disorder, bipolar disorder, delusional disorder, or auditory hallucinations), age < 18 or age > 67, lack of documentation of informed consent, or missing data for a matching variable (age, sex, or self-reported race). Cases were group-matched to controls by 5-year age band, sex, and self-reported race. Most cases (91.4%) were successfully matched to controls. The exception was for 66 cases (8.6%) that could not be matched due to a deficiency of African-American males aged 18–38 years in v4.0 of the control cohort. Rather than eliminate cases, African-American females in this age band were selected as controls.

Results
Candidate gene studies
In this section, we use the familiar format of a research abstract to summarize the results of the candidate gene studies we conducted using genetic samples from CATIE participants.

1. NCAM1 and neurocognition in schizophrenia [21]. OBJECTIVE: Alterations in neurocognition may be fundamental to schizophrenia and may be endophenotypes. Neural cell adhesion molecule 1 (*NCAM1*, aliases NCAM and CD56) may be a candidate gene for schizophrenia or for neurocognition in schizophrenia as supported by linkage and functional findings. METHODS: Subjects were 641 patients with schizophrenia who participated in the Clinical Antipsychotic Trials of Intervention Effectiveness (CATIE) clinical trial. Neurocognition was assessed at study baseline. Nine *NCAM1* single nucleotide polymorphisms (SNPs) were blindly genotyped. Analysis of covariance was used to test for single SNP associations and haplotype regression for multilocus associations. RESULTS: As there were suggestions of population stratification, all analyses were conducted stratified by inferred ancestry. In the "Europe only" stratum, there were nominally significant associations with five contiguous SNPs (rs1943620, rs1836796, rs1821693, rs686050, rs584427) with the strongest association at rs1836796 ($p = 0.007$). Via permutation testing, the probability of obtaining five consecutive statistically significant SNPs with p values $< = 0.05$ was $p = 0.0044$. These results were robust to examination of model assumptions. Haplotype analyses did not identify significant haplotype associations. CONCLUSIONS: Although it is essential to see if these findings replicate in additional samples, we suggest that *NCAM1* deserves further scrutiny for its relevance to clinical and etiological aspects of schizophrenia.

2. An SNP near INSIG2 (rs7566605) is not associated with body mass in CATIE [24]. OBJECTIVE: In a *Science* paper, Herbert *et al.* [25] provided compelling data supporting the association of the single nucleotide polymorphism (SNP) rs7566605 with body mass index (BMI) and obesity. The rs7566605 SNP was identified in an initial genomewide association screen and subsequently replicated in five of six samples (meta-analytic odds ratio with obesity 1.22, 95% confidence interval [CI] 1.05–1.42, $p = 0.008$ under a recessive model) [25]. METHODS: Using baseline and longitudinal data from the CATIE randomized clinical trial of schizophrenia, we first investigated whether rs7566605 was associated with BMI, and second, given the paucity of genotyping in the region of this SNP in the original report, whether other SNPs in the same haplotype block were associated. RESULTS: First, we did not replicate the association of rs7566605 with baseline BMI or for BMI change across all CATIE Phase 1/1A treatments under recessive and general association models. We observed a non-significant statistical trend similar in magnitude to that reported by Herbert *et al.* for a recessive model at rs7566605 (in subjects of European ancestry, mean BMI (SD) was 31.9 (0.94) for the CC genotype vs. 30.8 (0.43) for combined CG/GG genotypes). Second, rs7566605 lies in an apparently intergenic approximately 31.7-kb haplotype block; as Herbert *et al.* conducted limited genotyping in this region, we genotyped 10 additional tSNPs in the vicinity of rs7566605. There were no significant associations of these SNPs with BMI at CATIE baseline or longitudinally across CATIE Phase 1/1A. CONCLUSIONS: We were unable to replicate the reported association of rs7566605 with BMI. Explanations for our negative findings include the possibility that the initial report was false and that statistical power was insufficient. Alternatively, the nature of obesity may be different in individuals with schizophrenia than in more typical samples like those studied by Herbert *et al*—the association with rs7566605 with BMI may be true but the profoundly life-altering and obesogenic effects of schizophrenia and/or antipsychotic treatment may overwhelm any effect of rs7566605.

3. AKT1 and neurocognition in schizophrenia [26]. OBJECTIVE: Previous research has shown conflicting results for the significance of five v-akt murine thymoma viral oncogene homolog 1 (*AKT1*) single-nucleotide polymorphisms (SNPs) to the etiology of schizophrenia. Neurocognition is a plausible endophenotype for schizophrenia, and it was reasoned that the lack of agreement might be due to variability in neurocognition across studies. Therefore, the association of genetic variation in AKT1 with neurocognition was investigated in patients with schizophrenia. METHODS: The same five SNPs used in previous studies of the etiology of schizophrenia (rs2494732, rs2498799, rs3730358, rs1130241, and rs3803300) were genotyped in 641 individuals with schizophrenia who had participated in the Clinical Antipsychotic Trials of Intervention Effectiveness (CATIE) project. The primary dependent variable was a neurocognitive composite score and exploratory analyses investigated five domain scores (processing speed, reasoning, verbal memory, working memory, and vigilance). RESULTS: There were no significant asymptotic or empirical associations between any SNP and the neurocognitive composite score. The authors also investigated the association of five-SNP haplotypes with the neurocognitive composite score. A marginally significant association was observed for the neurocognitive composite score with one of the five-SNP haplotypes (global score statistic, 19.51; df $= 9$; permutation $p = 0.02$). Exploratory analyses of five domain scores (processing speed, reasoning, verbal memory, working memory, and vigilance) were non-significant for all five SNPs. CONCLUSION: Results published to date for an association between genetic variation in *AKT1* with schizophrenia are inconsistent. The results suggest that the *AKT1* markers studied are not associated with neurocognition in schizophrenia, and do not support unassessed variation in neurocognitive scores as a reason for this discrepancy.

4. Ethnic stratification of the association of RGS4 variants with antipsychotic treatment response in schizophrenia [27]. BACKGROUND: Genetic association studies, including a large meta-analysis, report association of regulator of G protein signaling 4 (*RGS4*) with schizophrenia in the context of heterogeneity. The central role of *RGS4* in regulating signaling via Gi/o coupled neurotransmitter receptors led us to hypothesize that there may be *RGS4* genotypes predictive of specific disease phenotypes and antipsychotic treatment responses. METHODS: Subjects were 678 individuals with schizophrenia who participated in the Clinical Antipsychotic Trials of Intervention Effectiveness (CATIE). Among the 678 subjects, the inferred ancestries were 198 (29%) "Africa only," 397 (59%) "Europe only," and 83 (12%) "Other." Eight single nucleotide polymorphisms (SNPs) spanning RGS4 were genotyped. Multiple linear regression was used to analyze association of *RGS4* markers with Positive and Negative Symptoms Scale (PANSS) scores at baseline and throughout antipsychotic treatment. RESULTS: Two consecutive markers within *RGS4*, rs2661319 and rs2842030, were associated with more severe baseline PANSS total score. Treatment with perphenazine was more effective than treatment with quetiapine ($p = 0.010$) or ziprasidone ($p = 0.002$) in individuals of inferred African ancestry and homozygous for the rs951439 C allele. CONCLUSIONS: *RGS4* genotypes predicted both the severity of baseline symptoms and relative responsiveness to antipsychotic treatment. Although these analyses are exploratory and replication is required, these data provide support for *RGS4* in schizophrenia pathogenesis and suggest a functional role for *RGS4* in differential antipsychotic treatment efficacy of schizophrenia.

5. Association of RGS2 and RGS5 variants with schizophrenia symptom severity [28]. BACKGROUND: Several lines of evidence indicate that Regulator of G Protein Signaling 4 (*RGS4*) contributes to schizophrenia vulnerability. *RGS4* is one of a family of molecules that modulate signaling via G-protein coupled receptors. Five genes encoding members of this family (*RGS2, RGS4, RGS5, RGS8* and *RGS16*) map to chromosome 1q23.3–1q31. Due to overlapping cellular functions and chromosomal proximity, we hypothesized that multiple RGS genes may contribute to schizophrenia severity and treatment responsiveness.

METHODS: Subjects were 750 individuals with schizophrenia who participated in the Clinical Antipsychotic Trials of Intervention Effectiveness (CATIE). Inferred ancestries were: 221 (30%) "Africa only," 422 (56%) "Europe only," and 107 (14%) "Other." Fifty-nine single nucleotide polymorphisms (SNPs) in or near the *RGS5, RGS16, RGS8* and *RGS2* genes were genotyped. Multiple linear regression was used to analyze association of markers with Positive and Negative Symptoms Scale (PANSS) total scores at baseline and throughout antipsychotic treatment. RESULTS: *RGS5* marker rs10799902 was associated with altered baseline PANSS total score in both the Africa only ($p = 0.0440$) and Europe only ($p = 0.0143$) strata, although neither association survived multiple comparisons correction. A common five-marker haplotype of the *RGS2* gene was associated with more severe baseline PANSS total score in the Europe only strata (global $p = 0.0254$; haplotype-specific $p = 0.0196$). In contrast to *RGS4*, none of the markers showed association with antipsychotic treatment response. CONCLUSIONS: RGS2 and RGS5 genotypes predicted severity of baseline symptoms in schizophrenia. Although these analyses are exploratory and replication is required, these data suggest a possible role for multiple RGS proteins in schizophrenia.

6. *The neuregulin 1 promoter polymorphism rs6994992 is not associated with chronic schizophrenia or neurocognition* [29]. BACKGROUND: The neuregulin 1 (*NRG1*) promoter single nucleotide polymorphism (SNP) rs6994992 has shown association with decreased activation of frontal and temporal lobe regions, increased risk of psychosis, and decreased pre-morbid IQ [30]. This SNP is part of a putative schizophrenia risk-associated haplotype and was associated with increased expression of the type IV transcript in postmortem tissue [31]. METHODS: We tested for association between rs6994992 and chronic schizophrenia by genotyping 738 cases from the Clinical Antipsychotic Trials of Intervention Effectiveness (CATIE) and 733 matched controls. We further tested for associations with age at onset and baseline neurocognition in cases with schizophrenia, reasoning that these phenotypes might yield results similar to those seen for pre-morbid IQ. RESULTS: Affection status was weakly associated with rs6994992 genotypes and trended toward association under a recessive model. This association did not survive correction for multiple comparisons and was in the opposite direction than has been reported. There was no association between rs6994992 and age at onset, an estimate of pre-morbid IQ, or neurocognition at study baseline. CONCLUSIONS: We were unable to replicate previous associations of rs6994992 with schizophrenia and, moreover, did not find significant associations with age of onset, an estimate of pre-morbid IQ, or neurocognition.

7. *Genetic determinants of variable metabolism have little impact on the clinical use of leading antipsychotics in the CATIE study* [32]. PURPOSE: To evaluate systematically in real clinical settings whether functional genetic variations in drug metabolizing enzymes influence optimized doses, efficacy, and safety of antipsychotic medications. METHODS: DNA was collected from 750 patients with chronic schizophrenia treated with five antipsychotic drugs (olanzapine, quetiapine, risperidone, ziprasidone, and perphenazine) as part of the Clinical Antipsychotic Trials of Intervention Effectiveness (CATIE) study. Doses for each of the medicines were optimized to 1, 2, 3, or 4x units in identically appearing capsules in a double blind design. We analyzed 25 known functional genetic variants in the major and minor metabolizing enzymes for each medication. These variants were tested for association with optimized dose and other relevant clinical outcomes. RESULTS: None of the tested variants showed a nominally significant main effect in association with any of the tested phenotypes in European-Americans, African-Americans, or all patients. Even after

accounting for potential covariates, no genetic variant was found to be associated with dosing, efficacy, overall tolerability, or tardive dyskinesia. CONCLUSION: There are no strong associations between common functional genetic variants in drug metabolizing enzymes and dosing, safety, or efficacy of leading antipsychotics, strongly suggesting merely modest effects on the use of these medicines in most patients in typical clinical settings.

Genomewide association studies

Background

In 2006, academic investigators from the NIMH-funded Clinical Antipsychotic Trials of Intervention Effectiveness project (CATIE) [19] entered into a scientific collaboration with Eli Lilly and Company to conduct individual GWAS genotyping and joint analyses on the CATIE samples. The collaboration contract required that genotype and phenotype data be made available to the scientific community with intellectual property rights consistent with NIH policies intended to maximize the public benefit resulting from the research. The genotype and phenotype data reported here were deposited with the controlled-access repository of the NIMH in June 2007 (http://www.nimhgenetics.org [accessed 28 June 2007]). Our 2008 publication [14] reported the primary analyses aimed at identifying SNPs associated with susceptibility to schizophrenia using 492,900 SNPs that were genotyped in 738 participants with schizophrenia and 733 group-matched controls from a United States population based sample.

For a complete description of the methods and quality control procedures used, please see the primary publication [14]. Briefly, peripheral venous blood samples were sent to Rutgers University Cell and DNA Repository (RUCDR) where cell lines were established via Epstein–Barr virus transformation. Individual genotyping was conducted by Perlegen Sciences (Mountain View, CA, USA) using three genotyping chips: Affymetrix 500K "A" chipset (Nsp I and Sty I chips; Santa Clara, CA, USA) and a custom 164K chip created by Perlegen to provide additional genome coverage. There were 500,568 SNPs on the Affymetrix 500K chips and 164,871 on the Perlegen custom chip (665,439 SNPs in total). Of these, 157,048 SNPs failed Perlegen's quality control (20.2% of the Affymetrix 500K and 33.9% of the Perlegen 164K SNPs). We used principal components to robustly control for stratification effects while preserving statistical power, using EigenSoft (http://www.genepath. med.harvard.edu/~reich/Software.htm, v1.0).

Results

We used logistic regression to test for association of the 492,900 SNPs in the GWAS data set with case/control status (with seven principal components [33] included as covariates to account for population stratification). The minimum p value obtained was 1.71×10^{-6}. There were 26,738 p values < 0.05: 6 p values in the 10^{-6} bin, 42 in the 10^{-5} bin, 486 in the 10^{-4} bin, 4,845 in the 10^{-3} bin, and 21,359 in the interval (0.01–0.05). The GWAS results are depicted in Figure 13.1. Panel A shows the QQ plot [34] for GWAS for case-control status. The QQ plot suggests that the observed p values do not strongly depart from the p value distribution expected by chance. Panel B shows the $-\log_{10}(p)$ for the 26,738 p values < 0.05 (5.425%) in the context of the human genome in order to make spatial clustering evident. For a false discovery rate threshold of 0.10, the proportion of all SNPs without true effects (p_0) can be estimated from the GWAS results and was found to be $p_0 = 0.9999904$. This result is consistent with the presence of ~5 SNPs with true effects in these GWAS data for

(a)

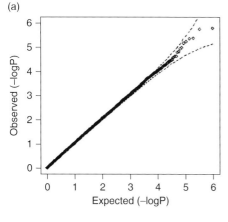

(b)

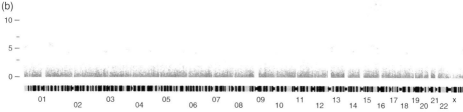

Figure 13.1. Results of single-marker association tests of case–control status for 492,900 SNPs. (a) Shows the QQ plot of the observed p values, $-\log10(P)$, versus those expected by chance, $-\log10(i/L + 1)$, where P is the asymptotic p value from the additive test that the SNP coefficient is 0, i is the rank for each SNP p value (1 = smallest, L = largest), and L is the number of SNPs. The dashed lines show the expected 95% probability interval for ordered p values. (b) Depicts $-\log10(P)$ by genomic location. The top 25 SNPs are indicated in green (online only).

schizophrenia. The q values were calculated for all p values under the conservative assumption that $p_0 = 1$, and no SNPs reached genomewide significance as the minimum q values of 0.45 (rs10911902 and rs16977195) did not exceed the pre-specified FDR threshold of 0.10.

Additional data about the SNPs with the 25 smallest p values are shown in Table 13.4. Most of the top 25 findings were not located within the transcript of a known gene and, for the 11 genes listed in Table 13.4, searches of PubMed and SZGene identified no published studies of schizophrenia, although prior linkage studies implicated these genomic regions. Of note, two pairs of SNPs in the top 25 were located near one another and 2 additional SNPs clustered with over 10 SNPs that were nominally significant and in relatively close proximity. Finally, Table 13.4 also presents SNP annotations: 2 SNPs were in copy number variant regions, 1 SNP was modestly conserved, 1 SNP was in a predicted transfactor binding site, and 17 of the top 25 SNPs were predicted to be in regions with regulatory potential.

We focused more closely on a consensus set of 15 candidate genes for schizophrenia with the best evidence of association—12 candidate genes were selected from a review [3], *CSF2RA* and *IL3RA* were from a published schizophrenia GWAS [15], and *PLXNA2* was from a large-scale candidate gene study for schizophrenia [35]. Of the 249 genes with one or more p values < 0.001 in this GWAS, only 1 was on this list of 15 candidate genes (*NRG1*). Although the GWAS platform we used had generally good coverage across the genome

247

Table 13.4. Top 25 results from GWAS for schizophrenia in the CATIE study*†

SNP data			Gene data	Logistic regression tests for association					Comments‡	SNP annotations			
SNP ID	Chr	Position	Transcripts in which SNP located	Odds ratio	p value	Rank	AFR odds ratio	EUR odds ratio		CNV	Conserved	Reg potential	TFBS
rs4846033	1	11,722,830		0.348	4.36E-06	3	0.401	0.146	1	No	No	Yes	No
rs10911902	1	183,363,974		0.560	1.85E-06	2	0.627	0.523		No	No	Yes	Yes
rs9309325	2	60,492,482		0.727	4.58E-05	22	0.704	0.770		Yes	Yes	Yes	No
rs1569351	3	60,287,457	FHIT	0.697	2.39E-05	1	0.609	0.729		Yes	No	Yes	No
rs4568102	3	72,070,679		4.118	4.08E-05	19	4.947	0.663	1, 2	No	No	Yes	No
rs1380272	4	21,431,975	KCNIP4	0.522	1.10E-05	7	0.425	0.610	6	No	No	Yes	No
rs1495716	4	177,103,725	GPM6A	1.423	2.41E-05	12	1.915	1.277		No	No	No	No
rs9295938	6	31,061,084	C6orf205	1.642	3.51E-05	16	1.288	1.769		No	No	No	No
rs9400690	6	114,453,545		1.534	5.08E-05	24	1.588	1.635		No	No	No	No
rs16917897	10	52,856,709	D45864 PRKG1 Y07512 BC062688	2.750	4.55E-05	21	2.864	1.650	1, 6	No	No	Yes	No
rs297257	10	127,298,704		0.689	3.64E-05	17	0.727	0.705		No	No	Yes	No
rs9512730	13	26,975,144		1.515	4.52E-06	4	1.724	1.385		No	No	No	No
rs942348	13	26,976,147		0.718	2.74E-05	14	1.641	1.399		No	No	Yes	No
rs17070578	13	78,431,983		1.903	4.72E-05	23	1.560	1.589	6	No	No	No	No
rs17095545	14	58,555,364		1.648	2.62E-05	13	1.501	1.746		No	No	No	No
rs7144633	14	58,582,146		1.784	1.64E-05	10	1.246	1.987		No	No	No	No

rs16977195	15	84,785,244	AGBL1	6.005	1.71E-06	1	2.028	6.801	1	No	No	No	Yes	No
rs234993	16	20,555,145	ACSM1 BUCS1	0.524	5.44E-05	25	0.263	0.596		No	No	No	Yes	No
rs151222	16	20,581,993	ACSM1 BUCS1	0.477	6.08E-06	5	0.310	0.549		No	No	No	No	No
rs17455133	18	49,719,513		0.643	3.44E-05	15	0.357	0.713		No	No	No	Yes	No
rs2824301	21	17,738,145		0.720	4.09E-05	20	1.917	1.386		No	No	No	Yes	No
rs10521865	X	146,501,918		0.550	3.70E-05	18	0.809	0.304	1, 3, 4, 6	No	No	No	Yes	No
rs2159767	X	147,086,567		0.752	6.94E-06	6	0.288	0.753	5	No	No	No	Yes	No
rs2536589	X	147,099,127		0.757	1.21E-05	8	0.285	0.762	5	No	No	No	Yes	No
rs952515	X	147,142,998		0.759	1.56E-05	9	0.337	0.711	5	No	No	No	Yes	No

Notes: *Table adapted from: Sullivan PF, Lin D, Tzeng JY, et al. Genomewide association for schizophrenia in the CATIE study: results of stage 1. *Mol Psychiatry* 2008;**13**:570–84 [14].

†All allele frequency data were standardized to the same reference alleles. Yellow boxes highlight issues of concern.

Although SNPs with overall MAF < 0.01 were dropped in the QC process, subgroups may have MAF < 0.01.

Some MAF > 0.5 as the reference allele may be different in subgroups.

EUR = European ancestry; AFR = African ancestry;

‡1 = rare allele; 2 = direction of effects different in AFR and EUR subgroups; 3 = low mean SNP quality scores; 4 = greater SNP missing in cases than controls; 5 = frequency difference of >10% versus HapMap; 6 = suboptimal clustering of genotype groups on manual inspection of scatterplots.

(1 SNP/6.2 kb on average), 6 of these 15 genes had inadequate coverage and 9 genes had SNP densities better than the GWAS average (2.2–5.0 SNPs/kb). For this subset of the GWAS data, the proportion of SNPs without true effects (p_0) was estimated at 0.997 for an FDR threshold of 0.10 and the minimum q value was 0.30. In comparison to all GWAS SNPs, these results suggest that these candidate regions may be enriched for genetic variants influencing susceptibility to schizophrenia.

Although no SNPs in the set of 15 candidate genes for schizophrenia survived FDR multiple comparison correction, we investigated a few of these results further. Of the 146 SNPs in the vicinity of *DISC1* (minimum p value 0.001), the significant findings clustered around the chr1 (1;11)(q42;q14.3) translocation break point [10]. These data are not conclusive, but the locations of the significant *DISC1* SNPs coincide very closely with the *DISC1* breakpoint [10] and the HEP1 haplotype implicated in the etiology of schizophrenia [36] and reduced prefrontal cortex gray matter density [37]. Of the 401 SNPs in the vicinity of *NRG1* (minimum p value 0.0009), there were 15 SNPs (6 with $p < 0.05$ including the most significant *NRG1* SNP, rs16879809) in a cluster at the 3' end of *NRG1*. This cluster was 875 kb from the 5' portion of NRG1 that has been of particular interest [8,30,31]. Three of 53 SNPs in the "HapIce" haplotype [8] had p values between 0.01 and 0.05. The SNP rs6994992 [30,31] was not genotyped in this GWAS but had been done in these samples previously: rs6994992 was weakly associated with schizophrenia but in the opposite direction than has been reported [29]. Of the 13 SNPs in the vicinity of *COMT*, 2 consecutive exonic SNPs 1 kb apart both had $p = 0.02$. These were rs4633 (synonymous) and rs4680 (val158met), which has been widely studied as a genetic risk factor for schizophrenia and other disorders [38]. Finally, of the 84 SNPs in the vicinity of *PLXNA2*, the significant SNPs were 80 kb away from those highlighted in the initial report [35] and whose most notable SNP (rs752016) was not significant in this GWAS ($p = 0.90$). It is important to stress that none of these findings met genomewide significance and the overlap with prior studies could have been merely due to chance.

Conclusions and future directions

The CATIE GWAS had multiple notable features. It was the second published GWAS for schizophrenia, and the first for which all individual genotype and phenotype data were made freely available to the research community. In addition, this project was conceptualized from the beginning as a two-stage study with the present report constituting the first stage. As anticipated, there are no definitive findings that meet genomewide significance; however, it is very possible that there exist true findings in these results that may not be impressive in any single study but that only emerge by comparing multiple large GWAS. It is hoped that the process of gene-finding for schizophrenia will mirror that of type 2 diabetes mellitus (T2DM). In 2006, three genes had accumulated strong evidence in support of association; after the publication of six T2DM GWAS in 2007, there are now eight (and perhaps as many as 11) genes with highly compelling support [13]. Notably, several of the initial T2DM GWAS had QQ plots very similar to that in Figure 13.1a, and only after data sharing across studies and additional genotyping in thousands of additional samples did multiple high confidence findings emerge [13]. Indeed, some of the findings that eventually proved to be highly significant had p values in the first study that were not even in the top 1,000 strongest p values.

Therefore, these data from the CATIE GWAS will be part of an inclusive meta-analysis of individual phenotype and genotype data from all available schizophrenia GWAS that was be finished at the end of 2008 under the auspices of the Psychiatric GWAS Consortium (http://pgc.unc.edu). There are currently over 10,000 cases and 13,000 controls available for meta-analysis—particularly large-scale projects include the GAIN schizophrenia samples [39] and a consortium led by Dr. Pamela Sklar at the Broad Institute. Members of the consortium will soon conduct large-scale Stage 2 genotyping to confirm and refine results from the schizophrenia meta-analysis. The CATIE samples are being used for deep re-sequencing of candidate genes under an award from the Medical Re-sequencing/Allelic Spectrum project supported by the NHGRI and can be used to discover variants not previously identified.

Additional notable features of this project include that, at the time genotyping was conducted, the GWAS platform used here had the best genomic coverage for common genomic variation with $r^2 \geq 0.8$ for 86% of the genome in subjects with European ancestry, 79% for East Asian ancestry, and 49% for African ancestry [40]. The CATIE sample was ascertained from diverse sites across the continental United States in order to accrue a "real-world" sample of patients in treatment for chronic schizophrenia and a rich set of phenotypes are available for all CATIE subjects, i.e., treatment response in a randomized, double-blind clinical trial, multiple assessments of tardive dyskinesia, and repeated assessments of neurocognition.

The principal finding of the CATIE GWAS was that no SNP or multi-marker combination of SNPs achieved genomewide significance. Moreover, there was no important overlap of our findings with those from published GWAS for schizophrenia [15–17] or bipolar disorder [41]. However, some findings with uncorrected p values < 0.05 overlapped with regions of *DISC1* and *COMT* that have been highlighted in prior studies. Of the 146 SNPs in the vicinity of *DISC1* (minimum genewise p value 0.001), the significant findings clustered around the chr1 translocation break point [10] and the HEP1 haplotype implicated in the etiology of schizophrenia [36] and associated with reduced prefrontal cortex gray matter density [37]. Whether the observed overlap is merely due to chance [42] or reflects genetic influences on liability to schizophrenia will require the meta-analyses described above.

In general, there are three explanations for the pattern of findings outlined above. The first is that this sample was underpowered to identify strong, true findings and that these data will first need to be combined with other data sets before definitive loci are found. This is also perhaps the most likely explanation when one considers the fact that most of the strong GWAS hits from other fields of biomedicine required data sharing. The sample size of 738 schizophrenia cases and 733 group-matched controls and a genomewide set of 492,900 SNPs provided the capacity to detect genetic effects of moderate size for reasonably common polymorphisms (i.e., minor allele frequencies exceeding 10%). True genetic effects influencing case-control status might not have been detected in this study for reasons predictable from the design of this study. Non-detection could have occurred if the genotypic effect size was below the detection threshold, if the effect was located in a genomic region for which there was poor SNP coverage, if the effect was a genetic variant other than an SNP (e.g., a copy number variant) and if there was low LD with genotyped SNPs, or in the presence of excessive phenotypic or locus heterogeneity. Additionally, it is possible that the heterogeneous nature of this sample acted to obscure true positive findings by the use of principal components analysis, particularly for SNPs in strongly stratified genomic regions.

The second possibility is that there are true genetic effects for schizophrenia but assumptions fundamental to GWAS are incorrect. It is possible that current definitions of schizophrenia lack validity. If true, attempting to identify genetic variants associated with "caseness" in a GWAS may prove fruitless as case classifications based on signs and symptoms are poorly correlated with genetic etiological factors. It is possible that the fundamental model is incorrect—GWAS are predicated under the common disease/common variant model whereby prevalent human diseases are caused by polymorphisms of relatively modest effects. If schizophrenia is caused by multiple rare variants (causation due to multiple quite uncommon genetic variants of very strong effect) [43], then the GWAS design is inappropriate to the fundamental genetic phenomenon. It is possible that liability to schizophrenia is mostly or entirely due to interactions between genomic regions or between genomic regions and environmental factors and that these must be explicitly modeled in order to be detected. Each of these instances provides an explanation why true effects were not detected.

Finally, the least optimistic possibility is that there exists no true genetic effects causal to schizophrenia. This seems highly unlikely in the face of convincing indirect evidence from family, adoption, and twin studies and a sizeable body of genetic epidemiological data. However, data from small experimental studies do not constitute proof of the involvement of specific genetic variants in the etiopathology of schizophrenia.

It is likely that meta-analyses will help determine which of these three possibilities were dominant in this study. Therefore, these analyses have been interpreted with caution and the individual phenotype and genotype data made available to the scientific community. There is an urgent need for greater knowledge of schizophrenia genetics, as replicable findings have ramifications for diagnosis, guided therapy, and drug development. We believe these data from the CATIE trial will help to usher in a new era in the knowledge of schizophrenia etiology.

References

1. Sullivan PF. Schizophrenia genetics: The search for a hard lead. *Current Opinion in Psychiatry* 2008;**21**:157–60.

2. Sullivan PF, Kendler KS and Neale MC. Schizophrenia as a complex trait: Evidence from a meta-analysis of twin studies. *Archives of General Psychiatry* 2003;**60**:1187–92.

3. Sullivan PF. The genetics of schizophrenia. *PLoS Medicine* 2005;**2**:e212.

4. Lohmueller KE, Pearce CL, Pike M, Lander ES and Hirschhorn JN. Meta-analysis of genetic association studies supports a contribution of common variants to susceptibility to common disease. *Nature Genetics* 2003;**33**:177–82.

5. Ioannidis JP. Commentary: Grading the credibility of molecular evidence for complex diseases. *International Journal of Epidemiology* 2006;**35**:572–8; discussion 593–6.

6. Lewis CM, Levinson DF, Wise LH, *et al.* Genome scan meta-analysis of schizophrenia and bipolar disorder. II: Schizophrenia. *American Journal of Human Genetics* 2003;**73**:34–48.

7. Li D, Collier DA and He L. Meta-analysis shows strong positive association of the neuregulin 1 (NRG1) gene with schizophrenia. *Human Molecular Genetics* 2006;**15**:1995–2002.

8. Stefansson H, Sigurdsson E, Steinthorsdottir V, *et al.* Neuregulin 1 and susceptibility to schizophrenia. *American Journal of Human Genetics* 2002;**71**:877–92.

9. Straub RE, Jiang Y, MacLean CJ, *et al.* Genetic variation in the 6p22.3 gene DTNBP1, the human ortholog of the mouse dysbindin gene, is associated with

schizophrenia. *American Journal of Human Genetics* 2002;**71**:337–48.

10. Millar JK, Wilson-Annan JC, Anderson S, *et al.* Disruption of two novel genes by a translocation co-segregating with schizophrenia. *Human Molecular Genetics* 2000;**9**:1415–23.

11. Frayling TM, Timpson NJ, Weedon MN, *et al.* A common variant in the FTO gene is associated with body mass index and predisposes to childhood and adult obesity. *Science* 2007;**316**:889–94.

12. Risch N and Merikangas K. The future of genetic studies of complex human diseases. *Science* 1996;**273**:1516–7.

13. Frayling TM. Genome-wide association studies provide new insights into type 2 diabetes aetiology. Nature Reviews. *Genetics* 2007;**8**:657–62.

14. Sullivan PF, Lin D, Tzeng JY, *et al.* Genomewide association for schizophrenia in the CATIE study: Results of stage 1. *Molecular Psychiatry* 2008;**13**:570–84.

15. Lencz T, Morgan TV, Athanasiou M, *et al.* Converging evidence for a pseudoautosomal cytokine receptor gene locus in schizophrenia. *Molecular Psychiatry* 2007;**12**:572–80.

16. Kirov G, Zaharieva I, Georgieva L, *et al.* A genome-wide association study in 574 schizophrenia trios using DNA pooling. *Molecular Psychiatry* 2009;**14**:796–803.

17. Shifman S, Johannesson M, Bronstein M, *et al.* Genome-wide association identifies a common variant in the reelin gene that increases the risk of schizophrenia only in women. *PLoS Genetics* 2008;**4**:e28.

18. Stroup TS, McEvoy JP, Swartz MS, *et al.* The National Institute of Mental Health Clinical Antipsychotic Trials of Intervention Effectiveness (CATIE) project: Schizophrenia trial design and protocol development. *Schizophrenia Bulletin* 2003;**29**:15–31.

19. Lieberman JA, Stroup TS, McEvoy JP, *et al.* Effectiveness of antipsychotic drugs in patients with chronic schizophrenia. *New England Journal of Medicine* 2005;**353**:1209–23.

20. Kay SR, Fiszbein A and Opler LA. The positive and negative syndrome scale (PANSS) for schizophrenia. *Schizophrenia Bulletin* 1987;**13**:261–76.

21. Sullivan PF, Keefe RS, Lange LA, *et al.* NCAM1 and neurocognition in schizophrenia. *Biological Psychiatry* 2007;**61**:902–10.

22. American Psychiatric Association. *Diagnostic and Statistical Manual of Mental Disorders.* 4th ed. Washington, DC: American Psychiatric Association; 1994.

23. First MB, Spitzer RL, Gibbon M and Williams JBW. *Structured Clinical Interview for DSM-IV Axis I Disorders–Administration Booklet.* Washington DC: American Psychiatric Press Inc; 1994.

24. Skelly T, Pinheiro AP, Lange LA and Sullivan PF. Is rs7566605, a SNP near INSIG2, associated with body mass in a randomized clinical trial of antipsychotics in schizophrenia? *Molecular Psychiatry* 2007;**12**:321–2.

25. Herbert A, Gerry NP, McQueen MB, *et al.* A common genetic variant is associated with adult and childhood obesity. *Science* 2006;**312**:279–83.

26. Pinheiro AP, Keefe RS, Skelly T, *et al.* AKT1 and neurocognition in schizophrenia. *The Australian and New Zealand Journal of Psychiatry* 2007;**41**:169–77.

27. Campbell DB, Ebert PJ, Skelly T, *et al.* Ethnic stratification of the association of RGS4 variants with antipsychotic treatment response in schizophrenia. *Biological Psychiatry* 2008;**63**:32–41.

28. Campbell DB, Lange LA, Skelly T, Lieberman J, Levitt P and Sullivan PF. Association of RGS2 and RGS5 variants with schizophrenia symptom severity. *Schizophrenia Research* 2008;**101**:67–75.

29. Crowley JJ, Keefe RS, Perkins DO, Stroup TS, Lieberman JA and Sullivan PF. The neuregulin 1 promoter polymorphism rs6994992 is not associated with chronic schizophrenia or neurocognition. *American Journal of Medical Genetics. Part B, Neuropsychiatric Genetics* 2008;**147B**:1298–300.

30. Hall J, Whalley HC, Job DE, *et al.*
    A neuregulin 1 variant associated with
    abnormal cortical function and psychotic
    symptoms. *Nature Neuroscience*
    2006;**9**:1477–8.

31. Law AJ, Lipska BK, Weickert CS, *et al.*
    Neuregulin 1 transcripts are differentially
    expressed in schizophrenia and regulated
    by 5′ SNPs associated with the disease.
    *Proceedings of the National Academy of
    Sciences of the United States of America*
    2006;**103**:6747–52.

32. Grossman I Sullivan PF, Walley N, *et al.*
    Genetic determinants of variable
    metabolism have little impact on the
    clinical use of leading antipsychotics in
    the CATIE study. *Genetics in Medicine*
    2008;**10**:720–9.

33. Pritchard JK, Stephens M, Rosenberg NA
    and Donnelly P. Association mapping in
    structured populations. *American Journal
    of Human Genetics* 2000;**67**:170–81.

34. Balding DJ. A tutorial on statistical
    methods for population association studies.
    Nature Reviews. *Genetics* 2006;**7**:781–91.

35. Mah S, Nelson MR, Delisi LE, *et al.*
    Identification of the semaphorin receptor
    PLXNA2 as a candidate for susceptibility
    to schizophrenia. *Molecular Psychiatry*
    2006;**11**:471–8.

36. Hennah W, Varilo T, Kestila M, *et al.*
    Haplotype transmission analysis provides
    evidence of association for DISC1 to
    schizophrenia and suggests sex-dependent
    effects. *Human Molecular Genetics*
    2003;**12**:3151–9.

37. Cannon TD, Hennah W, van Erp TG, *et al.*
    Association of DISC1/TRAX haplotypes
    with schizophrenia, reduced prefrontal
    gray matter, and impaired short- and
    long-term memory. *Archives of General
    Psychiatry* 2005;**62**:1205–13.

38. Shifman S, Bronstein M, Sternfeld M, *et al.*
    A highly significant association between a
    COMT haplotype and schizophrenia.
    American Journal of Human Genetics
    2002;**71**:1296–302.

39. Manolio TA, Rodriguez LL, Brooks L, *et al.*
    New models of collaboration in
    genome-wide association studies: The
    Genetic Association Information Network.
    Nature Genetics 2007;**39**:1045–51.

40. Barrett JC and Cardon LR. Evaluating
    coverage of genome-wide association
    studies. *Nature Genetics* 2006;**38**:659–62.

41. Genome-wide association study of 14,000
    cases of seven common diseases and 3,000
    shared controls. *Nature* 2007;**447**:661–78.

42. Sullivan PF. Spurious genetic associations.
    Biological Psychiatry 2007;**61**:1121–16.

43. McClellan JM, Susser E and King MC.
    Schizophrenia: A common disease caused
    by multiple rare alleles. *Br J Psychiatry*
    2007;**190**:194–9.

Human subjects considerations

T. Scott Stroup and Paul Appelbaum

Although much has been learned about the etiology, genetics, epidemiology, and treatment of schizophrenia in recent decades, there remains a great need for research requiring the participation of affected individuals to further elucidate its neurobiology, to identify means of prevention, and to improve and personalize treatments. Because schizophrenia impacts cognitive processes that could hinder affected individuals' abilities to protect their own interests, research involving people with schizophrenia has gotten considerable attention from research ethicists. Concerns about research involving individuals with schizophrenia include questions about their abilities to provide informed consent, the durability of such abilities, the possible need for more than usual protections of human research subjects, and the nature of such protections. The CATIE schizophrenia trial provided the opportunity to implement and evaluate innovative approaches to these human subjects concerns. Because of these concerns, and given the study's large scale, long duration, and high visibility as a major initiative of the National Institute of Mental Health, an Ethics Committee was convened and made several recommendations regarding the evaluation of consent-related abilities and procedures to protect the interests of research participants. This chapter will describe the special human subjects procedures used in CATIE and will summarize research results.

Assessment of decision-making capacity

All prospective research participants were screened for decision-making capacity using the MacArthur Competence Assessment Tool-Clinical Research (MacCAT-CR) [1]. Those individuals receiving study treatment also received the MacCAT-CR at month 6, month 18, and at any time a study antipsychotic medication was discontinued. The MacCAT-CR evaluates the following four abilities related to capacity to consent to research: (1) Understanding – the ability to comprehend relevant information; (2) Appreciation – the ability to be aware of the situation and its likely consequences; (3) Reasoning – the ability to manipulate information rationally; and (4) Choice – the ability to communicate a choice about participation [1]. Each ability is assessed by specific questions with answers rated on a 0–2 scale with 0 reflecting no comprehension, 1 partial comprehension, and 2 indicating full comprehension of the relevant concept. The Understanding scale has 13 questions (range 0–26), the Appreciation Scale has three questions (range 0–6), the Reasoning scale has four questions (range 0–8), and the Choice scale has only one question (range 0–2). The MacCAT-CR has been widely used in research [1–5], and is the most widely used and best validated of the competence assessment instruments, including

Antipsychotic Trials in Schizophrenia, ed. T. Scott Stroup and Jeffrey A. Lieberman. Published by Cambridge University Press. © Cambridge University Press 2010.

with subjects with schizophrenia [6]. Its content is adapted for specific research protocols. The MacCAT-CR Understanding subscale adapted for use in CATIE can be seen in Table 14.1

The MacCAT-CR was administered by research personnel who participated in training sessions at investigators' meetings that were held before the study began and again 15 months later. An Understanding score of 16 or higher on the 26-point scale was required as a minimum for study randomization, although clinical judgment was the final determinant of competence to consent even if a subject achieved this threshold. The selected threshold score reflected an *a priori* judgment by the CATIE investigators of minimally adequate understanding of this research study. An independent, post hoc analysis of MacCAT-CR interviews conducted among individuals with a broad range of schizophrenia illness severity to determine the appropriate trade-offs of sensitivity and specificity suggested that this was an appropriate threshold for the subjects who enrolled in the CATIE study [7]. The Understanding scale was used to establish the threshold of capacity because Understanding scores generally correlate highly with Appreciation scores and moderately with Reasoning scores, and it has the strongest psychometric properties of the three scales due to its greater range [7,8].

During the screening phase of the study, persons who demonstrated adequate decision-making capacity to participate in the study were randomized to study treatment if all other eligibility criteria were met. Persons who were initially assessed not to have the capacity to make an informed decision but who still wished to participate were offered a brief educational program designed to help improve the person's level of functioning to the point where a competent decision could be made about participation. After this program was completed, capacity was again assessed using the MacCAT-CR, and those individuals who demonstrated adequate decision-making capacity were able to continue in the study.

Subject advocate procedures

Because the decision-making capacity of individuals with schizophrenia may fluctuate, additional protections for such persons who enroll in long-term research studies may be needed. At the outset of research studies, potential subjects must have an adequate level of decision-making capacity to provide valid consent to participate. After subjects have given consent and are enrolled, their decision making capacity remains important because they must continue to be able to look out for their interests as the study proceeds. Little is known about how to deal with subjects who are competent when they enter a research study, but whose competence may fluctuate or disappear as the study proceeds. Without the capacity to recognize changes in their circumstances, subjects may lose the ability to protect their interests and become vulnerable to harms that they would not otherwise endure.

When faced with subjects who have lost the ability to protect themselves, investigators may withdraw subjects if they believe further participation would not be in their interests. But the interests of investigators and subjects may diverge when it comes to decisions about continuation in a project, making it hard for the investigator to act objectively. We developed the subject advocate procedures to help ensure objective consideration of a subject's interests.

At the time of enrollment in the CATIE schizophrenia trial, all participants were asked to designate a person to serve as their "subject advocate" to be involved with the informed consent discussion and to assist the subject with deciding about participation. Ideally,

Table 14.1. MacCAT-CR Understanding Scale adapted for the CATIE schizophrenia trial [1]

Rating guidelines

Score

2   Subject recalls the content of the item and offers a fairly clear version of it. A verbatim repetition of the interviewer's description is not required; in fact, paraphrase in the subject's own words is preferred.

1   Subject shows some recollection of the item content, but describes it in a way that renders understanding uncertain, *even after the clinician has made efforts to obtain clarification from the subject.*

[Examples include responses that could possibly indicate understanding but are too broad or vague for one to be sure (e.g., for purpose of research, "They want to see what will happen"), or responses that contain some specific and correct piece of information but lack some other part of the critical content.]

0   Subject (a) does not recall the content of the item; or (b) describes it in a way that is clearly inaccurate; or (c) describes it in a way that seriously distorts its meaning, *even after the clinician has made efforts to obtain clarification from the patient*; or offers a response that is unrelated to the question or unintelligible.

Disclosure 1 (Nature of Project)*

"The purpose of this study is to compare antipsychotic medicines for schizophrenia. Each person will be in the study for up to 18 months."

a)   Purpose of project

Ask: "What is the purpose of the study I described to you?"

b)   Duration of project

Ask: "How long will the study last?"

Disclosure 2 (Procedural elements)

"Every day, each person in the study will take medicines. Monthly, each person will have an appointment to answer questions."

c)   Daily medicine (Procedural element No. 1)

Ask: "What will people in the study do each day?"

Monthly interviews (Procedural element No. 2)

Ask: "What will people in the study do every month?"

Disclosure 3 (Purpose of research studies)

"It is important to understand that this is a research study. Its purpose is to help the doctors compare medicines for most people with schizophrenia. The purpose is not to find out the best medicine for each person in the study."

Ask: "What is the main purpose of the study?"

Disclosure 4 (Effect of research methods on individualized care)

"Because this is a research study, the doctors will be doing things differently. For example, each person's medicine will be decided by chance, like the flip of a coin. Neither the doctors nor the subjects will know which medicine is selected. Only the pharmacist will know which medicine is selected. If a medicine doesn't work well for a person, then he or she will be assigned to another medicine."

Table 14.1. (*cont.*)

a) Random assignment

Ask: "How will medicines be assigned to persons in the study?"

b) Double blind

Ask: "Who will know which medicine each person in the study is getting?"

c) New medicines when one doesn't work well

Ask: "What happens if one medicine doesn't work well?"

Disclosure 5 (Benefits of participation)

"There are several possible benefits of the study. First, the doctors will learn more about medicines for people with schizophrenia. Second, people in the study may get a medicine that works well for them."

a) Societal benefit

Ask: "What might doctors learn about the treatment of schizophrenia from this study?"

b) Personal benefit

Ask: "How might people who volunteer be better off by being in this study?"

Disclosure 6 (Risks/discomforts of participation)

"There are several possible risks and discomforts for people in the study. People may get a medicine that doesn't work well for them and their symptoms may get worse. Antipsychotic medicines can cause side effects like abnormal movements and weight gain."

c) Risk of getting ineffective medicine

Ask: "What might happen if a person gets a medicine that doesn't work well for them?"

d) Abnormal movements and weight gain

Ask: "What side effects can the medicine cause in some people?"

Disclosure 7 (Ability to withdraw/receive ordinary care)

"No one has to be in this study. People who agree to be in this research study can change their minds at any time. If they don't agree to be in this study or if they decide to stop, they will get the usual treatment for schizophrenia."

Ask: "What will happen if a person refuses to be in the research study, or decides to stop after starting?

Note: *After each disclosure patients are given the opportunity to ask questions.

patients chose someone who knew them well, for example a family member or close friend. If such a person was not available, researchers at the clinical research sites designated a person not otherwise involved with the project (e.g., a social worker or case manager) to serve in this role. If subsequently the participant was believed to have impaired ability to protect his or her own interests, then the subject advocate decided whether the patient should leave the study. That determination was based on whether the benefit-risk ratio for an individual participant had changed so adversely and substantially that the assumptions on which the participant's original decision to enter the study were no longer valid. Because consent was obtained at the outset for all treatment phases of the study, subject advocate involvement was especially important when new treatments were begun at entry into Phases 2 and 3.

The primary goal of the subject advocate was to ensure that the interests of research participants with schizophrenia were protected in the context of a multi-phase clinical trial. A secondary goal was to help the study achieve its aims, including the evaluation of the effectiveness of serial treatment strategies for "real-world" patients with schizophrenia, including those whose decision-making capacity might change over the course of illness.

Analysis 1: predictors of MacCAT-CR scores at baseline

The ability to determine predictors of decision-making capacity at the time patients enroll in studies should be useful to investigators who could then identify groups at highest risk of problems related to consent for careful screening and evaluation of decision-making abilities. We examined the relationship between symptoms of schizophrenia, comprehensive measures of neurocognitive functioning, and decision-making capacity in the large group of individuals with schizophrenia who enrolled in the screening phase of the CATIE schizophrenia trial. Initially, we explored relationships between measures of psychopathology, neurocognitive functioning, and demographic characteristics and the MacCAT-CR subscale scores using correlation coefficients. We modeled the relationship between the MacCAT-CR subscale scores and clinical parameters and demographic characteristics using stepwise linear regression models.

We measured psychopathology using the Positive and Negative Syndrome Scale (PANSS), which includes positive, negative, and general psychopathology subscales [9]. Neurocognitive functioning was measured by separate test scores, described in Chapter 6, that were converted to z-scores and combined to construct five separate scales that were themselves averaged to form a Neurocognitive Composite Score. Subjective attitudes toward treatment were measured using the Drug Attitude Inventory [10,11]. Symptoms of depression were measured using the Calgary Depression Scale for Schizophrenia [12].

Only 4% of individuals who entered the screening phase of the study were found to be ineligible due to inadequate decision-making capacity [13]. There were no significant correlations (Pearson's r) between the scores on the PANSS Positive Symptom Subscale and any of the MacCAT-CR scales (Table 14.2). (We did not examine the Choice scale because there was little variation in the score, with almost all subjects fully capable of expressing a choice.) The PANSS Negative Symptom Subscale scores had small inverse correlations with scores on the Understanding, Appreciation, and Reasoning scales (r = −0.09 to −0.14). The PANSS General Psychopathology Subscale score had very small inverse correlations with the MacCAT-CR Appreciation (r = −0.06) and Understanding (r = −0.06) scale scores. The composite neurocognitive score had larger, moderate correlations with all three MacCAT-CR scale scores (r = 0.23 to 0.26). Each neurocognitive subscore was also weakly correlated with decision-making capacity as measured by the MacCAT-CR Understanding, Appreciation, and Reasoning scale scores.

Step-wise regression models of the Understanding, Appreciation, and Reasoning scales of the MacCAT-CR all included measures of neurocognitive functioning (Table 14.2). Better working memory was a predictor of higher scores on all three subscales. The PANSS Negative Symptom subscale score was a predictor of the Understanding and Appreciation subscale scores, with extremely small parameters indicating that more negative symptoms predicted poorer Understanding and Appreciation. For the Understanding subscale score, processing speed was an additional predictor. The final model of the MacCAT-CR

Table 14.2. Models predicting MacArthur Competence Assessment Tool for Clinical Research Understanding, Appreciation, and Reasoning scores at study entry* [13]

Understanding scale

Predictor variable	Parameter estimate	Standard error	Probability	Partial r^2
Working memory	0.70	0.10	<0.0001	0.071
Processing speed	0.24	0.12	0.0489	0.005
PANSS Negative symptoms	−0.03	0.01	0.0127	0.002

Appreciation score

Predictor variable	Parameter estimate	Standard error	Probability	Partial r^2
Working memory	0.24	0.04	<0.0001	0.031
PANSS Negative symptoms	−0.02	0.01	0.0014	0.006

Reasoning score

Predictor variable	Parameter estimate	Standard error	Probability	Partial r^2
Working memory	0.21	0.07	0.0015	0.029
Verbal memory	0.16	0.06	0.0076	0.005
Neurocognitive reasoning summary score	0.18	0.07	0.0073	0.004
Years of education	0.04	0.02	0.0454	0.002

Note: *Parameters representing the 57 research sites are omitted from this table. Site was a strong predictor, with partial r^2 ranging from 0.18 to 0.37.
Source: Reprinted from *Schizophrenia Research*, Copyright 2005, with permission from Elsevier.

Reasoning subscale included verbal memory, the neurocognitive reasoning summary score, and years of education as predictors along with working memory. Research site, included in the models to control for inter-site variation among subjects and raters, was a significant predictor in all three models.

Analysis 2: evaluation of subject advocate

To evaluate the impact of the subject advocates, we surveyed research personnel regarding the effectiveness and implementation of the procedures [14]. Responses were received from 73 personnel at 49 research sites, representing 70% of possible respondents and 91% of eligible sites.

First, we assessed whether researchers understood the procedures. All research personnel who responded to the survey understood that the subject advocate had to be contacted if a participant had impaired decision-making capacity. All study coordinators and 91% of study principal investigators (PIs) understood that the subject advocate was supposed to be present or contacted at the time the participant consented to the study. We learned that

Table 14.3. Research personnel views of subject advocate procedures [14]

At your site, what effect did the subject advocate procedures have on enrolling people in the study (i.e., recruitment)?

Greatly helped	N = 2	3%
Somewhat helped	12	16%
Had no discernible effect	43	59%
Somewhat hindered	16	22%
Greatly hindered	0	0%

At your site, what effect did the subject advocate procedures have on keeping subjects in the study (i.e., retention)?

Greatly helpful	3	4%
Somewhat helpful	25	34%
Had no discernible effect	44	60%
Somewhat hindered	1	1%
Greatly hindered	0	0%

At your site, what effect did the subject advocate procedures have on the subject's ability to make his or her own decisions (i.e., autonomy)?

Very positive effect	2	3%
Somewhat positive effect	25	34%
No discernible effect	42	58%
Somewhat negative effect	4	5%
Very negative effect	0	0%

Overall, the effort required to obtain subject advocates for each subject was worthwhile.

Strongly Agree	16	22%
Agree	33	45%
Neither Agree nor Disagree	14	19%
Disagree	10	14%
Strongly Disagree	0	0%

Source: Used by permission of Oxford University Press.

respondents also contacted subject advocates in other circumstances. A total of 15% of respondents said it was helpful to contact subject advocates if the participant was upset with research staff, and 31% said this was helpful when the participant requested to leave the study. Forty-three percent of respondents reported it was useful to contact subject advocates whenever participants required a change in antipsychotic medicines.

Table 14.3 shows how research personnel perceived the effectiveness of the subject advocate procedures in achieving their main goals. A total of 61% of respondents thought the procedures had no effect on retention of subjects in the study, while 38% thought they were helpful and one person (1%) thought they hindered retention. A total of 37% of respondents indicated that the subject advocate procedures had a positive effect on subjects' abilities to make their own decisions, while 58% thought there was no discernible effect and 5% thought there was a negative effect on subject autonomy. A majority of respondents agreed that the effort to obtain subject advocates was worthwhile and thought the procedures had no effect on subject recruitment.

The phase of the evaluation involving surveys of subjects and subject advocates was implemented late in the course of the CATIE schizophrenia trial. A convenience sample of 41 subjects and 24 subject advocates provided responses at 10 sites. Subject advocates (42% were parents of subjects, 21% were friends or other relatives, 33% were clinicians whose patients or clients were enrolled in the study, and 4% were someone else designated by the site) had a positive view of their role. Seventy-six percent of advocates agreed or strongly agreed that the procedures allowed research participants greater freedom to make their own decisions. Seventy-nine percent agreed or strongly agreed with the statement that serving as subject advocate improved their opinion of schizophrenia research. None of the subject advocates who responded thought that serving as advocate was a burden. Ninety-six percent agreed or strongly agreed that all schizophrenia research studies should include "someone like a CATIE subject advocate."

Subject respondents also had a favorable view of the subject advocate mechanism. More than half of respondents (54%) agreed that having the subject advocate procedures positively influenced their decision to participate in the study. A total of 32% of respondents were neutral, 7% disagreed, and 7% did not respond. On the other hand, some study participants thought the procedures interfered with their autonomy. Two people (5%) strongly agreed and three (7%) agreed with the statement, "My subject advocate got in the way of my ability to make my own decisions." Most respondents, however disagreed (32%) or strongly disagreed (39%) with this statement; 5% were neutral.

Analysis 3: longitudinal course of consent-related abilities

If consent-related abilities fluctuate along with the course of schizophrenia, participants in long-term studies may not be able to judge or protect their own interests. For example, they may not be able to recognize or report to the investigators the occurrence of side effects, or to decide when it is in their best interests to withdraw from the study. We investigated changes in consent-related abilities over time to identify correlates of change and examined the frequency of lost abilities so that the need for additional protections might be better assessed.

The longitudinal analyses included MacCAT-CR data on 1,158 participants with a baseline MacCAT-CR and at least one post-baseline measure. The mean duration of study participation for the included subjects was 12.5 months. Those included were more likely to be Caucasian and had slightly higher baseline scores on the MacCAT-CR Reasoning scale than participants who were not included in the analysis because they provided no follow-up data. There were no differences in levels of symptoms or any other clinical or demographic variables.

Examinations of correlates of MacCAT-CR subscale score changes produced mostly consistent results for Understanding, Reasoning, and Appreciation scores, but with certain variations for the different subscales. For the Understanding subscale, better neurocognitive functioning at baseline was associated with improvement during the trial, while deteriorating positive and negative symptoms were predictors of deteriorating scores. For the

Table 14.4. Predictors of lost capacity

1	Marginal capacity at study entry.
2	Higher levels of positive symptoms at baseline.
3	Lower levels of neurocognitive functioning at baseline.
4	Worsening overall psychopathology during the study.
5	Worsening negative symptoms during the study.

Note: Lost capacity refers to falling below our threshold score for decision–making capacity.

Reasoning subscale, better neurocognitive functioning at baseline and increasing scores on the Drug Attitude Inventory, indicating a more favorable attitude toward antipsychotic medications, predicted more improvement in the Reasoning score. Worsening psychopathology was associated with deteriorating Reasoning scores. Better neurocognitive functioning at baseline was associated with more Appreciation score improvement, while worsening positive symptoms were associated with declining Appreciation scores.

The analysis to predict patients at risk of falling below the critical decision-making capacity threshold was done using logistic regression with a MacCAT-CR Understanding score below 16 as the target event. During the trial, 43 (4%) participants fell below this *a priori* decision-making capacity threshold, which was required for randomization to a study medication. Predictors of lost capacity are shown in Table 14.4. Lower baseline Understanding scores predicted higher likelihood of falling below the threshold, meaning that proximity to inadequate capacity at baseline predicted loss of capacity later. Poorer baseline neurocognitive functioning and higher levels of positive symptoms at baseline also predicted falling below the threshold. Worsening overall psychopathology, and worsening negative symptoms in particular, during the course of the trial also predicted falling below our threshold score for adequate decision-making capacity.

Discussion

In this large, longitudinal research study involving over a thousand individuals with schizophrenia, we found that few individuals (4%) formally enrolled for screening were judged to have inadequate decision-making capacity to participate in the study. Investigators seemed to invest the necessary effort for formal screening only in persons they deemed likely to be able to provide valid informed consent, arguably an important—if unanticipated—consequence of having a testing process in place. Presumably most individuals deemed not capable to participate were identified in a pre-screening process. A limitation of this finding is that in CATIE the persons administering the MacCAT-CR and making the assessment of adequate capacity were not independent of the study.

We identified predictors of capacity at baseline and of adverse changes during the course of the trial, as well as predictors of lost capacity during the trial. At baseline, neurocognition was the clinical factor most associated with decision-making capacity. Negative but not positive symptoms correlated with decision-making capacity for research participation, but the inverse correlations between negative symptoms and the Understanding, Appreciation, and Reasoning scores of the MacCAT-CR were small. All five neurocognitive domains measured, as well as the composite neurocognitive score, correlated with scores of the three subscales. In regression models adjusting for site variation, working memory was a predictor of all three subscales. For the critical Understanding scale, processing speed and the PANSS negative subscale were also predictors.

The association of working memory and decision-making capacity is not surprising. Working memory is a fundamental aspect of cognition that involves the encoding and manipulation of information over brief periods of time [15,16], and is an important component of the pattern of cognitive deficits in schizophrenia [17,18]. To generate responses about the relevant aspects of the study design the MacCAT-CR requires patients to encode and manipulate information, a process that clearly depends upon working memory. The relationship between MacCAT-CR Understanding scale and processing speed may be a reflection of the correlations between MacCAT-CR and general cognitive performance, which has been reported previously [2]. The relative importance of working memory and processing speed compared to verbal memory, reasoning, and problem solving in predicting MacCAT-CR scores may be due to the greater importance of encoding, manipulating, and delivering pertinent information relative to simpler skills in our neurocognitive testing battery such as recalling a list of words or learning from previous errors. In summary, the CATIE results confirmed earlier work with smaller samples [2,8,19] that found that persons with schizophrenia with higher degrees of cognitive difficulties and negative symptoms are at greater risk for decision-making impairment regarding research participation.

The MacCAT-CR was developed based on a thorough analysis of components of consent-related abilities. The resulting four-part scale has strong validity and reliability and was useful for the research reported here. Because the MacCAT-CR is somewhat time consuming and some interviewers and subjects have problems with its detailed questions, others have developed simpler screening tools to guide investigators regarding the capacity to participate in research studies. The University of California, San Diego, Brief Assessment of Capacity to Consent (UBACC) is one such 10-item instrument that we are using in our current investigations [20].

The subject advocate procedures as implemented in CATIE were generally well-received [14]. Research personnel understood the purposes of subject advocate procedures but some viewed the advocate's role as broader than intended (although some of these creative uses of subject advocates arguably reflect salutary efforts to assist subjects in making key, study-related decisions). Most researchers thought the effort to obtain subject advocates was worthwhile. Some reported that the procedures helped by engaging family members and promoting a positive view of schizophrenia research. A majority thought that similar arrangements would be useful in future longitudinal research studies. Non-specific benefits included good public relations and engagement of family members. A majority felt that such procedures should be used in future longitudinal studies involving subjects with schizophrenia, although a few strongly disagreed with this.

It is unclear whether the primary goals of the subject advocate procedures, to help protect the rights of research participants whose decision-making capacity may have fluctuated and to retain such subjects who wanted to continue in the study, were achieved. A third of respondents thought the procedures aided retention in the study, but most felt there was no effect. However, since only a small number of subjects (N = 43, 4%) lost capacity during the course of the study, most respondents may not have had the opportunity to test the efficacy of the subject advocate process. Somewhat more than a third of respondents thought the procedures had a positive effect on subject autonomy but most felt there was no discernible effect. On the other hand, almost no researchers discerned negative effects on subjects' rights or retention.

In spite of these opinions, reports from some research personnel that they contacted subject advocates when subjects wanted to leave the study, and from some subjects that having a subject advocate interfered with their autonomy, suggest that better specification of the role of the subject advocate—for subjects, researchers, and the advocates themselves—was needed. A need for better training procedures was widely endorsed by research personnel.

Although sites rarely reported that having to find subject advocates interfered with study recruitment, any such interference could have had an adverse effect on study generalizability. And although most research personnel thought the effort to get subject advocates was worthwhile, we cannot certify that the benefits of the CATIE procedures outweighed the costs of the efforts.

The longitudinal analyses of decision-making capacity also yielded useful empirical information. Study participants with marginal capacity at the time of enrollment and with worsening psychopathology during the study were at risk of lost capacity. We recommend that investigators conducting research involving individuals with schizophrenia pay special attention to participants with these risk factors so that their interests can be protected.

References

1. Appelbaum P and Grisso T. *The MacArthur Competence Assessment Tool-Clinical Research*. Sarasota, FL: Professional Resource Press; 2001.

2. Carpenter WT Jr, Gold JM, Lahti AC, *et al.* Decisional capacity for informed consent in schizophrenia research. *Archives of General Psychiatry* 2000;**57**:533–8.

3. Moser DJ, Reese RL, Hey CT, *et al.* Using a brief intervention to improve decisional capacity in schizophrenia research. *Schizophrenia Bulletin* 2006;**32**:116–20.

4. Moser DJ, Reese RL, Schultz SK, *et al.* Informed consent in medication-free schizophrenia research. *American Journal of Psychiatry* 2005;**162**:1209–11.

5. Palmer BW, Nayak GV, Dunn LB, *et al.* Treatment-related decision-making capacity in middle-aged and older patients with psychosis: A preliminary study using the MacCAT-T and HCAT. *The American Journal of Geriatric Psychiatry* 2002;**10**:207–11.

6. Dunn LB, Nowrangi MA, Palmer BW, *et al.* Assessing decisional capacity for clinical research or treatment: A review of instruments. *American Journal of Psychiatry* 2006;**163**:1323–34.

7. Kim SY, Appelbaum PS, Swan J, *et al.* Determining when impairment constitutes incapacity for informed consent in schizophrenia research. *British Journal of Psychiatry* 2007;**191**:38–43.

8. Kovnick JA, Appelbaum PS, Hoge SK, *et al.* Competence to consent to research among long-stay inpatients with chronic schizophrenia. *Psychiatric Services* 2003;**54**:1247–52.

9. Kay SR, Fiszbein A and Opler LA. The positive and negative syndrome scale (PANSS) for schizophrenia. *Schizophrenia Bulletin* 1987;**13**:261–76.

10. Awad AG. Subjective response to neuroleptics in schizophrenia. *Schizophrenia Bulletin* 1993;**19**:609–18.

11. Hogan TP, Awad AG and Eastwood R. A self-report scale predictive of drug compliance in schizophrenics: Reliability and discriminative validity. *Psychological Medicine* 1983;**13**:177–83.

12. Addington D, Addington J and Schissel B. A depression rating scale for schizophrenics. *Schizophrenia Research* 1990;**3**:247–51.

13. Stroup S, Appelbaum P, Swartz M, *et al.* Decision-making capacity for research participation among individuals in the CATIE schizophrenia trial. *Schizophrenia Research* 2005;**80**:1–8.

14. Stroup TS and Appelbaum PS. Evaluation of "subject advocate" procedures in the Clinical Antipsychotic Trials of Intervention Effectiveness (CATIE)

schizophrenia study. *Schizophrenia Bulletin* 2006;**32**:147–52.

15. Baddeley A. Working memory. *Science* 1992;**255**:556–9.

16. Goldman-Rakic PS. Circuitry of primate prefrontal cortex and regulation of behavior by representative memory. In: F. Plum (ed.), *Handbook of Physiology. The Nervous System. Higher Functions of the Brain.* Bethesda, MD: The American Physiological Society; 1987. pp 373–417.

17. Gold JM, Carpenter C, Randolph C, *et al.* Auditory working memory and Wisconsin Card Sorting Test performance in

schizophrenia. *Archives of General Psychiatry* 1997;**54**:159–65.

18. Park S and Holzman PS. Schizophrenics show spatial working memory deficits. *Archives of General Psychiatry* 1992;**49**:975–82.

19. Moser DJ, Schultz SK, Arndt S, *et al.* Capacity to provide informed consent for participation in schizophrenia and HIV research. *American Journal of Psychiatry* 2002;**159**:1201–7.

20. Jeste DV, Palmer BW, Appelbaum PS, *et al.* A new brief instrument for assessing decisional capacity for clinical research. *Archives of General Psychiatry* 2007;**64**:966–74.

Chapter 5

Population pharmacokinetics of antipsychotics

Kristin L. Bigos, Robert R. Bies, Stephen R. Marder, and Bruce G. Pollock

Introduction

Response to antipsychotics is highly variable, which may be due in part to differences in drug exposure. The CATIE trials reported overall high rates of discontinuation due to lack of efficacy and/or intolerable side effects for all antipsychotics [1,2]. Overall, 74% of patients with schizophrenia (SZ) discontinued the study medication before 18 months; 64% of those assigned to olanzapine, 75% of those assigned to perphenazine, 82% of those assigned to quetiapine, 74% of those assigned to risperidone, and 79% of those assigned to ziprasidone [1]. Similarly, the majority of patients with Alzheimer's disease (AD) discontinued their assigned treatment, and in fact the adverse effects offset advantages in the efficacy of atypical antipsychotic drugs for the treatment of psychosis, aggression, or agitation. In the AD trial, there were no significant differences among treatments with regard to the time to discontinuation of treatment for any reason: olanzapine (median, 8.1 weeks), quetiapine (5.3 weeks), risperidone (7.4 weeks), and placebo (8.0 weeks) [2].

One reason for the high rates of discontinuation may relate to the wide variability in the pharmacokinetics of these drugs, which often results in differences in the pharmacodynamics, both in the response to a drug and the incidence of adverse effects. For example, if a patient clears a drug faster than average, they will experience lower drug levels and may not respond as well at the same dose. Conversely, if a patient clears the drug slower than average, they will have higher drug levels and may be at a higher risk of experiencing adverse effects. Therefore, in order to limit the variability in response to a drug, it is often necessary to limit or control for the variability in the pharmacokinetics.

The CATIE trials afforded a unique opportunity to study a large number of patients treated with antipsychotics. This ancillary study to the CATIE trials aimed to evaluate the magnitude and variability of concentration exposure of antipsychotics using mixed-effects population pharmacokinetic methodologies. Population pharmacokinetics provide a means of estimating the magnitude of drug exposure in a large number of patients in a minimally invasive way, using sparse sampling [3]. These methodologies can also be used to identify factors that contribute to variability in drug exposure as well as detect potential pharmacokinetic drug interactions [3]. In this study, we constructed separate population pharmacokinetic models for each drug and evaluated specific covariates as potential contributors to variability in drug exposure.

Methods

Patients with AD were treated with oral olanzapine, risperidone, quetiapine, or citalopram. Patients with SZ were treated with oral olanzapine, risperidone, quetiapine,

Antipsychotic Trials in Schizophrenia, ed. T. Scott Stroup and Jeffrey A. Lieberman. Published by Cambridge University Press. © Cambridge University Press 2010.

perphenazine, ziprasidone, clozapine, aripiprazole, or fluphenazine decanoate, or a combination of medications. Demographic information was collected at study visits (i.e., height, weight, age, sex, smoking status, and concomitant medications). Race was self-reported and included the following categories: American-Indian, Asian alone, Black/African-American, Native Hawaiian, White alone, and two or more races. Subjects also reported if they were of Hispanic ethnicity, as a separate category from race.

Plasma samples were collected during the study visits, and time of last dose and time of sample was recorded. Each subject provided between one and six plasma samples for determination of drug concentrations. The CATIE AD trial contributed 795 samples in 260 patients (230 concentrations of olanzapine, 223 of quetiapine, 210 of risperidone, and 132 of citalopram). The CATIE SZ trial contributed 5,660 samples in 1,212 patients (1,528 concentrations of olanzapine, 1,137 of quetiapine, 1,274 of risperidone, 681 of ziprasidone, 641 of perphenazine, 216 of clozapine, 69 of aripiprazole, 18 of fluphenazine, and 96 of combination therapy). Data were excluded for missing (or incorrect) dose, time of dose, blood sample, or time of blood sample. Drug analyses and population pharmacokinetic modeling was supported by R01MH064173 "Atypical Antipsychotics: Determinants of Concentration," an ancillary study to the CATIE trials. As part of this project, analytic methods were developed for olanzapine [4], quetiapine (unpublished), and perphenazine (unpublished) and ziprasidone [5].

Non-linear mixed effects modeling was used for the population pharmacokinetic analysis using NONMEM® (Version 5, Level 1.1; GloboMax, Ellicott City, MD) [6,7]. The population pharmacokinetic analysis included the development of a structural base model, which defines the pharmacokinetic parameters and describes the plasma concentration-time profile for each drug. Drug dose, time of dose, time of sample, and drug concentration were entered into the model for each sample for each subject.

Pharmacokinetic parameters, including apparent oral clearance (CL) and volume of distribution (Vd), as well as inter-individual (IIV; between-subject) and intra-individual (within-subject) variability were estimated. The population analysis calculates both "population" characteristics (e.g. the population average CL and Vd for the group analyzed) as well as individual specific CL and Vd that are conditioned on the population characteristics and estimated using a Bayesian approach. The IIV model describes the unexplained random variability in individual values of structural model parameters. It was assumed that the IIV of the pharmacokinetic parameters was log-normally distributed. The residual variability, which was composed of, but not limited to, IIV, experimental errors, process noise, and/or model misspecifications, was modeled using additive, proportional, and combined error structures.

The developed models were evaluated using both statistical and graphical methods. The likelihood ratio test was used to discriminate between alternative models. The likelihood ratio test is based on the property that the ratio of the NONMEM objective function values (-2 log-likelihood) are asymptotically chi-square distributed. The objective function value is the sum of squared deviations between the predictions and the observations. An objective function decrease of 3.84 units was considered significant (chi-square, df $= 1$, $p < 0.05$).

The initial base model provided the basis for exploring subpopulations based on whether or not those individual specific characteristics or covariates could explain and reduce the population variance estimated in the group. The final model was then developed by testing the effects of subject-specific covariates on pharmacokinetic parameter estimates. Continuous covariates (e.g., age, height, weight) and discrete covariates (e.g., sex, race, smoking status) were introduced into each parameter in a step-wise fashion.

Covariates for inclusion in the model were first identified using a graphical method comparing the individual Bayesian estimates for that parameter versus the covariate. The step-wise incorporation of the covariates on a particular parameter is analogous to a multiple regression on the particular parameter (i.e., the incorporation of an effect on CL in a step-wise fashion). The approach provides for what would be returned from a classical multiple linear regression of the post hoc values, but has the significant advantage of preserving the data structure and uncertainty when evaluating the covariate effect. A covariate was retained in the model if it improved the model fit (objective function decrease of 3.84 units). A combination of covariates was only included if there was a significant additional reduction in the objective function value indicating a substantially improved goodness-of-fit. Covariate influence on IIV was also examined. Standard errors for all parameters were obtained using the covariance option in NONMEM. This modeling approach is used to determine the most parsimonious model that adequately describes the data.

Linear regression was performed to determine the magnitude of contribution to the variability of a parameter for multiple significant covariates. Unpaired t-tests were done for each significant covariate. Analysis of variance (ANOVA) was used to compare the parameters for each of the race categories, and Bonferroni's multiple comparison test was used to correct for multiple comparisons.

Olanzapine

Patients (N = 523) were treated with oral olanzapine [8] (2.5 to 20 mg/day taken once a day for AD and 7.5 to 30 mg/day taken once or twice a day for SZ, with the exception of one patient in the SZ trial who received up to 80 mg/day). Overall, 63% of patients were male (71% in SZ and 37% in AD) [8]. Patients identified themselves as White (N = 346), Black/African-American (N = 149), Asian (N = 19), American-Indian (N = 5), or two or more races (N = 4). More than half of the patients with SZ were active smokers (66%), while only 6% of patients with AD were active smokers.

Plasma levels of olanzapine were determined using liquid chromatography tandem mass spectrometry (LC-MS-MS) [4]. Patients with AD (N = 117) and SZ (N = 406) provided 1,527 plasma olanzapine concentrations (200 samples from AD and 1,327 from SZ) that were usable for the population pharmacokinetic analyses.

One- and two-compartment models were evaluated using NONMEM with the subroutines ADVAN2 TRANS2 (one-compartment model) and ADVAN4 TRANS4 (two-compartment model). First-order conditional estimation method (FOCE) with interaction was used for both the base and the final models. A one-compartment pharmacokinetic model with additive error best described the data [8]. The population mean CL and Vd were 16.1 L/h and 2150 L, respectively. The first-order absorption rate constant K_a was fixed at 0.5 h^{-1} based on previous literature reports [9].

Elimination of olanzapine varied nearly 10-fold (range 6.66 to 67.96 L/h) [8]. The best model fit included sex, smoking, and race as contributors to variability in olanzapine CL. Each covariate (sex, smoking, and race) independently contributed to a better model fit (i.e., when the covariates were added in a step-wise fashion, the model continued to improve).

Smoking status, sex, and race accounted for 26%, 12%, and 7% of the variability, respectively ($p < 0.0001$) [8]. Smokers cleared olanzapine 55% faster than non/past-smokers

($p < 0.0001$, unpaired t-test). Men cleared olanzapine 38% faster than women ($p < 0.0001$, unpaired t-test). Patients who identified themselves as Black or African-American cleared olanzapine 26% faster than other races (ANOVA overall $p < 0.05$). Olanzapine CL was significantly higher in Black/African-American patients compared to White patients (ANOVA mean difference 6.141, $p < 0.001$) and Asian patients (mean difference 7.738, $p < 0.05$), and was also higher than American-Indian patients and those who identified with two or more races (mean differences 4.514 and 7.995, respectively, $p > 0.05$), although these did not reach significance likely due to small sample sizes. The difference between Black/African American men who smoke and non-Black/African-American women who do not smoke (35.70 L/h $\pm$ 10.70 vs. 16.70 L/h $\pm$ 4.662, $p < 0.0001$ unpaired t-test) highlights the combined effect of sex, race, and smoking status. Hispanic ethnicity did not have an effect on olanzapine CL.

The AD and SZ populations were also analyzed separately. Differences in CL between these groups were explained entirely by differences in sex and smoking status between these groups, and not by age or any other factor. Neither age, height, nor weight had an effect on olanzapine CL.

Concomitant medications that had an incidence of approximately 1% or greater were also individually tested as discrete covariates to identify potential pharmacokinetic drug interactions with olanzapine. None of the 41 concomitant medications tested had an effect on olanzapine CL. None of the covariates (including concomitant medications) had an effect on the Vd of olanzapine.

The extensive pharmacokinetic variability reported in this study likely contributes to the wide variability in response to olanzapine. Polyaromatic hydrocarbons in cigarette smoke are known to induce the liver enzyme cytochrome P450 (CYP) 1A2 [10,11], which is the major metabolizing enzyme for olanzapine [12]. This is a potentially serious problem due to the fact that many patients with SZ smoke. In this population, 66% of patients with SZ were active smokers. Due to faster clearance, it may be necessary to increase the dose in patients who smoke. Conversely, doses may need to be decreased following smoking cessation.

Sex differences in pharmacokinetics have been reported for many psychotropic medications [13,14], including olanzapine [9,15–17]. Estrogen is a known inhibitor of CYP1A2, which could explain the slower olanzapine CL found in women [18]. Other possible mechanisms include sex differences in blood flow and liver size, as well as differences in expression of metabolizing enzymes and transporters [13,14]. The difference in olanzapine CL between men and women is not a result of differences in body weight, given that body weight was not a significant covariate.

This was the first study to find racial differences in olanzapine CL [8]. Patients who identified themselves as Black or African-American cleared olanzapine faster than patients of other races. There are many possible factors underlying these racial differences, potentially arising from both the sociologic (i.e., partial adherence) and possible biologic realms [19]. One possible explanation for racial differences in pharmacokinetics is the known genotypic differences in metabolizing enzymes [20–23].

In summary, sex, race, and smoking status impact olanzapine CL and therefore impact drug exposure. This 10-fold difference in CL may account for some of the variability in response to olanzapine, in terms of efficacy as well as the frequency of side effects. Therefore, an insufficient or undesirable response to olanzapine might be explained by a patient's sex, race, or smoking status. It is important for treating physicians to be aware of the potential impact of smoking on olanzapine CL. If a patient quit smoking and experienced increased side effects, their dose of olanzapine may have to be reduced by about 1/3 (given that smoking increases CL by more than 50%). Conversely, they may experience a relapse when restarting smoking due to insufficient olanzapine concentrations. Contrary to the label recommendations, our data suggests that smoking may well have a clinical impact and therefore dosing adjustments may be warranted. While we also found significant differences due to sex and race, we believe that the underlying reasons for their potential contributions to affecting olanzapine CL are worthy of further exploration and that the combined effect of smoking, sex, and race is substantial and therefore should be taken into consideration when deciding an appropriate dose.

Risperidone

Patients (N = 490) were treated with oral risperidone [24] (0.5 to 6 mg/day). Most of the patients had a single daily dose (N = 313), and 177 patients had two daily doses of risperidone. Patients age ranged from 18 to 93 years, and approximately half were male (47% for AD and 73% for SZ). Patients identified themselves as White (N = 328), Black/African-American (N = 140), Asian (N = 12), American Indian (N = 5), or Native Hawaiian (N = 1).

Risperidone and 9-OH-risperidone plasma concentrations were determined using a highly sensitive and specific LC-MS-MS method with a detection limit of 0.1 ng/ml [25]. Patients with AD (n = 110) and SZ (n = 380) provided 1236 plasma risperidone and 9-OH-risperidone concentrations (168 samples from AD and 1068 samples from SZ) that were usable for the population pharmacokinetic analyses.

The population pharmacokinetics were modeled simultaneously for risperidone and its 9-OH-risperidone to describe parent drug and its 9-OH metabolite concentrations. The FOCE method was used for both the base and the final models. A covariate was retained in the model if it decreased the objective function value by 7.88 (chi-square, $p < 0.005$, df = 1).

In order to describe the pharmacokinetics for both risperidone and its major active metabolite, 9-OH-risperidone, three pharmacokinetic disposition models were tested using NONMEM: 1) a standard one-compartment model with subroutine ADVAN2 TRANS2 (risperidone parent only); 2) a standard two-compartment model with subroutine ADVAN4 TRANS4 (risperidone parent only); 3) a mixture model to distinguish subpopulations related to CYP2D6 polymorphisms with subroutine ADVAN5 (a one-compartment model for both risperidone and 9-OH-risperidone). In the mixture model, risperidone CL, and fraction of risperidone to 9-OH-risperidone (KF) were separately estimated for CYP2D6 subpopulations (poor metabolizers [PM], intermediate metabolizers [IM], and extensive metabolizers [EM]).

A one-compartment model with first-order absorption and first-order elimination best described the base model for risperidone and 9-OH-risperidone [24]. The following parameters were estimated based on that model: CL for risperidone, Vd, K_a, KF, and CL for 9-OH-risperidone (CLM).

Among the three disposition models, the one-compartment model with mixture structure to distinguish CYP2D6 polymorphism-related subpopulations provided the best description of risperidone and 9-OH-risperidone concentration data [25], based on the Akaike information criterion (AIC) [26] and diagnostic plots. The IIV on CL, Vd, and CLM were described by the log-normal IIV model. Residual errors were separately estimated for parent and metabolite. The best residual error model was a combined additive and proportional model.

The KF was estimated in PM, IM, and EM subpopulations. The model with estimation of all three parameters was unstable; thus, KF for subjects in the IM group was fixed to stabilize the model estimation of KF in the PM and EM populations. The mixture model with two subpopulations (PM and EM) resulted in a 187-point increase in objective function value, suggesting that the mixture model with three subpopulations (PM, EM and IM) significantly improved the goodness of fit. The model with a mixture structure was selected as the final base model and was used in the subsequent evaluation of covariates.

Estimated CL was 12.9 L/h for PM, 65.4 L/h for EM, and fixed at 36 L/h for IM [24]. The Vd was 444 L. The K_a was fixed at 1.7 h^{-1}. The CLM was 8.83 L/h. The KF was 0.96 for PM and 0.595 for EM.

Age was the only significant covariate that impacted CLM. The inclusion of age on CLM resulted in a 68.1-point decrease in objective function value ($p < 0.005$). Compared to the base model, the IIV on CLM decreased 6.3% in the final model. None of the covariates had an impact on risperidone CL.

Age was identified as a statistically significant and clinically relevant covariate (with more than a 20% effect) on 9-OH-risperidone elimination [27]. Other studies have found that older subjects taking oral risperidone had higher plasma concentrations than younger subjects [28]. Metabolite clearance decreased as age increased; the average CLM estimate in a 45-year-old subject is 6.1 L/h compared to 4.9 L/h in a 70-year-old subject. Creatinine CL in this same age range for an individual weighing 70 kg and having a serum creatinine measurement of 1 mg/dL would be reduced from 92 mL/min to 68 mL/min, a decrease of approximately 25%. This is similar to the 20% decrease observed in the elimination of 9-OH-risperidone across this age range. The result of the age effect on 9-OH-risperidone elimination is consistent with previous reports [29,30]. Thus, older individuals may have a higher exposure to the active metabolite of risperidone, which may be a significant contributor to adverse drug reactions in this population [31].

The estimated risperidone half-life in PM, IM, and EM subpopulations was 25 h, 8.5 h, and 4.7 h. The percentage of subjects in the PM and EM groups was estimated to be 41.2% and 52.4%. CYP2D6 is the major metabolizing enzyme for risperidone. More than 80 allelic variants have been identified for the CYP2D6 gene among different ethnic populations [32], which result in variable enzymatic activity [33,34]. CYP2D6 polymorphisms influence metabolism of other drugs, including paroxetine [35].

In this analysis, race was a significant covariate on risperidone CL, when a mixture approach for CL was not incorporated in the model [35,36]. Race was no longer a significant covariate in the model with mixture structure when risperidone CL was estimated separately in three different CL subpopulations (possibly reflecting the CYP2D6 metabolizer phenotype). These results suggest that, due to the differential expression of CYP2D6 phenotype across race, the use of the mixture analysis approach has accounted for the differences in CYP2D6 activity. In addition, these differences are not present when tested within each of the subpopulations.

Additionally, sex and concomitant administration of paroxetine or fluoxetine were found to be significant covariates affecting risperidone CL when a one-compartment pharmacokinetic model without the mixture model structure was used as a base model for covariate screening. Subjects taking paroxetine or fluoxetine appear to have lower risperidone CL compared to those not taking these medications. Paroxetine and fluoxetine are both potent CYP2D6 inhibitors. Other studies have reported higher risperidone and/or 9-OH-risperidone concentrations during co-administration of paroxetine [37] or fluoxetine [38]. Paroxetine and fluoxetine were not significant covariates in the mixture model, where risperidone CL was separately estimated in CYP2D6 polymorphism-related subpopulations, again suggesting that differences are accounted for in the different CYP2D6 subpopulations. Additionally, significant differences in the proportion of individuals assigned to a particular metabolizer subpopulation were observed between African-American and White subjects ($p < 0.001$) with and without concomitant paroxetine ($p < 0.002$). The differences across sex and individuals taking fluoxetine in assignment to a metabolizer subpopulation were not significant.

In summary, risperidone CL is predicted by metabolizer phenotype, which likely reflects CYP2D6 genotype. Additionally, age is a significant predictor of CLM. Age of the patient should be taken into consideration when dosing risperidone. Although paroxetine and fluoxetine did not impact the final model, co-administration of these drugs should also be done with caution.

Quetiapine

Patients were treated with oral quetiapine for AD (N = 79) or SZ (N = 326). The total dose per day (administered once daily or in divided doses twice daily) was 25 to 200 mg for AD and 200 to 800 mg for SZ. Overall, 70% of patients were male (75% male in SZ and 47% in AD). Patients identified themselves as White (N = 286), Black/African-American (N = 105), Asian (N = 9), American-Indian (N = 2), Native Hawaiian (N = 1), or two or more races (N = 2). Approximately one third of patients (32%) were active smokers (39% in SZ and 5% in AD).

Plasma levels of quetiapine were determined using reverse phase high performance liquid chromatography (HPLC) using ultraviolet detection (analytical method unpublished). A total of 943 concentrations from 405 patients were available for the population pharmacokinetic analyses.

One- and two-compartment pharmacokinetic models with various statistical forms for IIV and residual variability were tested during model development using NONMEM. The subroutines ADVAN2 TRANS2 (one-compartment model) and ADVAN4 TRANS4 (two-compartment model) were used. The FOCE method with interaction was used for both the base and the final models. A one-compartment linear model with additive error best described the data. The population mean CL (IIV) and Vd (IIV) were 104 L/h (78%) and 653 L (100%), respectively. Given the limited number of blood samples taken shortly following dosing and the instability of this parameter in the models tested, the absorption constant K_a was fixed to 2.0 h^{-1} based on model fit and values reported in the literature [39]. The estimated IIV of K_a was 141%.

Elimination of quetiapine varied more than 12-fold (range 17.6 to 222.4 L/h). Patients with SZ had a larger range in estimated CL than the AD population (17.6 to 222.4 L/h as compared to 33.6 to 112.8 L/h). However, the arithmetic median was similar between the two cohorts (102.9 L/h for SZ and 104.2 L/h for AD). None of the covariates tested (e.g., age, race, sex, smoking status, or weight) had any significant effects on the CL of quetiapine.

The estimated apparent Vd of quetiapine varied more than 37-fold (range 59 to 2215 L). Similar to CL, patients with SZ had a larger range in estimated values than patients with AD (59 to 2,215 L compared to 92 to 942 L). The arithmetic median was similar between the two cohorts (649.8 for SZ and 653.5 L for AD). The subjects' weight had a significant effect on the Vd ($p < 0.001$). None of the other covariates tested (e.g., age, race, sex, or smoking status) had significant effects on Vd.

Concomitant medications that had an incidence of approximately 1% or greater were also individually tested as discrete covariates to identify potential pharmacokinetic drug interactions with quetiapine. Subjects receiving concomitant bupropion (N = 31 SZ, N = 0 AD) had a significantly higher CL ($p < 0.001$) when tested in the base model and when weight was added as a covariate on Vd based on a significant change in objective function value. Bupropion has been suggested in previous studies to cause mild induction of P450 metabolism [40–42]. None of the remaining 52 medications tested had significant effects on CL or Vd.

These findings are similar to those reported in other studies [39,43–46]. No effects of race, sex, or smoking status on CL and/or Vd have been reported [39,43,45,47–49]. Age has been reported by some groups [39,50] but not others [48,51] to be associated with decreasing CL. It is important to note that all of the studies investigating the effects of age on quetiapine CL were limited by small sample size and/or a limited number of individuals greater than 60 years of age.

Given the short half-life of quetiapine (approximately 6 hours) [39], adherence and accurate recording of previous dose administration times are especially important in the estimation of pharmacokinetic parameters. Adherence and poor recollection of last dose could be partially contributing to the large estimates of IIV in CL and Vd, particularly in patients with SZ. It is also possible that specific concomitant medications may be contributing to the individual variability in CL and/or Vd, but did not reach significance in this model given the small number of subjects receiving each concomitant medication.

In summary, a one-compartment linear model with additive error adequately described the data. A large IIV was evident with CL, Vd, and the absorption rate K_a with significant effects of bupropion on CL and weight on Vd. This model can be used for future pharmacokinetic–pharmacodynamic studies investigating effectiveness and tolerability of quetiapine.

Perphenazine

Patients with SZ (N = 156) were treated with oral perphenazine (8 to 32 mg once daily or in divided doses twice daily). Approximately 73% of the patients were male (N = 115) and were on average 40 years old. Subjects identified themselves as White (N = 102), Black/African-American (N = 46), or Asian (N = 6), or two or more races (N = 2). Subjects were categorized into two groups, Black/African-American (N = 46) and all other races (N = 110) for the purposes of these analyses. More than half of the patients were active smokers (67%, N = 104).

Plasma concentrations of perphenazine were determined using reverse phase HPLC using electrochemical detection, a method developed by the Clinical Pharmacology Lab at the University of Pittsburgh (unpublished). There were 421 concentrations available for population pharmacokinetic analyses, with an average of 2.7 samples per patient.

One- and two-compartment models were evaluated using NONMEM with the subroutines ADVAN2 TRANS2 (one-compartment model) and ADVAN4 TRANS4 (two-compartment model). Both base model and final models were estimated using the FOCE with interaction method. A one-compartment model with first-order elimination and proportional error best described the perphenazine pharmacokinetics in this patient population. The population mean CL and Vd for perphenazine were 483 L/h and 18,200 L, respectively.

Race and smoking were identified as significant covariates affecting perphenazine CL. The population estimate for CL was 48% higher in African-Americans than the other race group (512 L/h vs. 346 L/h). Patients who smoked in the past week eliminated perphenazine on average 159 L/h faster than non-smokers. The combined effect of these two covariates is that smoking African-American patients (N = 38) clear perphenazine 94% faster than non-smoking non-African-American patients (N = 44) (671 L/h vs. 346 L/h).

The estimated population pharmacokinetic parameters in this study are consistent with other literature reported values [52,53]. Estimated population mean CL of perphenazine was 48% higher in African-Americans than that in other races. Perphenazine is extensively metabolized by CYP2D6 [54], and CYP2D6 genotype has been previously identified as a significant predictor of perphenazine CL [53]. As discussed with risperidone, there are differences in the frequencies of CYP2D6 polymorphisms between African-Americans and other racial groups [34,55–58]. African-Americans have higher frequencies of the reduced-function allele CYP2D6*17 and the non-functional allele CYP2D6*5, but a lower allele frequency of the non-functional allele CYP2D6*4. Therefore it is likely that differences in frequency of CYP2D6 polymorphisms contribute to racial differences in perphenazine CL.

Smoking was also identified as a predictor of perphenazine CL in patients with SZ. An in vitro metabolism study showed that in addition to CYP2D6, CYP1A2, 3A4, and 2C19 are involved in the N-dealkylation of perphenazine as well [59]. Smoking has been shown to be a potent inducer of the hepatic CYP1A [60], and therefore metabolism of a CYP1A2 substrate like perphenazine may be increased in smokers, as also found with olanzapine.

In summary, a one-compartment model with first-order elimination and proportional error best described perphenazine pharmacokinetics. Race and smoking were found to be significant covariates affecting CL, which results in the combined effect that smoking African-American patients clear perphenazine 94% faster than non-smoking non–African-American patients.

Discussion

Many studies have shown a relationship between plasma concentrations and clinical response to antipsychotics in patients with SZ [61–66]. Most of the previous studies on the pharmacokinetics of antipsychotics have been conducted in a small number of subjects and, therefore, cannot identify contributors of variability or adequately measure the magnitude of effect of the covariates. Identifying factors that contribute to the variability in the pharmacokinetics of a drug is not only important in predicting a clinical response but also in order to avoid possible adverse events.

In the SZ trial, approximately 10% of patients experienced a serious adverse event, and more than 65% of subjects experienced a moderate or severe adverse event [1]. Additionally, almost 15% of subjects discontinued treatment owing to intolerability [1]. In the AD trial, there were no overall differences between drug and placebo in the incidence of adverse events (71% on olanzapine, 63% on quetiapine, 73% on risperidone, compared with 58% on placebo) [2]. However, the rate of discontinuation for intolerability, adverse effects, or death was much higher for drug compared to placebo (24% on olanzapine, 16% on quetiapine,

Table 15.1. Summary of covariates impacting antipsychotic exposure

	Olanzapine	Risperidone	Quetiapine	Perphenazine
Sex	↑ Clearance in men	None	None	None
Race	↑ Clearance in African-Americans	↑ Clearance in African-Americans	None	↑ Clearance in African-Americans
Smoking	↑ Clearance in active smokers	None	None	↑ Clearance in active smokers
Age	None	Age decreases clearance of 9-OH-risperidone (active metabolite)	None	None
Weight	None	None	Weight affects volume of distribution but not clearance	None
Metabolizer phenotype	Not tested	CYP2D6 metabolizer phenotype predicts risperidone clearance	Not tested	Not tested
Drug interactions	None	Potential for interaction with paroxetine and fluoxetine	Bupropion increases quetiapine clearance	None

18% on risperidone, and 5% on placebo) [2]. The high rates of toxicity in these studies may be a result of the variable pharmacokinetics identified in this study.

This study identified several contributors to variability to the pharmacokinetics in both typical and atypical antipsychotics, which are summarized in Table 15.1. Sex, race, and smoking accounted for some of the variability in olanzapine exposure [8]. Men cleared olanzapine faster than women, African-Americans cleared olanzapine faster than other races, and active smokers cleared olanzapine faster than non-smokers. Metabolizer phenotype predicted risperidone CL and CLM decreased with increasing age [24]. Additionally co-administration of paroxetine and fluoxetine may impact the CL of risperidone. While none of the covariates tested had an impact on quetiapine CL, the variability in the CL of quetiapine was the largest of any drug and ranged 12-fold, which may have impacted on its effectiveness. Additionally, coadministration of bupropion increased the CL of quetiapine. Similar to olanzapine, perphenazine CL was impacted by race and smoking. African-Americans cleared perphenazine faster than other races, and smokers cleared perphenazine faster than non-smokers. In summary, it may be necessary to take these factors into consideration when prescribing individual antipsychotics and make appropriate dosage adjustments. Further research is necessary to determine whether these covariates, which impact the pharmacokinetics, also predict the clinical response to antipsychotics.

References

1. Lieberman JA, Stroup TS, McEvoy JP, *et al.* Effectiveness of antipsychotic drugs in patients with chronic schizophrenia. *New England Journal of Medicine* 2005; **353**:1209–23.

2. Schneider LS, Tariot PN, Dagerman KS, *et al.* Effectiveness of atypical antipsychotic drugs in patients with Alzheimer's disease. *New England Journal of Medicine* 2006; **355**:1525–38.

3. Bigos KL, Bies RR and Pollock BG. Population pharmacokinetics in geriatric psychiatry. *American Journal of Geriatric Psychiatry* 2006;**14**:993–1003.

4. Aravagiri M and Marder SR. Determination of olanzapine in plasma by liquid chromatography/electrospray tandem mass spectrometry and its application to plasma level monitoring in schizophrenic patients. *AAPS PharmSci* 2002;**4**:Abstract W5016.

5. Aravagiri M, Marder SR and Pollock BG. Determination of ziprasidone in human plasma by liquid chromatography-electrospray tandem mass spectrometry and its application to plasma level determination in schizophrenia patients. *Journal of Chromatography. B. Analytical Technologies in the Biomedical and Life Sciences* 2007;**847**:237–44.

6. Sheiner LB, Rosenberg B and Marathe VV. Estimation of population characteristics of pharmacokinetic parameters from routine clinical data. *Journal of Pharmacokinetics and Biopharmaceutics* 1977;**5**:445–79.

7. Beal SL and Sheiner LB, eds. *NONMEM Users Guides.* Hanover, MD: GloboMax, LLC; 1989–98.

8. Bigos KL, Pollock BG, Coley KC, *et al.* Sex, race, and smoking impact olanzapine exposure. *Journal of Clinical Pharmacology.* 2008;**48**:157–65.

9. Callaghan JT, Bergstrom RF, Ptak LR and Beasley CM. Olanzapine: Pharmacokinetic and pharmacodynamic profile. *Clinical Pharmacokinetics* 1999;**37**:177–93.

10. Carrillo JA, Herráiz AG, Ramos SI, Gervasini G, Vizcaíno S and Benítez J. Role of the smoking-induced cytochrome P450 (CYP)1A2 and polymorphic CYP2D6 in steady-state concentration of olanzapine. *Journal of Clinical Psychopharmacology* 2003;**23**:119–27.

11. Bozikasa VP, Papakostab M, Niopasb I, Karavatosa A and Mirtsou-Fidanic V. Smoking impact on CYP1A2 activity in a group of patients with schizophrenia *European Neuropsychopharmacology* 2004;**14**:39–44.

12. Ring BJ, Catlow J, Lindsay TJ, *et al.* Identification of the human cytochromes P450 responsible for the in vitro formation of the major oxidative metabolites of the antipsychotic agent olanzapine *Journal of Pharmacology & Experimental Therapeutics* 1996;**276**:658–66.

13. Bies RR, Bigos KL and Pollock BG. Gender differences in the pharmacokinetics and pharmacodynamics of antidepressants. *The Journal of Gender-Specific Medicine* 2003;**6**:12–20.

14. Bies RR, Bigos KL and Pollock BG. *Gender and Antidepressants.* Vol 2. New York: Elsevier Academic Press; 2004.

15. Gex-Fabry M, Balant-Gorgia AE and Balant LP. Therapeutic drug monitoring of olanzapine: The combined effect of age, gender, smoking, and comedication. *Therapeutic Drug Monitoring* 2003;**25**:46–53.

16. Kelly DL, Conley RR and Tamminga CA. Differential olanzapine plasma concentrations by sex in a fixed-dose study. *Schizophrenia Research* 1999;**40**:101–4.

17. Kelly DL, Richardson CM, Yu Y and Conley RR. Plasma concentrations of high-dose olanzapine in a double-blind crossover study. *Human Psychopharmacology in Clinical Experience* 2006;**21**:393–8.

18. Pollock BG, Wylie E, Stack JA, *et al.* Inhibition of caffeine metabolism by estrogen replacement therapy in postmenopausal women. *Journal of Clinical Pharmacology* 1999;**39**:936–40.

19. Krieger N. Stormy weather: Race, gene expression, and the science of health disparities. *American Journal of Public Health* 2005;**95**:2155–60.

20. Ingelman-Sundberg M, Daly AK and Nebert DW, eds. Human Cytochrome P450 (CYP) Allele Nomenclature Committee. http://www.cypalleles.ki.se/. 2006.

21. Feng Y, Pollock BG, Reynolds C and Bies RR. Paroxetine pharmacokinetics in geriatric patients. *AAPS PharmSci* 2004: Abstract M1116.

22. Feng Y, Pollock BG, Ferrell RE, Kimak MA, Reynolds CF III and Bies RR. Paroxetine: Population pharmacokinetic analysis in late-life depression using sparse concentration sampling. *British Journal of Clinical Pharmacology* 2006;**61**:558–69.

23. Murayama N, Soyama A, Saito Y, *et al.* Six novel nonsynonymous CYP1A2 gene polymorphisms: Catalytic activities of the naturally occurring variant enzymes *Journal of Pharmacology & Experimental Therapeutics* 2004;**308**:300–6.

24. Feng Y, Pollock BG, Coley KC, *et al.* Population pharmacokinetic analysis for risperidone using highly sparse sampling measurements from the CATIE study. *British Journal of Clinical Pharmacology* 2008;**66**:629–39.

25. Aravagiri M, Marder SR, VanPutten T and Midha KK. Determination of risperidone in plasma by high-performance liquid chromatography with electrochemical detection: Application to therapeutic drug monitoring in schizophrenic patients. *Journal of Pharmaceutical Sciences* 1993;**82**:447–9.

26. Akaike H. A new look at the statistical model identification. *IEEE Transactions on Automatic Control* 1974;**AC-19**:716–23.

27. Green B and Duffull SB. Development of a dosing strategy for enoxaparin in obese patients. *British Journal of Clinical Pharmacology* 2003;**56**:96–103.

28. Aichhorn W, Weiss U, Marksteiner J, *et al.* Influence of age and gender on risperidone plasma concentrations. *Journal of Psychopharmacology* 2005;**19**:395–401.

29. Mannens G, Huang ML, Meuldermans W, Hendrickx J, Woestenborghs R and Heykants J. Absorption, metabolism, and excretion of risperidone in humans.

Drug Metabolism and Disposition 1993;**21**:1134–41.

30. Snoeck E, Van Peer A, Sack M, *et al.* Influence of age, renal and liver impairment on the pharmacokinetics of risperidone in man. *Psychopharmacology (Berl)* 1995;**122**:223–9.

31. Schneider L, Dagerman K and Insel P. Risk of death with atypical antipsychotic drug treatment for dementia: Meta-analysis of randomized placebo-controlled trials. *Journal of the American Medical Association* 2005;**294**:1934–43.

32. Human Cytochrome P450 (CYP) Allele Nomenclature Committee. http://www.imm.ki.se/CYPalleles/.

33. Kagimoto M, Heim M, Kagimoto K, Zeugin T and Meyer UA. Multiple mutations of the human cytochrome P450IID6 gene (CYP2D6) in poor metabolizers of debrisoquine. Study of the functional significance of individual mutations by expression of chimeric genes. *The Journal of Biological Chemistry* 1990;**265**:17209–14.

34. Bradford LD. CYP2D6 allele frequency in European Caucasians, Asians, Africans and their descendants. *Pharmacogenomics* 2002;**3**:229–43.

35. Feng Y, Pollock BG, Ferrell RE, Kimak MA, Reynolds CF, III and Bies RR. Paroxetine: Population pharmacokinetic analysis in late-life depression using sparse concentration sampling. *British Journal of Clinical Pharmacology* 2006;**61**:558–69.

36. Feng Y, Pollock B, Reynolds C and Bies R. Paroxetine pharmacokinetics in geriatric patients. *AAPS PharmSci* 2004; Abstract M1116.

37. Saito M, Yasui-Furukori N, Nakagami T, Furukori H and Kaneko S. Dose-dependent interaction of paroxetine with risperidone in schizophrenic patients. *Journal of Clinical Psychopharmacology* 2005;**25**:527–32.

38. Spina E, Avenoso A, Scordo MG, *et al.* Inhibition of risperidone metabolism by fluoxetine in patients with schizophrenia: A clinically relevant pharmacokinetic drug

interaction. *Journal of Clinical Psychopharmacology* 2002;**22**:419–23.

39. DeVane CL and Nemeroff CB. Clinical pharmacokinetics of quetiapine: An atypical antipsychotic. *Clinical Pharmacokinetics* 2001;**40**:509–22.

40. Tucker WE Jr. Preclinical toxicology of bupropion: An overview. *Journal of Clinical Psychiatry* 1983;**44**(Pt. 2):60–2.

41. Hesse LM, Sakai Y, Vishnuvardhan D, Li AP, von Moltke LL and Greenblatt DJ. Effect of bupropion on CYP2B6 and CYP3A4 catalytic activity, immunoreactive protein and mRNA levels in primary human hepatocytes: Comparison with rifampicin. *The Journal of Pharmacy and Pharmacology* 2003;**55**:1229–39.

42. Schroeder DH. Metabolism and kinetics of bupropion. *Journal of Clinical Psychiatry* 1983;**44**(Pt. 2):79–81.

43. Kimko HC, Reele SS, Holford NH and Peck CC. Prediction of the outcome of a phase 3 clinical trial of an antischizophrenic agent (quetiapine fumarate) by simulation with a population pharmacokinetic and pharmacodynamic model. *Clinical Pharmacology and Therapeutics* 2000;**68**:568–77.

44. Mauri MC, Volonteri LS, Colasanti A, Fiorentini A, De Gaspari IF and Bareggi SR. Clinical pharmacokinetics of atypical antipsychotics: A critical review of the relationship between plasma concentrations and clinical response. *Clinical Pharmacokinetics* 2007;**46**:359–88.

45. Nemeroff CB, Kinkead B and Goldstein J. Quetiapine: Preclinical studies, pharmacokinetics, drug interactions, and dosing. *Journal of Clinical Psychiatry* 2002;**63**(Suppl. 13):5–11.

46. Cheer SM and Wagstaff AJ. Quetiapine. A review of its use in the management of schizophrenia. *CNS Drugs* 2004;**18**:173–99.

47. Small JG, Hirsch SR, Arvanitis LA, Miller BG and Link CG. Quetiapine in patients with schizophrenia. A high- and low-dose double-blind comparison with placebo. Seroquel Study Group. *Archives of General Psychiatry* 1997;**54**:549–57.

48. Hasselstrom J and Linnet K. Quetiapine serum concentrations in psychiatric patients: The influence of comedication. *Therapeutic Drug Monitoring* 2004;**26**:486–91.

49. Thyrum PT, Wong YW and Yeh C. Single-dose pharmacokinetics of quetiapine in subjects with renal or hepatic impairment. *Progress in Neuro-Psychopharmacology & Biological Psychiatry* 2000;**24**:521–33.

50. Jaskiw GE, Thyrum PT, Fuller MA, Arvanitis LA and Yeh C. Pharmacokinetics of quetiapine in elderly patients with selected psychotic disorders. *Clinical Pharmacokinetics* 2004;**43**:1025–35.

51. Kimko HC, Reele SS, Holford NH and Peck CC. Prediction of the outcome of a phase 3 clinical trial of an antischizophrenic agent (quetiapine fumarate) by simulation with a population pharmacokinetic and pharmacodynamic model. *Clinical Pharmacology and Therapeutics* 2000;**68**:568–77.

52. Eggert Hansen C, Rosted Christensen T, Elley J, *et al.* Clinical pharmacokinetic studies of perphenazine. *British Journal of Clinical Pharmacology* 1976;**3**:915–23.

53. Jerling M, Dahl ML, Aberg-Wistedt A, *et al.* The CYP2D6 genotype predicts the oral clearance of the neuroleptic agents perphenazine and zuclopenthixol. *Clinical Pharmacology and Therapeutics* 1996;**59**:423–8.

54. Schering Corporation. *Product Information: Trilafon(R), perphenazine.* Kenilworth, NJ: Schering Corporation; 07/2002.

55. Wan YJ, Poland RE, Han G, *et al.* Analysis of the CYP2D6 gene polymorphism and enzyme activity in African-Americans in southern California. *Pharmacogenetics* 2001;**11**:489–99.

56. Leathart JB, London SJ, Steward A, Adams JD, Idle JR and Daly AK. CYP2D6 phenotype-genotype relationships in African-Americans and Caucasians in Los Angeles. *Pharmacogenetics* 1998;**8**:529–41.

57. Wennerholm A, Dandara C, Sayi J, *et al.* The African-specific CYP2D617 allele encodes an enzyme with changed substrate

specificity. *Clinical Pharmacology and Therapeutics* 2002;**71**:77–88.

58. Masimirembwa C, Persson I, Bertilsson L, Hasler J and Ingelman-Sundberg M. A novel mutant variant of the CYP2D6 gene (CYP2D6*17) common in a black African population: Association with diminished debrisoquine hydroxylase activity. *British Journal of Clinical Pharmacology* 1996;**42**:713–9.

59. Olesen OV and Linnet K. Identification of the human cytochrome P450 isoforms mediating in vitro N-dealkylation of perphenazine. *British Journal of Clinical Pharmacology* 2000;**50**:563–71.

60. Kroon LA. Drug interactions with smoking. *American Journal of Health-System Pharmacy* 2007;**64**:1917–21.

61. Mauri MC, Volonteri LS, Colasanti A, Fiorentini A, De Gaspari IF and Bareggi SR. Clinical pharmacokinetics of atypical antipsychotics: A critical review of the relationship between plasma concentrations and clinical response. *Clinical Pharmacokinetics* 2007;**46**:359–88.

62. Perry PJ, Lund BC, Sanger T and Beasley C. Olanzapine plasma concentrations and clinical response: Acute phase results of the North American Olanzapine Trial. *Journal of Clinical Psychopharmacology* 2001;**21**:14–20.

63. Perry PJ, Sanger T and Beasley C. Olanzapine plasma concentrations and clinical response in acutely ill schizophrenic patients. *Journal of Clinical Psychopharmacology* 1997;**17**:472–7.

64. Lane HY, Guo SC, Hwang TJ, *et al.* Effects of olanzapine plasma concentrations on depressive symptoms in schizophrenia: A pilot study. *Journal of Clinical Psychopharmacology* 2002;**22**:530–2.

65. Fellows L, Ahmad F, Castle DJ, Dusci LJ, Bulsara MK and Ilett KP. Investigation of target plasma concentration-effect relationships for olanzapine in schizophrenia. *Therapeutic Drug Monitoring* 2003;**25**:682–9.

66. Mauri MC, Steinhilber CPC, Marino R, *et al.* Clinical outcome and olanzapine plasma levels in acute schizophrenia. *European Psychiatry* 2005;**20**:55–60.

Implications for research design and study implementation

T. Scott Stroup and Jeffrey A. Lieberman

As a complex, highly visible, and controversial project intended to address a multitude of questions and to satisfy many constituencies, the design and implementation of the CATIE schizophrenia trial required many choices with significant implications. In this chapter, we will discuss lessons learned and aspects of study conduct that may be of value to other researchers seeking to implement large, multi-site clinical trials and to those seeking to better understand the study design and results.

Ongoing involvement of NIMH and vetting of the protocol

To ensure accountability, the National Institute of Mental Health (NIMH) chose to conduct CATIE through a contract mechanism that had extensive reporting requirements and allowed close oversight. NIMH program and operations personnel were involved in the project in an ongoing way, were influential in critical decisions, and provided operational expertise that helped the project meet its objectives.

The NIMH arranged multiple vetting processes to ensure scientific rigor, contemporary relevance, and stakeholder support. Each of these vetting processes led to important decisions. For example, NIMH scientific advisors agreed that individuals with tardive dyskinesia (TD) could be included in the study but recommended that they not be allowed to receive perphenazine because of its presumed risk of worsening involuntary movements. This led to perphenazine having a smaller sample size than the other main treatment arms of the study. A second group of stakeholders, advocacy groups, influenced the protocol with a strong recommendation that participants be allowed to make some choices in the protocol. This led to allowing participants to choose between the efficacy and tolerability arms of Phase 2 in an effort to bring "shared decision-making" to the study. Allowing a choice of the Phase 2 studies may have been helpful in encouraging some individuals to participate, and resulted in the study replicating something known in clinical practice—patients and clinicians tend to be reluctant to consider a trial of clozapine treatment. Another group of stakeholders, the pharmaceutical companies that made the study medications, were informed about the study design and were only allowed to make suggestions regarding use of their own medication. All of the pharmaceutical companies were greatly interested in the study but in only one instance did a company recommend a dosage range different from what was proposed; Janssen recommended a range of 1.5–6 mg/day for risperidone rather than the 2–8 mg/day proposed by the study designers.

Antipsychotic Trials in Schizophrenia, ed. T. Scott Stroup and Jeffrey A. Lieberman. Published by Cambridge University Press. © Cambridge University Press 2010.

Staying on a medication vs. switching to a different one

The inclusion of people who could be randomized to stay on the medication they were taking when they entered the study led to a finding that is important for people designing studies. Essock and colleagues examined the impact of "staying versus switching" in Phase 1 of the trial [1]. Patients randomized to olanzapine and risperidone who stayed on the antipsychotic they were taking at study entry had significantly longer times until discontinuation than did those who had switched from other antipsychotics. When these "stayers" were removed, the original pattern of treatment discontinuations in Phase 1 remained, although differences seen in the original analyses were attenuated. The authors and some commentators concluded that comparisons of medication effectiveness should take into account whether the medications being compared were each newly started [2]. The CATIE findings strongly suggest that, if people can enter a study on a medication to which they can be randomized, then the randomization should be stratified by incoming medication so that bias can be minimized. The importance of the specific medication individuals were taking at the time of study entry in CATIE also suggests that stratification on this variable may be needed in other situations too. For example, if evaluating the impact of a weight loss intervention, then it might be important to stratify according to the entry medication's liability for weight gain.

Multiple phases

The CATIE design included multiple phases to answer questions beyond those that could be answered in the initial randomization. Three of the follow-up phases (1B, 2E, and 2T) provided information, with the benefit of randomized treatment assignments, about specific clinical situations. Phase 1B examined the best treatment following the discontinuation of a single agent, perphenazine. Phase 2E examined the best treatment for individuals who had gotten poor symptom response from an SGA. Phase 2T in many ways resembled Phase 1 but everyone who entered received a new medication. Results of these phases have helped move toward the goal of personalized care in that they provide guidance for medication selection in specific clinical situations.

A downside of multiple phases, according to some critics, is that this may have encouraged early discontinuation of the preceding medication. But for a study meant to be applicable to typical treatment situations, the option for another medication when one is not optimal may better imitate usual care than studies in which only a single treatment phase is offered. Some benefits of having multiple phases included answering questions about patients in different clinical situations and the ability to evaluate optimal treatment sequences. The possibility of developing evidence-based "adaptive treatment strategies" based on information from the sequential medication trials in CATIE is now being pursued through an ancillary study led by Susan Murphy, PhD, of the University of Michigan.

Assessment of substance use

Because the study was intended to imitate real-world practice so that CATIE results could be widely generalizable, we did not exclude individuals with substance use disorders. As described in Chapter 11, we carefully measured substance use so we could fully characterize our sample, examine the effects of substance use on treatment outcomes, and determine whether treatments had differential effects on substance use. Because of problems with reliability and validity of self-report measures of alcohol and illicit drug use, we also used urine drug testing combined with radioimmunoassay of hair (RIAH) specimens to improve rates of detection. Urine drug

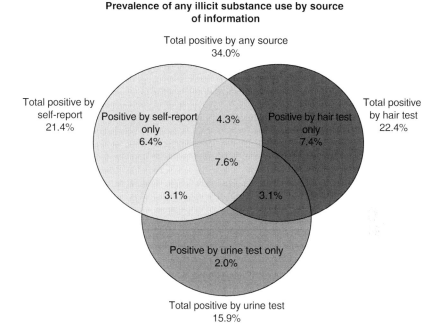

Prevalence of any illicit substance use by source of information

Total positive by any source
34.0%

Total positive by self-report
21.4%

Positive by self-report only
6.4%

4.3%

Positive by hair test only
7.4%

Total positive by hair test
22.4%

7.6%

3.1%

3.1%

Positive by urine test only
2.0%

Total positive by urine test
15.9%

Note: Positive lab tests for medications where there is a prescription are excluded from this figure.

Figure 16.1. Prevalence of any illicit substance use by source of information.

testing generally detects substance use in the past 24 hours, whereas RIAH can detect 90 days or more of use, depending on the length of hair sampled. Figure 16.1 demonstrates how RIAH and urine drug testing allowed recognition of substance use far beyond what would have been detected using self-report alone. Multiple sources of information, from laboratory tests as well as collateral informants, greatly reduced the under-reporting of substance use that is common when only self-report measures are used.

Screening for capacity to consent to participate in research

As discussed in Chapter 14, we introduced new measures to protect research participants and conducted empirical ethics research that may inform future investigations. We used a structured interview, the MacArthur Competence Assessment Tool-Clinical Research (MacCAT-CR), to guide decisions regarding capacity to consent at the time prospective participants enrolled in the study. We also used the MacCAT-CR to evaluate the longitudinal course of consent-related abilities and to help identify individuals who may have lost ability to protect their own interests. In addition, we introduced a "subject advocate" mechanism, in which a designated person not involved in the research (ideally a friend or family member of the research participant) was consulted to help determine objectively whether the continued participation of the subject was in the individual's best interests if their consent-related abilities declined substantially.

We learned that investigators rarely brought in for formal screening patients who were later determined to be ineligible due to inadequate consent-related abilities. One reason for this may be that investigators use effective prescreening methods to determine who might be eligible and are unwilling to invest time in individuals who are probably not capable of competently consenting to research participation; in this scenario, the presence of a competence-evaluating instrument has the favorable impact of keeping people without adequate competence to consent out of the research process. However, this may limit the generalizability of the research findings. A less favorable possibility is that researchers are not unbiased in administering the MacCAT-CR and in their assessment of competence, with the result that they err toward including individuals with marginal or inadequate competence in the study. To eliminate this bias, in high-risk studies for which it is deemed necessary to formally assess capacity to consent, it would be preferable for raters to be independent of the research.

Statistical issues

The statistical approach in CATIE is described in detail in Chapter 2. For the primary outcome, a final statistical analysis plan was developed and disseminated before any data was unblinded. The primary analysis followed this plan and its adjustments for multiple comparisons. We also examined many adverse events and attempted to present these results descriptively but learned that journal editors and reviewers expect and often require that data are presented with statistical testing.

The study also had multiple phases and many secondary outcomes of interest, including neurocognition, costs, substance use, violence, many of which are subjects of chapters in this book. This led to a substantial opportunity for Type I errors, or finding statistically significant differences when there were none. While these secondary analyses might best be considered exploratory and hypothesis generating, the results are nevertheless informative for researchers, clinicians, patients, and policy makers.

Project management

The CATIE investigators decided that the best way to ensure successful completion of the study was to engage a collaborator experienced in implementing large scale, multi-site trials. We chose to work with Quintiles Inc., a large and well-respected contract research organization (CRO), to implement the study. CATIE investigators designed the study, selected outcomes measures, trained site investigators, served as medical officers, and maintained close contact with the sites. Quintiles provided project management, data management (including development of web-based data entry), statistical analyses, reporting to the NIMH Data and Safety Monitoring Board (DSMB), drug supply and randomization, and site monitoring. Quintiles also provided expertise in reporting of serious adverse events (SAEs) and managed the process to make sure that all SAEs were reported fully and in compliance with regulatory requirements.

Difficulty of predicting site productivity

We learned it was very difficult to predict site performance. Even with an elaborate site selection process and the experience of our CRO, factors affecting site productivity, including illness, death, and changing priorities in the work places of our investigators were quite unpredictable. As might be expected, sites with experienced researchers and access to large numbers of individuals with schizophrenia tended to be most effective at recruiting subjects and implementing the protocol.

Desirability of avoiding protocol modifications

An important lesson learned is that protocols, which require multiple approvals (e.g., DSMBs and Institutional Review Boards [IRBs]) before a study begins and when any modification is proposed, should contain only the details necessary for conducting the study. Operational details that affect only the coordinating center should not be included. For example, if a vendor is mentioned in the protocol changes, this may require updating the protocol, which is time consuming and adds little or no value.

Adapting to the changing world required several protocol modifications while the study was under way. Some protocol modifications, for example when the FDA issued a black box warning citing risk of myocarditis with clozapine, were necessary and unavoidable. The addition of ziprasidone after the study began, to make the study results as up-to-date as possible, however, led to a number of difficulties including cohort effects and diminished sample size described above. We strongly recommend avoiding discretionary protocol changes.

Observations regarding institutional review boards

We developed the following process intended to expedite approvals by local IRBs. First we developed a protocol and a template for consent forms. We then submitted this to our local IRB, made appropriate revisions based on this initial review, and then simultaneously resubmitted the protocol and consent form to our IRB and to the NIMH DSMB. IRBs varied considerably between sites on a number of issues. One point of variability was how IRBs preferred to have the known risks of study medications described in consent forms, with a few requiring the known adverse effects of each drug to be listed by drug and others allowing these to be listed as a group. Another point of variability was whether subjects were allowed to consent for all phases of the study at the outset or were required to re-consent at the beginning of each phase. Regarding the subject advocate procedures described in Chapter 14, one site's IRB insisted that, if a study participant did not have a family member or friend to choose as subject advocate and thus one had to be provided, then the designated advocate could not be in the same department as the researcher. Other IRBs did not address this issue or allowed members of the same department to serve as subject advocate so long as they were not directly involved in the research, as recommended by the study procedures. In each of these examples, the vast majority of sites were able to use our usual procedures and consent form with only minimal modifications; only a small minority of sites had to make significant adjustments to satisfy the concerns of a local IRB.

The variability of IRBs and their ideosyncracies argue strongly, for the sake of efficiency, to attempt to put multi-site studies under the control of a single IRB that is ultimately responsible. Additional oversight by a Data and Safety Monitoring Board should adequately protect research participants. Unfortunately, few institutions now allow their IRBs to defer to others.

Ancillary studies

We developed an ancillary studies process that allowed investigators to propose complementary studies that could add to the project's overall scientific merit. Proposed ancillary studies were reviewed by the Ancillary Study Committee (ASC) if the study involved: 1) patients currently participating in CATIE, 2) patients of interest because of previous participation in CATIE, or 3) patients who are defined by their relationship to the CATIE study (e.g., family members of the population of patients who were approached to participate in CATIE and refused). The ASC also reviewed 4) requests for data collected as part of CATIE for secondary analyses and 5) studies that involve use of CATIE personnel, equipment, or other resources, or that systematically draw on the network of sites participating in CATIE (e.g., provider surveys). The Ancillary Studies Committee, which included members of the CATIE Executive Committee and representative site investigators, reviewed applications to make sure they had merit, did not conflict with existing plans, and did not unnecessarily burden research participants or study resources.

Ancillary studies that significantly extended the scientific productivity of the study included the genetics studies described in Chapter 13 [3], a study of the determination of decision-making capacity described in Chapter 14 [4], and the population pharmacokinetics work described in Chapter 15.

Some recommendations

Based on our experience carrying out the CATIE study and lessons learned in the process, we offer the following suggestions that might be beneficial for investigators planning large-scale studies:

1. *Keep it simple*: A major recommendation to those seeking to conduct large, multi-site studies is to resist complexity. Not only do complex design features cause confusion and make results less interpretable, in CATIE efforts to accommodate the late availability of ziprasidone and to avoid the presumed increased risk of tardive dyskinesia of perphenazine led to suboptimal statistical power for some important analyses. We sought and accepted the input of several outside groups to make the study scientifically rigorous and acceptable to relevant stakeholders. The process was time consuming, added complexity, and rather than protect the study from later criticisms the results of our vetting process opened the study to questions even from the scientific advisors and stakeholder groups that had offered input.

2. *Consider baseline treatment status*: In CATIE, individuals were allowed to be randomly assigned to the same medication they were taking upon study entry. We learned in post hoc analyses that incoming medication is a moderator of treatment effects and, therefore, recommend that study designers carefully consider stratifying the randomization scheme by medication taken at the time of study entry.

3. *Invest in good study management*: The use of an experienced CRO was invaluable for this large, complex trial. The ability to program a complex randomization scheme, package and deliver multiple medications to more than 50 sites, to monitor study performance at those sites, to develop a web-based data entry system and a database that captured a huge amount of data from multiple sources would not have been feasible at our academic institution when the study was designed and developed.

4. *Consider all aspects of the study as research opportunities*: We recommend creation of an ancillary studies process to maximize scientific yield. The ancillary studies process allowed new collaborations and facilitated systematic study of many aspects of the study. For example, we examined the consent-related abilities of all participants during our screening process to determine eligibility for randomization. Only 4% of those tested during screening were found to be ineligible due to poor decision-making capacity. Targeted screening of consent-related abilities may be more useful than universal

testing. In addition, we speculate that independent evaluations are likely less subject to biases than are evaluations conducted by the research team. If a study decides to formally assess the capacity of some individuals, it would be preferable to have independent assessors. In addition, residual blood samples were subsequently analyzed for inflammatory markers that were not considered when the protocol was first designed. The CATIE genetic and pharmacokinetic analyses were also part of add-on studies that added to the scientific output of the original study.

5. *Write a publication policy and plan*: Creating a data analysis plan and then developing a publication policy and plan based on it will avoid future confusion and disputes. It also will enable you to publish the results more efficiently.

6. *Choose your collaborators carefully and establish an organizational structure and plan*: Finally, we are grateful that we had a talented team of investigators and administrators at the academic institutions that ran the program and a talented group of collaborators at Quintiles, the CRO that was instrumental in the successful implementation of the study. Without a dedicated and competent team, no study the size and scope of CATIE can succeed. We established an organizational structure and operations plan at the beginning of the study and then refined it early on. This plan meant that each person knew their role and responsibilities and the schedule of activities for the project.

References

1. Essock SM, Covell NH, Davis SM, Stroup TS, Rosenheck RA and Lieberman JA. Effectiveness of switching antipsychotic medications. *American Journal of Psychiatry* 2006;**163**:2090–5.

2. Leucht S, Heres S, Hamann J and Kissling W. Pretrial medication bias in randomized antipsychotic drug trials. *American Journal of Psychiatry* 2007;**164**:1266; author reply -7.

3. Sullivan PF, Lin D, Tzeng JY, *et al.* Genomewide association for schizophrenia in the CATIE study: Results of stage 1. *Molecular Psychiatry* 2008;**13**:570–84.

4. Kim SY, Appelbaum PS, Swan J, *et al.* Determining when impairment constitutes incapacity for informed consent in schizophrenia research. *British Journal of Psychiatry* 2007;**191**: 38–43.

17 Conclusion and implications for practice and policy

Robert A. Rosenheck, T. Scott Stroup, and Jeffrey A. Lieberman

The CATIE schizophrenia trial was among the largest, longest, most comprehensive, studies of psychotropic medication ever undertaken. The federal government and NIMH made a major investment in CATIE because schizophrenia is a major cause of disability and even small benefits could have important ramifications for patients and their families and savings for the country. Antipsychotics under patent protection usually cost $10 or more per day of treatment. Much of their huge annual cost falls to taxpayers since most people with schizophrenia and other severe mental illnesses receive their health care or health insurance through the public sector. There was thus understandable interest in evaluating the effectiveness and cost-effectiveness of these medicines. As we conclude this volume, the following five key questions remain:

- What, in sum, are the major results of this large complex study?
- Do these results alter what we know about these medications when they are considered in the context of the literature of this field and clinical practice?
- Do methodological limitations temper the credibility of the study findings?
- How has CATIE been received by stakeholder communities and has it changed clinical practices?
- What are the implications of CATIE findings for clinical practice, for mental health policy, and for psychiatric education?

Summary of results

The important methodological strengths of the CATIE trial are the following: 1) that all treatment choices were made through random assignment, ensuring that differences in outcomes between drugs were caused by the drugs themselves and not by other confounding differences between treatment groups; 2) that all assessments were made under double-blind conditions to ensure that no rater biases in favor of one drug or another could distort the assessment of primary and secondary outcomes; and 3) the study was conducted in a wide range of "real-world" sites and enrolled a broad sample of subjects with clinical characteristics that allow for the generalizability of the study's results. The results highlighted below, with a few exceptions, all rest on this firm methodological foundation.

Primary outcome

On the primary outcome, time to all-cause discontinuation, olanzapine did better than the other treatments, with some variability across the different phases of the study. In Phase 1,

Antipsychotic Trials in Schizophrenia, ed. T. Scott Stroup and Jeffrey A. Lieberman. Published by Cambridge University Press. © Cambridge University Press 2010.

patients continued on olanzapine for significantly longer than on risperidone or quetiapine. In Phase 2T, among patients who had not tolerated the second-generation antipsychotic (SGA) to which they were first assigned, olanzapine and risperidone were both superior to quetiapine and ziprasidone. Among patients who had discontinued perphenazine (Phase 1B), both olanzapine and quetiapine did better than risperidone. In Phase 2E, among patients whose first drug did not prove efficacious, patients assigned to clozapine stayed on their treatment longer than those assigned to quetiapine or risperidone, but there was no significant difference between clozapine and olanzapine. However, Phase 2E was not conducted under double-blind conditions, and this could have given clozapine an advantage since it is widely believed by clinicians to be the most effective drug in patients who have not responded to other medications. It is all the more impressive, therefore, that patients did not stop taking olanzapine significantly sooner than clozapine in this phase of the study.

On the primary outcome of CATIE, therefore, olanzapine was superior to other agents, with the possible exception of clozapine. What was most surprising in these results was that the first-generation antipsychotic (FGA), perphenazine, appeared similar in effectiveness to three of the four SGAs to which it was compared (risperidone, quetiapine, and ziprasidone). When CATIE was designed, it was expected that all of the SGAs would be better tolerated than perphenazine, and at least some would be more effective. Some of the study investigators were so confident of these results that they questioned whether there was any need to include one of the older drugs in the study at all. This input led to the decision not to include perphenazine in subsequent phases of the trial.

A caveat to the superiority of olanzapine that was determined in post hoc analyses is that, in spite of the use of random assignment, both olanzapine and risperidone had an advantage at baseline over the other drugs on the primary outcome. Substantial numbers of patients randomly assigned to these medications had actually been taking them previously and thus were assigned to stay on the same medication they had been taking prior to the trial. While many experts would have thought that switching to a new medication would be advantageous [1], analysis of CATIE data showed that, for patients on risperidone and olanzapine, switching to a new medication led to worse outcomes on the measure of time to all-cause discontinuation [2]. While the effect of changing medications in schizophrenia has not been extensively studied, CATIE patients who stayed on their pre-CATIE medication stayed on their assigned medication longer than those who switched. When this advantage was eliminated by excluding "stayers" from the analysis, the advantage of olanzapine was attenuated but still present.

Secondary outcomes

The results of CATIE extend well beyond the primary outcome. The primary outcome of CATIE, time to all-cause discontinuation, integrates several important goals of treatment (e.g., reduced symptoms, improved quality of life, greater tolerability) without being a direct measure of these outcomes. Although the ultimate goal of pharmacotherapy is not that a patient continues on medication for as long as possible, the CATIE primary outcome was expected to both reflect and result in other important outcomes such as superior efficacy, fewer side effects, and greater global satisfaction among both patients and their clinicians. Numerous direct measures of these outcomes were also collected at regular intervals during the trial, and for the most part, confirmed the findings on the primary outcome. With the exceptions of weight gain, measures of glucose and lipids, and cost, there were few differences between any of the treatments on these myriad measures, as follows:

- On measures of change in psychopathology, olanzapine was significantly superior to risperidone and quetiapine, but differences were of small magnitude (Chapter 3).
- On measures of psychosocial functioning including social relationships, role functioning (e.g. work or housekeeping), there were no significant differences between any treatments at any of several times points that were examined (Chapter 5).
- On neurocognitive measures, which are viewed as the most direct measures of brain function, there were no differences between treatments after 2 months. Perphenazine was superior to olanzapine at 18 months, but this difference was small in magnitude (Chapter 6).
- On multiple standardized measures of side effects including akathisia, pseudoparkinsonism, and tardive dyskinesia (TD), there were also no significant differences between treatments (Chapter 9). However, patients assigned to perphenazine were more likely to discontinue that medication because of extrapyramidal side effects (EPS) (8% for perphenazine vs. 4% for ziprasidone and 2% for olanzapine) and to receive more adjunctive anticholinergics for EPS (10% for perphenazine vs. 3% for quetiapine and 7–9% for the other medications).
- However, when considering all patients who discontinued medication due to adverse effects, there was no significant difference between perphenazine and any of the other drugs.
- As one might expect from the lack of robust difference on the previous measures, there were also no significant differences between treatments on days of employment, family burden, or violent behavior (Chapters 7, 8, and 12).
- Finally on a measure of quality adjusted life years (QALYs), which combines symptom and side effect indicators, the preferred outcome measure in cost-effectiveness analysis, perphenazine did significantly better than risperidone, but the difference was small (0.016 on a 1–100 scale) and there were no other significant differences between other treatments on either QALYs or on three other patient-centered measures of quality of life.
- Patients assigned to olanzapine showed significantly greater weight gain per month than other treatments. Weight gain was observed with risperidone and quetiapine, the magnitudes were far smaller, and perphenazine and ziprasidone were associated with weight loss.
- Olanzapine, and to a lesser extent quetiapine, were associated with increases in blood glucose and triglycerides, suggesting a clinically meaningful increase in cardiovascular risk for patients.
- Finally, cost findings showed that virtually none of the higher costs of the patented drugs was offset by reductions in other types of health service use. Even after including the cost of patented drugs prescribed to perphenazine patients after their initial medication switch, total monthly costs for the perphenazine group were $300–$500 lower than for the newer antipsychotics, or $3,600–$6,000 less per year.

Summary

On the primary outcome, the essential finding of CATIE is that patients continued on olanzapine longer than on other drugs, although this finding was not statistically significant in comparisons with perphenazine and ziprasidone. However, the superiority of olanzapine on time to all-cause discontinuation did not translate into any advantage on a broad array of secondary outcome assessments of health status and quality of life. In addition, potential clinical advantages of olanzapine may be offset by weight gain and increased risk of cardiovascular disease. Perhaps the most important finding of the study, because it was unexpected, was that perphenazine did no worse than any other study medication on any measure of clinical status, quality of life, or tolerability. Due to its substantially lower cost, perphenazine was the most cost-effective treatment in CATIE and cost-benefit analysis showed there to be little uncertainty about this overall result.

CATIE in the context of other research

While we were engaged in the conduct of the CATIE study, colleagues around the world were carrying out related studies, reviews, and analyses of published data that bear on the interpretation of the CATIE results. In 2003 and again in 2009, meta-analyses suggested that four SGAs, clozapine, olanzapine, risperidone, and amisulpride (which is not marketed in the United States) were more effective at reducing symptoms of schizophrenia [3,4] than older drugs, although several other atypicals did not show such superiority. It was also widely believed that newer drugs uniformly caused fewer neurological side effects, with an especially lower risk of TD [5]. Some studies also reported that these drugs could save enough in inpatient costs to pay for their considerable costs even while under patent protection [6]. Through the 1990s, a number of prominent industry-sponsored trials had evoked great enthusiasm, especially for olanzapine and risperidone [7–9].

Other reviews and meta-analyses, including those conducted by the independent Cochrane Collaborative in recent years, have not supported the conclusion that SGAs are superior to FGAs [10]. A systematic overview and meta-regression analysis published in 2000 found that the superiority of SGAs over FGAs was largely attributable to comparisons with high doses of haloperidol [11] and concluded that they were not generally superior to FGAs. As early as 1996, an attempted meta-analysis of risperidone trials, found a "bewildering array of disaggregation (when results from a multicentre trial are presented in several publications) as well as . . . redundant reporting," [12, p. 1024] which, along with changing authorship of the same data, was thought to perhaps misleadingly "give an artificial impression of wide support for the efficacy of the drug." [12 p. 1025].

Then, in 2003, a 12-month, multi-site, Veterans Administration (VA) Cooperative Study found no significant differences between olanzapine and haloperidol on measures of symptoms, quality of life, or most side effects [13]. One possible explanation for these unexpected findings (in addition to the dose effect subsequently presented by Geddes *et al.* [11] was that haloperidol was given with prophylactic anticholinergics. About two-thirds of industry-sponsored trials had used haloperidol without such medicines [14], and often at higher than FDA recommended doses [15], posing a high risk of neurological side effects that could be mistaken for negative symptoms of schizophrenia or depression, a suggestion that was consistent with the meta-analysis by Geddes *et al.* [11]. In stark contrast to these findings, however, an additional meta-analysis by Davis *et al.* [16], found no effects associated with extrapyramidal symptoms, use of prophylactic anticholinergics, industry sponsorship, or study quality, and made no mention of the disaggregation or redundant reporting found previously.

In 2005, the first CATIE publication reporting study results [17] again found little or no advantage of four SGAs over perphenazine. Soon thereafter, the Cost Utility of the Latest Antipsychotic Drugs in Schizophrenia Study (CUtLASS 1), a prominent government-funded 12-month trial in the United Kingdom, similarly found no advantage of second-generation antipsychotics over first-generation drugs on symptoms, side effects, or quality of life [18].

These three government-sponsored trials [13,17,18] also found no cost savings in health service use associated with SGAs and that the greater costs of these drugs resulted in increased costs to society. The VA trial found olanzapine increased total health care costs (including drugs) by $3,000–10,000/patient/year [13]. CATIE found all SGAs to have significantly greater costs than perphenazine by $2,400–$6,000/year (see Chapter 4), and CUtLASS found FGAs to be more cost-effective than second-generation antipsychotics, which were still under patent protection [19].

A review of cost-effectiveness research prior to CATIE reported no evidence of cost savings or greater cost-effectiveness for SGAs [20]. A naturalistic analysis of data from California Medicaid, furthermore, found that the six-fold increase in antipsychotic spending for schizophrenia attributable to SGAs did not generate savings in other health care costs and concluded that the drugs did not "pay for themselves" [21]. Thus, the cost and cost-effectiveness data are far less mixed than the clinical outcome data, with the older generic drugs having an advantage because of the clearly higher cost of SGAs under patent protection.

What the three recent independent studies seemed to have in common was that they were large, randomized, double-blind, clinical trials conducted under the auspices of government agencies and used somewhat different comparators from prior trials. More recently an industry-sponsored trial that compared aripiprazole and perphenazine in patients who had failed to respond to olanzapine or risperidone also found no substantial benefit for the newest SGA over perphenazine [22,23].

Most recently, a large multisite study of first-episode psychosis comparing SGAs to low dose haloperidol [24] found that SGAs had lower rates of treatment discontinuation than haloperidol but did not differ on measures of psychopathology. This report was followed by a study of adolescent schizophrenia comparing molindone (the intermediate potency FGA that causes the least weight gain), olanzapine, and risperidone and found comparable therapeutic efficacy among the three medications, whereas olanzapine followed by risperidone produced substantially greater weight gain and increase in metabolic indices [25]. Finally, two large meta-analyses reported findings that were generally consistent with the CATIE study and the lack of substantial and consistent differences in effectiveness between the SGAs and FGA medications save clozapine [4,26].

Summary

Although we are faced with conflicting results from numerous clinical trials and meta-analyses published in major journals, the CATIE results are consistent with and reinforce much of what is known about pharmacotherapies for chronic schizophrenia. First, the findings of CATIE do not represent an anomalous event reflecting "just one trial" that stands out from most others. Rather, there have been a number of large randomized trials that have reported results similar to those of CATIE, even for neurological side effects.

Second, consideration of the magnitude of effects shows that the results of CATIE are not substantially different even from the large meta-analysis that favored some SGAs [3,16].

Thus, even the results of studies that appear to be in conflict with CATIE are actually not very inconsistent in that no studies have found even moderately large effect sizes for SGAs as compared to FGAs [3,4,26].

Third, CATIE and related studies, taken together, suggest that differences between SGAs and FGAs are either negligible or so small that they may fluctuate from study to study, perhaps in response to small differences in choice of comparator, study design, or in the population studied. Some have declared that there is little remaining justification for even considering FGAs and SGAs to be distinctive drug classes [4,27]. The CATIE results found considerable heterogeneity among the newer medications. CATIE thus is best seen as having re-framed the way we understood previous findings that, when examined closely, consistently show either no or small differences between FGAs and SGAs.

Methodological limitations

However, the CATIE study was not without methodological limitations that have been highlighted in many commentaries and that require review. These limitations can be summarized under eight headings: 1) low follow-up rates, 2) inadequate study duration, 3) idiosyncratic sample characteristics, 4) unusual outcome measures, 5) exclusion of patients with TD from the randomization that included perphenazine, 6) choice of study drugs and doses, 7) biasing differences in treatments used before randomization, and 8) inadequate statistical power to determine equivalence of treatments and an overly complex design resulting in suboptimal statistical power for some drug comparisons. Many of these limitations have been addressed in detail previously [28], and we will briefly summarize the principal points here.

Follow-up rates

Although the 18-month follow-up rates on initially assigned treatments in CATIE were only 18%–36% across treatments, CATIE actually achieved higher follow-up rates on the initially assigned treatment at comparable time points to most of the studies that had established the efficacy of SGAs. For example, at 8 weeks, CATIE follow-up rates on the initially assigned study drug were 69%–77% across treatments [17], somewhat better than the 67% follow-up rate for olanzapine patients in the International Collaborative Trial at only 6 weeks [8] and substantially superior to the 52%–56% follow-up rates at 8 weeks among patients assigned to risperidone in the major registration trial of that drug [7]. Data presented from a 28-week study of olanzapine, show follow-up rates of 42%–59% across groups at 28 weeks, not substantially different from the 40%–60% follow-up rates at the equivalent time point in CATIE [29].

In one study, the risperidone relapse trial [9], 12-month follow-up rates were substantially better than in CATIE with over 70% of risperidone patients and almost 60% of haloperidol patients still participating at 12 months. Unlike CATIE, however, this study specifically targeted stable patients with PANSS scores that were lower by a clinically significant amount (10 points).

Study duration and longer-term outcomes

Although longer than other studies, CATIE may not have been long enough to compare long-term side effects such as TD, diabetes, and cardiovascular morbidity that develop from cumulative treatment exposure [30]. The risk of weight gain and probably diabetes with some SGAs is well-established, especially for olanzapine and clozapine [31]. Olanzapine showed dramatic increases in weight, blood glucose, and triglycerides in CATIE, although the study was too short and too small to evaluate differences in incident cases of diabetes.

TD, a sometimes permanent movement disorder that often affects the mouth and tongue, is of greater concern since a lowered risk of this disorder may remain an important advantage of SGAs. A recent comprehensive review of past studies could identify only four 1-year randomized trials of TD [32]. These trials included 1,707 patients who were followed for an average median of 8.8 months across the studies. These studies, taken together, were not substantially different in duration from CATIE, in which patients assigned to perphenazine and to the best performing SGA, olanzapine, participated for a median of 5.6 and 9.2 months, respectively. While CATIE may not have been as long as desirable for a study of TD, it was not much shorter than the studies that are cited as suggesting SGA benefits on this outcome, and thus its "no difference" findings may be no less informative. A critical point is that CATIE used perphenazine at moderate doses rather than haloperidol, which is noted for causing EPS and TD.

Sample characteristics

When findings are unexpected, as in CATIE, it is natural to wonder whether some idiosyncratic feature of the sample may have obscured benefits of the SGAs. Available data, however, suggest that participants in CATIE were broadly comparable to those in seven other major trials of SGAs with similar mean age (41 years in CATIE vs. 36–43 in other trials) and duration of illness (16.6 years in CATIE vs. 14.7–16.3 in other trials), and no indication of greater "chronicity" or "refractoriness." Mean baseline PANSS total symptoms scores in CATIE averaged 76.1 (SD = 18.2), notably lower than both the 87.5 (SD = 15.4) mean score in the major registration trial of olanzapine [8] and the 92.2 (SD = 16.7) mean score in the comparable study of risperidone [7], but higher than the 65.0 (SD = 15.9) score in the "stable" cohort recruited for the risperidone relapse study [9].

Comparative data from two large non-experimental outcome studies of schizophrenia in the general population, presented previously [33 p. 492–493], showed similarities on gender, age, and education, symptoms levels, and quality of life, although CATIE had a lower proportion of minority patients. Comparisons have also been reported with data from the Schizophrenia PORT survey of 745 randomly sampled patients treated for schizophrenia in Ohio and Georgia [34] and further demonstrate that the CATIE sample was broadly representative of Americans with chronic schizophrenia.

It is important to acknowledge, however, that first-episode patients and geriatric patients were not a focus in CATIE and deserve additional study.

Choice of outcome measures

The primary outcome measure, time to all-cause treatment discontinuation, and the main effectiveness in the cost-effectiveness analysis, QALYs, have not been commonly used in clinical trials of schizophrenia. But the presence of more standard measures of symptoms, quality of life, and side effects, all of which gave similar results, suggests that the results of CATIE cannot be explained by the choice of measures. Time to all-cause treatment discontinuation stands out as a measure of a drug's enduring acceptability that reflects efficacy and tolerability and that has the distinct statistical advantage of having no missing data.

Exclusion of patients with tardive dyskinesia from the randomization that included perphenazine

The initial reason for excluding patients with TD from randomization to perphenazine was the belief among senior scientific advisors to the NIMH, in 2000, that patients with TD should not be exposed to any FGA. Within the non-TD stratum (85% of the sample), however, patients had an equal and unbiased chance of being assigned to each of the five available treatments—the essential feature of any randomization.

In view of the unexpected CATIE findings of no significant group differences on measures of tardive dyskinesia, it is relevant to reiterate a basic principle of risk assessment research—that patients who already have the outcome being studied should be excluded from the study cohort [35, page 88–89; 36 p. 82]. Since such patients already are "cases," they are not at risk for becoming "cases" and add uninformative variance that biases results toward the null. The exclusion of TD patients thus allows more precise comparison of TD incidence in CATIE than in studies that included mixed samples.

Choice of medications and doses

The central feature of the dosing regimens used in CATIE is that they were designed to allow flexible adjustment by physicians according to the clinical needs of each patient. Concern has been expressed that the mean modal dose of olanzapine was higher than in typical practice at the time of the CATIE study and that dosing of risperidone and ziprasidone were somewhat lower than in typical practice [37,38]. Since dosing was determined according to the individualized clinical judgment of each psychiatrist, and was thus based entirely on the manifest clinical needs of individual patients, it would seem that differences in outcome were not likely to have been attributable to differences in permissible dosing, but this possibility cannot be ruled out.

Concern has also been expressed that perphenazine was used at unusually low doses to avoid neurological side effects [37]. The mean modal dose of perphenazine in CATIE (20.8 mg) is toward the upper end of the recommended outpatient dose range (24 mg), and CATIE participants were outpatients for 95% of the trial. Because it is a mid-potency drug, perphenazine may be more representative of the class of FGAs than high-potency haloperidol, especially as it was used in many past FGA-SGA trials—at high doses and without prophylactic anticholinergics to prevent EPS.

Differences in pre-randomization treatment

As noted above, about 40% of CATIE patients were treated prior to study entry with either of two study drugs (olanzapine or risperidone) [17]. Thus, while most patients were assigned to a change in medication, about 20% of those assigned to olanzapine or risperidone were assigned to the same medication they had been taking before entering the study. The re-analysis of CATIE data showed that those who stayed on their prior medication did better on the primary study outcome [2] and that, when these patients were excluded, the differences between treated patients were attenuated, although the same general patterns in time to all-cause discontinuation were preserved.

Inadequate statistical power

The statistical analysis of the primary results of CATIE, which adjusted for multiple comparisons, found olanzapine superior to quetiapine and risperidone but not perphenazine and ziprasidone even though the median time to discontinuation was no longer for perphenazine or ziprasidone [17]. There was lower power to detect differences involving the perphenazine and ziprasidone arms of the study because individuals with TD were excluded from randomization to perphenazine and because ziprasidone was added to the protocol late and fewer participants took these drugs. As the CATIE study was originally conceived as a study to determine superiority of the SGAs, and was not statistically powered to determine equivalence or non-inferiority, the findings of no differences between perphenazine and the SGAs cannot be considered definitive in that regard.

While several design features in CATIE have been identified as potential methodological limitations, many of these turn out to have either not been important weaknesses or were in fact relative strengths after careful comparison with other studies. The remaining limitations are not substantially different from limitations that characterize the studies that highlighted the advantages of SGAs. Although many observers have pointed to methodological limitations to explain why CATIE results were different than some expected [37–40], the results of CATIE were, in fact, not as dramatically different from those that preceded it as has been portrayed.

Reception/reaction in the professional community and initial impact on prescribing

Science is often portrayed as an edifice built by individual investigators, one brick, or one study, at a time. However, medical science, in particular, is more aptly described as the collaborative construction of a learning community, which includes researchers, clinicians, pharmaceutical companies, health providers, consumers and their families, and other interested parties (e.g., insurers). An important part of the appraisal of a major research study such as CATIE is its reception by the community to which it was broadly addressed.

Initial critiques

The initial responses to CATIE were surprise, skepticism, and concern. For many involved in the world of antipsychotic pharmacotherapy, the CATIE results, with their implication that most SGAs had little advantage over an FGA in effectiveness and no advantage on neurological side effects came as a surprise. Some psychopharmacologists who had championed the SGAs over the years and many of whom had conducted landmark studies, emphasized the methodological limitations addressed earlier in this chapter, which they thought limited both the validity and generalizability of the results [37–40]. A common refrain was that treatment should always be individualized and development of more effective treatments is sorely needed. The fact that only 24% (range 18%–36%) of patients completed 18 months of treatment without changing medications was widely taken as evidence of the ineffectiveness of current treatment, although such a conclusion was one that CATIE was not designed to evaluate since there was no placebo treatment condition. Informally, many commented that CATIE was "just one study" and was not an occasion for revising the accepted assessment of SGAs.

Some of the strongest reactions were those of professional organizations and consumer groups whose press releases expressed less concern with the unexpected results of CATIE, and more apprehension that insurance companies and government funders would use (or perhaps misuse) the CATIE results to impose harmful restrictions on the ability of physicians to prescribe drugs as needed by individual patients on the basis of their unique needs. The Director of the American Psychiatric Association's Division of Research noted in response to CUtLASS that "clinicians have long recognized that SGAs were no more effective than FGAs in reducing psychotic symptoms" [40] but nevertheless cautioned against abrupt changes in practice or policy.

Early acceptance

Other researchers, perhaps reflecting the underlying consistency of CATIE with an emerging current of opinion [41], recognized that this major study in fact confirmed what many had suspected in recent years, that a fundamental reconsideration of SGAs was needed to guide both clinical practice and policy [42–45]. The president of the American Psychiatric Association expressed personal anger that the profession seemed to have been misled by corporate marketing [46].

The CATIE trial received widespread coverage by the press. An editorial in the *New York Times* [47] concluded that CATIE showed that "the system for approving and promoting drugs is badly out of whack" and that "The nation is wasting billions . . ." A *Washington Post* article on CATIE reported that "patients and policymakers can be blindsided by self-interested research by drugmakers" [48]. There were, however, no calls for draconian limits on access or any other policy initiatives. It is notable in this respect that CATIE was published almost exactly 1 year after Vioxx was withdrawn from the market because of concerns about its safety, a year in which a spate of books by highly respected physicians had been published documenting many apparently misleading methods used to promote patent medications to US physicians [49–52]. Although limited attention was focused on SGAs in these books, they reflected a climate that was more likely to accept empirical results that questioned established beliefs about patent medicines.

Shifting consensus

With time, as additional reports from CATIE showed that the initial pattern of results was repeated in clinical domains such as neurocognitive functioning, symptoms, quality of life, violent behavior, and employment, a consensus of opinion came to accept the study's results. In the Fall of 2007, the Texas Medication Algorithm Project (TMAP) group concluded that there was no reason to prefer SGAs over FGAs in chronic schizophrenia, although with considerable difference of opinion they continued to recommend SGAs in first-episode illness [53]. The Medical Directors of the National Association of State Mental Health Program Directors also completed a policy report which began by concluding that recent research had shown that SGAs should not be assumed to be markedly superior to FGAs and that new policy approaches are needed. In addition, in November 2007, following discussions with the FDA in which the CATIE results [54] figured prominently, Eli Lilly strengthened its warning about adverse metabolic consequences in their labeling.

Almost 3 years after the original CATIE paper was published, the May 2008 issue of the APA journal *Psychiatric Services*, was devoted almost entirely to current perspectives on antipsychotic medications and included a special section devoted to the CATIE study. Commentaries from experts and stakeholders seemed to uniformly accept the findings of CATIE, even on the subject of TD [55]. While the debate over the scientific meaning of CATIE seemed to have produced a new consensus, debate about issues like TD risk continues, and discussions about the implications of the CATIE consensus for changes, practice, and policy are just beginning.

Changes in prescribing

There have been only two studies of changes in prescribing practices of antipsychotics since the first CATIE publication. One study of antipsychotic prescription use in the VA showed declining use of olanzapine beginning about 2002, well before CATIE was published, and stabilization of the use of conventionals for about 15% of patients after 2003 [56]. A total of 1.8% of VA patients with schizophrenia were prescribed perphenazine during the year before CATIE was published and 1.8% in the year after. One other study also showed little change in patterns of FGA prescriptions before and after CATIE [57]. Citrome and colleagues reported that prescriptions for both clozapine and perphenazine increased among individuals with schizophrenia in inpatient units operated by the New York State Office of Mental Health in the year after the original CATIE report was published [58].

Summary

While initial reactions of surprise and skepticism were accompanied by an inclination to minimize the importance of the CATIE study, because of both methodological limitations and concern about restrictive formulary policies, a more recent consensus has emerged that has largely accepted the CATIE findings. While agreement on the science progressed over the initial years after the results were published, influence on practice was slower, and the debate about policy implications will be ongoing.

Implications for clinical practice

While clinical trials provide the most rigorous understanding of the benefits and risks of various treatments for populations of patients, they can only guide, not dictate, clinical practice since treatment must always be individualized for each unique patient. The results of CATIE, however, can help practicing clinicians tailor treatment for their patients. We single out seven issues as of particular relevance for practice.

Use of intermediate potency FGAs

The CATIE results suggest that the armamentarium for treating schizophrenia can be expanded to include perphenazine as well as three other intermediate potency drugs: loxitane, molindone, and thiothixene. The intermediate potency FGA perphenazine, when used at modest doses appeared to be as effective and to have no substantially greater neurological side effects than SGAs.

Clinical cost considerations

Whether cost should ever play a role in the clinical care of individual patients is controversial [59], but an important implication of CATIE is that clinicians should inquire as to whether each patient, or their family, is paying out-of-pocket for their medicines. About 20% of patients treated in CATIE had no health insurance, and the results of CATIE suggest that far less expensive treatment options are available, when needed, with similar effectiveness. Cost-saving strategies for patients who have either private or government insurance are left to the discussion of public policy options.

Minimizing metabolic adverse effects

Second, the substantial and distinct increase in metabolic risk with olanzapine and to a lesser extent quetiapine, should make them lower preference agents, but especially for those who are obese, or who are at high risk, by family history or blood chemistries, for diabetes or cardiovascular disease. The greater time to all-cause discontinuation for olanzapine did not translate into gains in quality of life, neurocognition, employment, or reduced violence; thus, the robust and sustained increase in metabolic risks for this drug may outweigh the limited evidence of relative benefit.

Clozapine for refractory illness

Among patients who have persistent psychotic symptoms in spite of adequate antipsychotic trials, clozapine may be useful because of its distinct advantages for refractory symptoms. However, clozapine also incurs an increased risk of weight gain, suggesting that caution is indicated for patients who are obese or at risk for diabetes or cardiovascular diseases. Effective strategies to mitigate metabolic side effects are needed.

Potential hazards of switching

One of the more unexpected findings of CATIE is that switching to a new drug may result in poorer outcomes than staying on the same drug [2]. It is widely believed that patients who do not respond to one treatment may have a better response to another, even when there are no demonstrated differences in effectiveness in head-to-head trials [1]. While the findings from CATIE tend to undermine that widely held belief, additional studies of this issue are needed. Perhaps more watchful waiting is indicated in the use of antipsychotic therapy.

Applicability to use of SGAs in illnesses other than schizophrenia

The greatest area of growth in the use of antipsychotics in recent years has not been in the treatment of schizophrenia but in bipolar disorder, the second illness for which most SGAs have received FDA approval, and in the off-label (i.e., not FDA approved) treatment of affective disorders, post-traumatic stress disorder, and dementia [60,61]. While a separate CATIE study found little evidence of benefit of SGAs as compared to placebo in treating agitation and psychosis in Alzheimer's disease [62], it is unclear how generalizable the results of CATIE are to the use of SGAs in bipolar disorder and in many other conditions for which they are currently prescribed. Narrowly considered, CATIE results would only apply to schizophrenia, but it would seem reasonable to apply data on side effects to other illnesses, although the generalizability of efficacy data has not been widely discussed. This is an important challenge since it is unlikely that studies like CATIE will ever be conducted on the many off-label uses of antipsychotics.

Implications for mental health policy and psychiatric education

Mental health policies are formal rules intended to shape behavior of administrators and clinicians within defined jurisdictions, whether government funded agencies, private health care systems, or insurance plans. While psychiatric care represents the application of medical science to the treatment of unique individuals, one at a time, mental health policies are intended to affect the behavior of many providers and patients simultaneously. Such policies are implemented when there are strong grounds for wanting to change behavior on a large scale and when it would be inefficient or impractical to do so through educational initiatives or case-by-case persuasion. The hazard of implementing policy initiatives in health, and especially in mental health care, is that they may reduce attentiveness to the unique needs of each individual patient.

In the previous section, we identified eight issues in clinical practice that could be shaped by the findings of CATIE along with other recent research. None of these issues would seem to be appropriate targets for a mental health policy because virtually all apply to highly individualized aspects of care. Several of the clinical implications discussed above, such as inquiring about insurance coverage for pharmacy benefits, or watchfully waiting before a medication change, would be cumbersome to monitor, and both costly and intrusive to enforce. Off-label polypharmacy with multiple antipsychotics has been a reasonable target for mental health policy in some state Medicaid programs, but these issues were not specifically addressed by CATIE.

Perhaps of greatest policy relevance are the cost and cost-effectiveness results of the CATIE study. CATIE, CUtLASS, and the earlier VA trial all suggested that the new drugs do not generate savings sufficient to offset their higher costs, and in view of their limited benefits, the cost of their use for the vast majority of patients with schizophrenia may not be a rational practice. The research reviewed here indicates there are likely many patients with schizophrenia who are treated with SGAs who could be treated just as successfully with an FGA. Now that risperidone is off-patent, there is now at least one lower cost SGA.

While it seems desirable to adopt policies that would increase the use of less expensive treatments when more expensive treatments are not medically necessary, it is challenging to identify specific policies that would achieve this goal without provoking a concern from stakeholder groups (e.g. clinicians, consumers, and advocacy groups) and posing a risk that some patients would be unintentionally deprived of needed access to more expensive drugs. The most immediately applicable approaches to this challenge are utilization management policies. Policies that would affect pricing mechanisms or changes in the government regulation of pharmaceuticals would not be specific to SGAs and will not be considered here (but see Hoadley) [63].

Utilization management

The most restrictive utilization management strategies would either exclude some expensive drugs from a formulary, or impose limits on the total number of prescriptions that can be prescribed. These approaches pose the greatest risk to patients with schizophrenia and cannot be recommended.

Less restrictive approaches such as step therapy or prior authorization would also restrict access to a drug or drug class unless other less costly or safer medications had been tried first and proved to be ineffective or intolerable. Such approaches have been strongly recommended in the treatment of hypertension where research showed generic drugs, like some FGAs, are no less beneficial than newer medications [64]. But recent studies have shown little cost savings from pre-authorization policies that limit access to some but not all SGAs [65], and there is some suggestion of poorer adherence when one such policy was implemented in Maine [66]. Prior authorization has been vigorously criticized by professional and consumer groups [67] and by some health services researchers [68,69].

Tiered formularies that require differential cost-sharing for generic, preferred brand-name, and non-preferred brand name drugs have also been used to create financial incentives for patients to use less expensive, but medically equivalent, drugs. Prescription cost-sharing can be in the form of a copayment (i.e., a fixed dollar amount per prescription filled, regardless of drug price) or coinsurance (i.e., a percentage of total drug price). Studies of implementation of three-tiered formularies have shown little adverse effect on utilization of antidepressants [70] or stimulants among children [71], but a draconian intervention that imposed a three-per-month payment limit on prescriptions under Medicaid was associated with an increase in emergency room use and partial hospitalization, offsetting all drug cost savings in patients with schizophrenia [72]. These approaches are less relevant to patients with schizophrenia who are often poor and whose medications are most often funded entirely by government agencies that do not charge co-payments.

More acceptable utilization management strategies are directed to providers rather than patients. In physician profiling, data are compiled on individual doctors' prescriptions for high cost drugs and/or polypharmacy, and either administrative feedback [68] or economic incentives are used to discourage costly prescribing practices. Less intrusive provider-oriented approaches include disease management, independent research reviews, educational interventions, or academic detailing based on provider-specific data [23] that impose less risk that needed drugs will not be available, but they are less likely to change provider behavior.

While the scientific evidence from CATIE and other studies suggests that it would be desirable and justifiable to realize greater efficiencies in the use of antipsychotic medications, there is insufficient evidence on the effects of any antipsychotic utilization policy to support the needed consensus of stakeholders [67]. As State Medicaid programs experiment with various arrangements [73], it can be hoped that safe and effective policies will emerge.

Issues for medical education

It has unfortunately not been unusual in recent years for treatments that, like SGAs, were initially believed to represent major advances to be found subsequently to be less effective or to have more serious adverse side effects than had been appreciated. Among the more widely publicized treatments of this type are Vioxx®, hormone replacement therapy for symptoms of menopause, the fen-phen combination of diet pills, and Neurontin® for migraine and bipolar disorder. In many cases, these reversals appear to have been a result of overzealous marketing and there has been growing concern about the influence of industry on the medical profession through gifts, sponsored symposia, office-based detailing, speakers' bureaus, and even, indirectly, through direct-to-consumer advertising [50,52]. More serious are concerns that the integrity of medical science has been jeopardized by the publication of ghost-written articles by commercial writers in leading medical journals [74], the suppression of negative trials [75], and by the disaggregation of data into multiple publications with different authors [12,76].

In response to these and other concerns, the clinical trials registry was implemented, and both AMA and PHRMA have adopted ethics guidelines for the interactions between industry representatives and physicians. These initiatives have not, however, solved this knotty problem and the Institute of Medicine recently convened a new committee on Conflict of Interest in Medical Research, Education and Practice to recommend additional approaches. A recent public hearing emphasized that, at a minimum, residents as well as more senior physicians, nurses, and other mental health professionals should be educated to think critically about industry-sponsored studies, continuing education programs, and marketing campaigns [77]. The story of research on SGAs over the past two decades, culminating in the CATIE trial and the large independently sponsored studies of the comparative effectiveness of antipsychotic drugs which followed, provide an illustrative example and perhaps a cautionary tale that may be useful in such educational initiatives.

A final word

With the publication of this volume, the complete results of CATIE have become available for the first time from a single accessible source. It is well known that changes in medical practice come slowly [78]. CATIE has helped to establish a new scientific foundation for the use of antipsychotic medications in psychiatric practice and we will all be experiencing the as yet unforeseen consequences of this new knowledge for many years to come.

References

1. Simon GE, Psaty BM, Hrachovec JB, *et al.* Principles for evidence-based drug formulary policy. *Journal of General Internal Medicine* 2005;**20**:964–8.

2. Essock SM, Covell NH, Davis SM, *et al.* Effectiveness of switching antipsychotic medications. *American Journal of Psychiatry* 2006;**163**:2090–5.

3. Davis JM, Chen N and Glick ID. A meta-analysis of the efficacy of second-generation antipsychotics. *Archives of General Psychiatry* 2003;**60**:553–64.

4. Leucht S, Corves C, Arbter D, *et al.* Second-generation versus first-generation antipsychotic drugs for schizophrenia: A meta-analysis. *Lancet* 2009;**737**:31–41.

5. Correll CU, Leucht S and Kane JM. Lower risk for tardive dyskinesia associated with second-generation antipsychotics: A systematic review of 1-year studies. *American Journal of Psychiatry* 2004;**161**:414–25.

6. Hamilton SH, Revicki DA, Edgell ET, *et al.* Clinical and economic outcomes of olanzapine compared with haloperidol for schizophrenia – results from a randomized clinical trial. *Pharmacoeconomics* 1999;**15**:469–80.

7. Marder SR and Meibach RC. Risperidone in the treatment of schizophrenia. *American Journal of Psychiatry* 1994;**151**:825–35.

8. Tollefson GD, Beasley CM Jr, Tran PV, *et al.* Olanzapine versus haloperidol in the treatment of schizophrenia and schizoaffective and schizophreniform disorders: Results of an international collaborative trial. *American Journal of Psychiatry* 1997;**154**:457–65.

9. Csernansky JG, Mahmoud R and Brenner R. A comparison of risperidone and haloperidol for the prevention of relapse in patients with schizophrenia. *New England Journal of Medicine* 2002;**346**:16–22.

10. Carpenter WT and Thaker GK. Editorial: Evidence based therapeutics: Introducing

the Cochrane Corner. *Schizophrenia Bulletin* 2007;**33**:633–4.

11. Geddes JR, Freemantle N, Harrison P, *et al.* Atypical antipsychotics in the treatment of schizophrenia – systematic overview and meta-regression analysis. *British Medical Journal* 2000;**321**:1371–6.

12. Huston P and Moher D. Redundancy, disaggregation, and the integrity of medical research. *Lancet* 1996;**347**:1024–6.

13. Rosenheck RA, Perlick D, Bingham S, *et al.* Effectiveness and cost of olanzapine and haloperidol in the treatment of schizophrenia. *Journal of the American Medical Association* 2003;**290**:2693–702.

14. Rosenheck RA. Efficacy vs. effectiveness of second-generation antipsychotics: Haloperidol without prophylactic anticholinergics as a comparitor. *Psychiatric Services* 2005;**56**:85–92.

15. Hugenholtz GW, Heerdink ER, Stolker JJ, *et al.* Haloperidol dose when used as active comparator in randomized controlled trials with atypical antipsychotics in schizophrenia: Comparison with officially recommended doses. *Journal of Clinical Psychiatry* 2006;**67**:897–903.

16. Davis JM, Chen N and Glick ID. Issues that may determine the outcome of antipsychotic trials: Industry sponsorship and extrapyramidal side effects. *Neuropsychopharmacology* 2007;**33**:971–5.

17. Lieberman JA, Stroup TS, McEvoy JP, *et al.* Effectiveness of antipsychotic drugs in patients with chronic schizophrenia. *New England Journal of Medicine* 2005;**353**:1209–23.

18. Jones PB, Barnes TRE, Davies L, *et al.* Randomized controlled trial of effect on quality of life of second-generation versus first-generation antipsychotic drugs in schizophrenia – CUtLASS1. *Archives of General Psychiatry* 2006;**63**:1079–87.

19. Davies LM, Lewis S, Jones PB, *et al.* Cost-effectiveness of first- v. second-generation antipsychotic drugs: results from a randomised controlled trial in schizophrenia responding poorly to previous therapy. *The British Journal of Psychiatry* 2007;**191**:14–22.

20. Polsky D, Doshi JA, Bauer MS, *et al.* Clinical trial-based cost-effectiveness analyses of antipsychotic use. *American Journal of Psychiatry* 2006;**163**:2047–56.

21. Duggan M. Do new prescription drugs pay for themselves? The case of second-generation antipsychotics. *Journal of Health Economics* 2005;**24**:1–31.

22. Kane JM, Meltzer HY, Carson WH, *et al.* Aripiprazole for treatment-resistant schizophrenia: Results of a multicenter, randomized, double-blind, comparison study versus perphenazine. *Journal of Clinical Psychiatry* 2007;**68**:213–23.

23. Rosenheck RA, Leslie DL, Busch S, *et al.* Rethinking antipsychotic formulary policy. *Schizophrenia Bulletin* 2008;**34**:375–80.

24. Kahn RS, Fleischhacker WW, Boter H, *et al.* Effectiveness of antipsychotic drugs in first-episode schizophrenia and schizophreniform disorder: An open randomised clinical trial. *Lancet* 2008;**371**:1085–97.

25. Sikich L, Frazier JA, McClellan J, *et al.* Double-blind comparison of first- and second-generation antipsychotics in early onset schizophrenia and schizoaffective disorder: Findings from the Treatment of Early-Onset Schizophrenia Spectrum Disorders (TEOSS) study. *American Journal of Psychiatry* 2008;**165**:1420–31.

26. Leucht S, Komossa K, Rummel-Kluge C, *et al.* A meta-analysis of head-to-head comparisons of second-generation antipsychotics in the treatment of schizophrenia. *American Journal of Psychiatry* 2009;**166**:152–63.

27. Owens DC. What CATIE did: Some thoughts on implications deep and wide. *Psychiatric Services* 2008;**59**:530–3.

28. Rosenheck R, Craner J, Xu W, *et al.* A comparison of clozapine and haloperidol in hospitalized patients with refractory schizophrenia. Department of Veterans Affairs Cooperative Study Group on clozapine in refractory schizophrenia. *New England Journal of Medicine* 1997;**337**:809–15.

29. Breier A, Berg PH, Thakore JH, *et al.* Olanzapine versus ziprasidone: Results of a

28-week double blind study in patients with schizophrenia. *American Journal of Psychiatry* 2005;**162**:1879–87.

30. Freedman R, Carpenter WT, Davis JM, *et al.* The cost of drugs for schizophrenia. *American Journal of Psychiatry* 2006;**163**:2029–31.

31. American Diabetes Association (ADA), American Psychiatric Association, American Association of Clinical Endocrinologists, North American Association for the Study of Obesity. Consensus development conference on antipsychotic drugs and obesity and diabetes. *Diabetes Care* 2004;**27**:596–601.

32. Correll CU, Leucht S and Kane JM. Lower risk for tardive dyskinesia associated with second-generation antipsychotics: A systematic review of 1-year studies. *American Journal of Psychiatry* 2004;**161**:414–25.

33. Swanson JW, Swartz MS, Van Dorn RA, *et al.* A national study of violent behavior in persons with schizophrenia. *Archives of General Psychiatry* 2006;**63**:490–9.

34. Rosenheck RA, Hoff RA, Steinwachs D, *et al.* Benchmarking treatment of schizophrenia: A comparison of service delivery by the national government and by state and local providers. *Journal of Nervous and Mental Disease* 2000;**188**:209–16.

35. Kelsey JL, Whittemore AS, Evans AS, *et al. Methods in Observational Epidemiology.* 2nd ed. New York: Oxford University Press; 1996. pp 88–9.

36. Last JM, ed. *A Dictionary of Epidemiology.* 3rd ed. New York: Oxford University Press; 1996.

37. Meltzer HY and Bobo WV. Interpreting the efficacy findings in the CATIE study: What clinicians should know. *CNS Spectrum* 2006;**11**(Suppl. 7):14–24.

38. Kane JM. Commentary on the Clinical Antipsychotic Trials of Intervention Effectiveness (CATIE). *Journal of Clinical Psychiatry* 2006;**76**:831–2.

39. Tandon R and Constaine R. Avoiding EPS is key to realizing "atypical benefits". *Current Psychiatry* 2006;**5**:35–45.

40. Rosack J. Experts say tread slowly when trying to interpret study results. *Psychiatric News* 2006;**41**:23.

41. Goode E. Leading drugs for psychosis come under scrutiny. *NY Times* May **20**, 2003, p. A1.

42. Freedman R. The choice of antipsychotic drugs for schizophrenia. *New England Journal of Medicine* 2005;**353**:1286–8.

43. Ganguli R, Strassnig M. Are older antipsychotic drugs obsolete: No. *British Medical Journal* 2006;**332**:1345–6.

44. Lewis S and Lieberman JA. CATIE and CUtLASS: Can we handle the truth? *British Journal of Psychiatry* 2008;**192**:161–3.

45. Nasrallah H. The role of efficacy, safety, and tolerability in antipsychotic effectiveness: Practical implications of the CATIE schizophrenia trial. *Journal of Clinical Psychiatry* 2007;**68** (Suppl. 1):5–11.

46. Sharfstein S. Antipsychotics, economics and the press. *Psychiatric News* 2005;**40**:3.

47. *New York Times.* Editorial: Comparing schizophrenia drugs. *New York Times*, 2005 September 21. http://www.nytimes.com/ 2005/09/21/opinion/21wcd3.html? ex=1183953600&en=1cadcb61b264f0c5& ei=5070.

48. Vedantam S. New antipsychotic drugs criticized Federal study finds no benefit over older, cheaper drug. *Washington Post*, September **20**, 2005, A0.

49. Abramson J. *Overdosed America: The Broken Promise of American Medicine.* New York, NY: Harper Collins; 2004.

50. Angel M. *The Truth About the Drug Companies: How They Deceive Us and What to do About It.* New York, NY: Random House; 2004.

51. Avorn J. *Powerful Medicines: The Benefits, Risks, and Costs of Prescription Drugs.* New York, NY: Knopf; 2004.

52. Kassirer J. *On the Take: How Medicine's Complicity with Big Business Can Endanger Your Health.* New York, NY: Oxford University Press; 2004.

53. Moore TA, Buchanan RW, Buckley PF, *et al.* The Texas medication algorithm

project antipsychotic algorithm for schizophrenia: 2006 update. *Journal of Clinical Psychiatry* 2007;**68**:1751–62.

54. Parks J, Radke A, Parker G, *et al.* Principles of antipsychotic prescribing for policy makers, circa 2008. Translating knowledge to promote individualized treatment. *Schizophrenia Bulletin* 2009;**35**:931–6.

55. Carpenter WT and Buchanan RW. Lessons to take home from CATIE. *Psychiatric Services* 2008;**59**:523–5.

56. Sernyak MJ, Leslie D and Rosenheck RA. Antipsychotic use in the treatment of outpatients with schizophrenia in the VA from fiscal years 1999 to 2006. *Psychiatric Services* 2008;**59**:567–9.

57. Cascade E and Kalali A. One of antipsychotics pre-and post dissemination of the CATIE data. *Psychiatry* 2007;**4**:21–3.

58. Citrome L, Jaffe A, Martello D, *et al.* Did CATIE influence antipsychotic use? *Psychiatric Services* 2008;**59**:476.

59. Ubel PA. *Pricing Life: Why Its Time for Health Care Rationing.* Cambridge, MA: MIT Press; 2001.

60. Domino ME and Swartz MS. Who are the new users of antipsychotic medications? *Psychiatric Services* 2008;**59**:507–14.

61. Briesacher BA, Limcangco MR, Simoni-Wastila L, *et al.* The quality of antipsychotic drug prescribing in nursing homes. *Archives of Internal Medicine* 2005;**165**:1280–5.

62. Schneider LS, Tariot PN, Dagerman KS, *et al.* CATIE-AD Study Group: Effectiveness of atypical antipsychotic drugs in patients with Alzheimer's disease. *New England Journal of Medicine* 2006;**355**:1525–38.

63. Hoadley J. *Cost Containment Strategies for Prescription Drugs: Assessing the Evidence in the Literature.* Health Policy Institute. Georgetown University; 2005. http://www.kff.org/rxdrugs/7295.cfm.

64. Weisfeldt ML and Zieman SJ. Advances in the prevention and treatment of cardiovascular disease. *Health Affairs (Millwood)* 2007;**26**:25–37 (cf. p. 29).

65. Law MR, Ross-Degnan D and Soumerai SB. Effect of prior authorization on second-generation antipsychotic agents on pharmacy utilization and reimbursements. *Psychiatric Services* 2008;**59**:540–6.

66. Soumerai SB, Zhang F, Ross-Degnan D, *et al.* Use of atypical antipsychotic drugs for schizophrenia in Maine Medicaid following a policy change. *Health Affairs (Millwood)* 2008;**27**:w185–w195.

67. Duckworth K and Fitzpatrick MJ. NAMI perspective on CATIE: policy and research indications. *Psychiatric Services* 2008;**59**:537–40.

68. Covell NH, Finnerty MT and Essock SM. Implications for CATIE for mental health services researchers. *Psychiatric Services* 2008;**59**:526–9.

69. Frank RG. Policy toward second-generation antipsychotic drugs: A cautionary note. *Psychiatric Services* 2008;**59**:521–2.

70. Goldman DP, Joyce GF, Escarce JJ, *et al.* Pharmacy benefits and the use of drugs by the chronically-ill. *Journal of the American Medical Association* 2004;**291**:2344–50.

71. Huskamp HA, Deverka PA, Epstein AM, *et al.* Impact of 3-tier formularies on drug treatment of attention-deficit/hyperactivity disorder in children. *Archives of General Psychiatry* 2005;**62**:435–41.

72. Soumerai SB, McLaughlin TJ, Ross-Degnan D, Casteris CS and Bollini P. Effects of a limit on Medicaid drug-reimbursement benefits on the use of psychotropic agents and acute mental health services by patients with schizophrenia. *New England Journal of Medicine* 1994;**331**:650–5.

73. Polinski JM, Wang PS and Fischer MA. Medicaid's prior authorization program and access to atypical antipsychotic medications. *Health Affairs (Millwood)* 2007;**26**:759–60.

74. DeAngelis CD and Fontanarosa PB. Impugning the integrity of medical science: The adverse effects of industry influence. *Journal of the American Medical Association* 2008;**299**:1833–5.

75. Turner EH, Matthews AM, Linardatos E, Tell RA and Rosenthal R. Selective publication of antidepressant trials and its influence on apparent efficacy. *New England Journal of Medicine* 2008;**358**:252–60.

76. Rennie D. Fair conduct and fair reporting of clinical trials. *Journal of the American Medical Association* 1999;**282**:1766–8.

77. Yan J. Experts disagree on impact of medicine, industry relationship. *Psychiatric News* 2008;**43**:1.

78. Peterson M. *Our Daily Meds.* New York: Sarah Crichton Books-Farrar, Straus and Giroux; 2008.

Index

Printed in the United States
by Baker & Taylor Publisher Services